Ong dex

AMCOEX @ MSN.com

Philip's Instructor.

Jan 13-23

Thur 6-27 next day..
if not convenient thu
Feb?

Case Studies in
ECHOCARDIOGRAPHY

a diagnostic workbook

RALPH D. CLARK, M.D.

Director, Echocardiography Laboratory,
Staff Cardiologist, Division of Cardiology,
Presbyterian Hospital, Pacific Medical Center,
San Francisco, California;

Assistant Clinical Professor of Medicine,
University of California School of Medicine,
San Francisco, California

With the assistance of

John S. Edelen, M.D.

Associate Director, Department of Cardiology,
Alta Bates Hospital,
Berkeley, California;

Clinical Instructor in Medicine,
University of California School of Medicine,
San Francisco, California

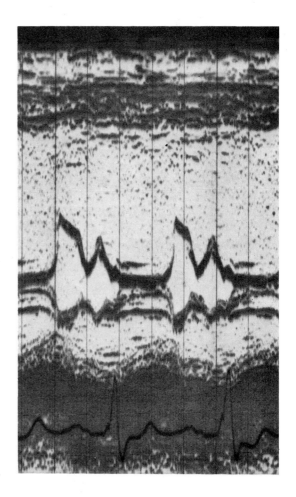

W. B. SAUNDERS COMPANY
Philadelphia, London, Toronto

W. B. Saunders Company: West Washington Square
Philadelphia, PA   19105

1 St. Anne's Road
Eastbourne, East Sussex BN21 3UN, England

1 Goldthorne Avenue
Toronto, Ontario M8Z 5T9, Canada

Library of Congress Cataloging in Publication Data

Clark, Ralph D

Case studies in echocardiography.

Includes bibliographical references and index.

1. Ultrasonic cardiography — Cases, clinical reports,
   statistics.   I. Edelen, John S., joint author.   II. Title.
   [DNLM: 1. Echocardiography — Case studies. WG 141
   C594c]

RC683.5.U5C56   616.1′2′0754   76–1212

ISBN 0–7216–2594–0

Case Studies in Echocardiography   ISBN   0–7216–2594–0

Last digit is the print number: 9   8   7   6   5   4

To

Arthur Selzer, M.D.

Preface

The purpose of this workbook is to teach the proper interpretation of M-mode echocardiography in adults and to discuss the many recent advances in this exciting field. It is designed to be used by physicians and technicians as a companion to standard texts and journal articles. Regardless of whether their experience is basic or extensive, it is hoped that these readers will find the format of 52 actual case histories with illustrative echocardiograms, questions, and subsequent extensive discussion of the points pertinent to each echocardiogram an informative and rewarding method of learning and of updating their knowledge of interpretative echocardiography.

Cases included cover all the major areas encountered in the clinical practice of adult cardiology, several cases having been used to illustrate particularly important areas. Multiple illustrations, summary diagrams and tables, and extensive references are included. Numerous technical hints for obtaining improved echo tracings are given. Emphasis is put on the importance of learning the many different echo patterns seen in cardiac disease, as well as on the need to make accurate measurements and calculations from the echo. After the proper method of making measurements is precisely defined and illustrated, multiple opportunities are given to measure, calculate, and evaluate the importance of these measurements in the case studies.

The importance is stressed of proceeding from observation and measurement to interpretation. The numerous clinical uses of echocardiography in the practice of medicine are discussed in the context of actual case histories and are summarized under clinical applications throughout the book. Particular attention is given to the basic principles and limitations of echo essential to the proper understanding and interpretation of clinical echocardiography.

Numerous line drawings of the echos from the case studies are included in the discussion to help the reader learn the many different echo patterns and details of measurement. It is central to the process of learning echocardiography that the mind should be trained to see those echoes that are important and that represent true structures, and to exclude extraneous ones. Such images probably are formed and stored in the mind as line drawings, and it is hoped that the illustrations included with these cases will facilitate this learning process.

For the best results, the reader should commit himself in writing to all the questions for each case before turning to the discussion. These questions are designed to emphasize pertinent interpretative and technical points illustrated by the echocardiograms, as well as the differential diagnosis of certain echo findings. By making all possible measurements and calculations on each case, the reader can test and further improve his skill in echocardiography.

All the echocardiograms shown were performed at Presbyterian Hospital, Pacific Medical Center in San Francisco, using an Ekoline 20 (Smith-Kline Instruments) ultrasonascope and 2.25 MHz transducers of 0.5-inch (13 mm) diameter focused at 5 cm or 7.5 cm. The echoes were recorded at 50 mm/sec, using an Electronics for Medicine DR6 or DR8 strip chart recorder.

The authors wish to acknowledge the outstanding contribution of Ms. Judith Burgess, who played such an essential part in our beginning experience in echocardiography and in obtaining many of the echoes in this workbook. She is truly a superstar of echocardiography. We also are especially indebted to Mr. James Brodale for his outstanding artistic skill and untiring effort in preparing the multiple illustrations.

RALPH D. CLARK, M.D.

Contents

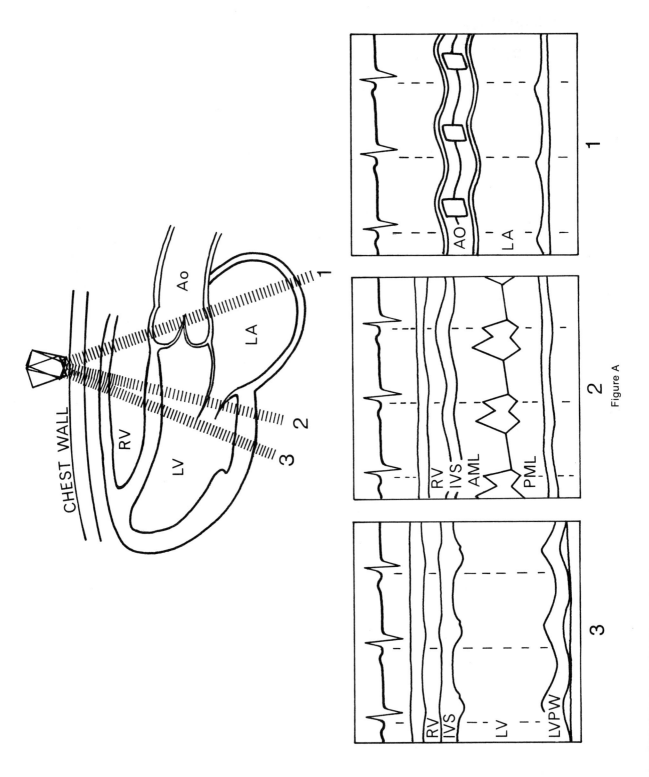

Figure A

DESCRIPTION OF THE NORMAL ECHOCARDIOGRAM

In echo *Position 1* (see Figure A) the aortic root, aortic valve, and left atrium are recorded. The echo of the normal aorta consists of two parallel lines — representing the anterior and posterior aortic walls — that move anteriorly during systole as blood is forcibly ejected from the left ventricle and posteriorly during diastole. A short plateau or delay occurs as the aortic root moves posteriorly in diastole. Within these parallel lines the thin aortic valve cusps are seen to open during ventricular systole, forming a box or parallelogram-like structure that almost reaches the aortic walls. These cusps normally may exhibit a fine, high-frequency shuddering during systole. The anterior part of this boxlike structure is thought to originate from the right cusp and the posterior part from the noncoronary cusp. Occasionally, a thin echo is recorded that moves through the center of this structure. This is thought by some to represent the left coronary cusp.

Directly posterior to the aorta lies the left atrium. The characteristic pattern of motion of the posterior left atrial wall is slightly posteriorly during ventricular systole. This posterior motion represents the enlargement of the left atrium as blood continues to flow from the pulmonary veins into the left atrium when the mitral valve is closed. The characteristic pattern of motion of the left atrium is the opposite of that of the left ventricular posterior wall. This difference aids in determining where the transducer is aiming. Occasionally, a small anterior motion of the posterior left atrial wall is recorded just following the P wave of the electrocardiogram.

Position 2 is used primarily to record the mitral valve. In this position the interventricular septum usually is seen to be horizontal, but it may show a slight posterior motion during systole. However, if the septum is recorded near its attachment to the aorta, it will have the anterior systolic motion characteristic of the adjacent aortic root. Because of this great variability in motion, Position 2 is not reliable for evaluating septal motion.

During ventricular systole, the normal mitral valve echo appears as a single line that moves slowly from a posterior position (C point) to an anterior position (D point). Normally it does not move sharply anteriorly or sag posteriorly; rather, it moves slowly anteriorly throughout systole. This slow anterior systolic motion is attributed to the forward motion of the mitral annulus as the left ventricle empties and the left atrium fills.

During ventricular diastole, the normal anterior mitral leaflet forms an "M"-shaped pattern. The first part of the "M" (E point) results from the rapid filling wave of blood rushing from the left atrium to the left ventricle at the beginning of diastole, opening the mitral valve and causing the anterior leaflet to move anteriorly toward the transducer. As this rapid filling wave subsides, the anterior leaflet begins to close and moves posteriorly (F point). If left atrial systole occurs, the anterior leaflet again is pushed anteriorly toward the transducer (A point). As atrial systolic flow subsides, the leaflet again drifts posteriorly, and with ventricular systole is promptly closed (C point). The distance between the A and C points is referred to as the "B segment." During diastole, the posterior mitral leaflet moves roughly opposite the anterior leaflet, forming a "W"-shaped pattern. Notice that normally the amplitude of the posterior mitral leaflet is considerably less than that of the anterior leaflet.

In echo *Position 3* the right ventricle, the interventricular septum, an approximation of the minor diameter of the left ventricular cavity, and the left ventricular posterior wall are recorded. The characteristic motion of the anterior right ventricular wall is posteriorly during ventricular systole at the time the left ventricular posterior wall is moving anteriorly. In systole, the characteristic motion of the left side of the septum is posteriorly as the left ventricular posterior wall moves anteriorly. As a result, normally the septum and left ventricular free wall move sharply toward each other during systole and away from each other during diastole. Sometimes, a slight posterior motion of the left ventricular free wall is recorded just before the left ventricle moves anteriorly with systole. This "thinning" of the ventricular free wall is thought to occur during isovolumic ventricular systole. The septum also may show a slight "thinning" at this same time. In addition, a small notch often occurs in the septum as it moves anteriorly at the end of systole. This septal notch is thought to be caused by the motion of the heart as a whole, and is so characteristic that it often is helpful in identifying the septum. The endocardium of the free left ventricular wall must be distinguished from the mitral supporting apparatus that lies just anterior to it, and from the left ventricular epicardium. Characteristically, the endocardium will move anteriorly in systole, with a steeper slope than either of these two structures. Directly posterior to the left ventricular free wall is the highly reflective interface of the epicardium, pericardium, pleura, and lung. This interface is recorded as an echo-dense structure. Occasionally, a small, relatively echo-free space or window is normally recorded between the epicardium and pericardium during ventricular systole, with these surfaces remaining in contact during diastole.

ECHOCARDIOGRAPHIC MEASUREMENTS AND CALCULATIONS

CALCULATION OF CALIBRATION FACTOR (cf)

With a ruler, measure the distance in centimeters of a certain number of calibration lines and calculate a calibration factor by the following formula:

$$cf = \frac{actual\ number\ of\ calibration\ spaces}{the\ distance\ these\ spaces\ measure\ in\ cm}$$

Measure the maximal number of calibration lines possible to minimize slight variation in the spacing of the lines.

$$Example\ (Position\ 1): \quad cf = \frac{10\ spaces}{7.6\ cm} = 1.32$$

All measurements made from the echo tracings in millimeters or centimeters must be multiplied by a calibration factor to convert them to true measurements.

An alternative method of making measurements that does not require calculation of a calibration factor involves the use of calipers. The calipers are placed directly on the distance to be measured, then transferred to the calibration marks, and the measurement estimated to the nearest millimeter. With experience and careful attention to detail, this method is accurate within a few millimeters and is satisfactory for most routine echo reading.

AORTIC ROOT (Position 1 – Figure B)

A. Aortic (Ao) Diameter (Normal adult range = (20–37 mm)[1]

At the level of the aortic valves, measure the vertical distance between the anterior and posterior aortic walls, using the outermost boundary of the anterior wall and the inner boundary of the posterior wall during ventricular systole when the aorta is in its maximal anterior position. Use the minimal distance recorded for this diameter to avoid increases due to transducer angulation.

$$Example\ (Position\ 1): \quad Ao\ diameter = 21 \times 1.32 = 28\ mm$$

3

B. Aortic (Ao) Amplitude (Normal adult range = 5–16 mm)[11]

Measure the anterior motion of the posterior aortic wall during ventricular systole. First, draw a horizontal line between the external boundaries of the posterior aortic wall during diastole (line x, Position 1); then measure the maximal vertical distance from this line to the external boundary of the aortic wall during ventricular systole (line y, Position 1).

Example (Position 1): Ao amplitude = 6 mm × 1.32 = 8 mm

C. Aortic Valve Opening (Normal adult range = 1.5–2.6 cm)[1]

Measure the maximal openings of the aortic valve cusps during the initial part of ventricular systole, using the *internal* borders of the aortic cusp echoes. The distance between the cusps may decrease slightly during systole.

Example (Position 1): Ao leaflet opening = 1.1 cm × 1.32 = 1.5 cm

LEFT ATRIAL (LA) SIZE (Position 1 – Figure B)

(Normal adult range = 1.9–4.0 cm)[183]
(LA index   = 1.2–2.1 cm/m²)[183]

Measure the greatest vertical distance between the anterior side of the posterior aortic wall and the posterior left atrial wall during ventricular systole when the aorta is in its maximal anterior position.

Example (Position 1): LA = 2.6 cm × 1.32 = 3.4 cm

POSITION 1

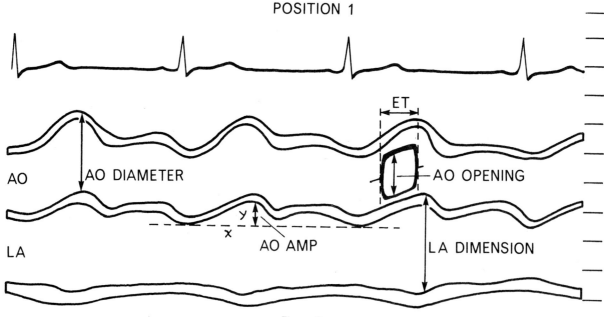

Figure B

The left atrial index is obtained by dividing the left atrial size by the patient's body surface area.

The ratio of left atrial to aortic root dimension (LA/Ao ratio) has been proposed as an improved method of evaluating left atrial size.[184] For calculation of this ratio, the end-diastolic dimension of the aortic root, measured from the outer edge of the anterior aortic wall to the inner edge of the posterior aortic wall, and the end-systolic dimension of the left atrium, measured from the anterior edge of the posterior aortic wall to the posterior left atrial wall, are taken. In normals, the ratio is 0.87 to 1.11, whereas in patients with known left atrial enlargement it is 1.17 or greater. A limitation of this ratio is that it introduces into the assessment of the left atrial size another variable, i.e., aortic root dimension. For example, normal LA/Ao ratios may be obtained in patients with large left atria and dilated aortic roots.

MITRAL VALVE (MV) (Position 2—Figure C)

Make all measurements on a recording of the anterior mitral leaflet (AML) that shows the maximal amplitude of motion and is well recorded with the transducer perpendicular to the chest wall. Slight medial and superior angulation of the transducer usually is required to record the mitral valve as a continuous echo. The very slightest lateral and inferior angulation may be necessary to record the posterior mitral leaflet.

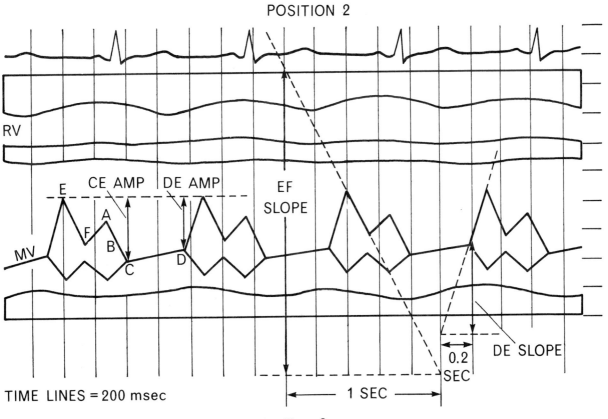

Figure C

A. C-E Amplitude (Normal adult range = 20–32 mm)[45, 70]

Measure the vertical distance from the point where the anterior and posterior mitral leaflets coapt at the beginning of ventricular systole (C point) and an imaginary horizontal line that marks the maximal anterior motion of the anterior mitral leaflet in the beginning of ventricular diastole (E point).

Example (Position 2): C-E Amplitude = 17 mm × 1.30 = 22 mm

B. D-E Amplitude (Normal adult range = 17–30 mm)[70]

Measure the vertical distance from the point where the anterior and posterior mitral leaflets separate at the end of ventricular systole (D point) and an imaginary horizontal line that marks the maximal anterior motion of the anterior mitral leaflet in the beginning of ventricular diastole (E point).

Example (Position 2): D-E Amplitude = 14 mm × 1.30 = 18 mm

C. D-E Slope (Normal adult range = 240–380 mm/sec)[70]

This slope is obtained by constructing a triangle with the following three steps:
(1) Draw a diagonal line through the D-E portion of the anterior mitral leaflet.

(2) Draw a horizontal line near the bottom of the tracing rightward beginning at a point where line 1 intersects one of the time lines on the tracing.

(3) Construct a vertical line perpendicular to line 2 at a point along line 2 that is exactly 0.2 sec from the intersection of lines 1 and 2. (Note the distance between time lines on the tracing.) The length of this line 3, measured in mm, from line 2 to where it intersects line 1, multiplied by 5 and then multiplied by the calibration factor is the D-E slope of the anterior mitral leaflet in mm/sec.

Example (Position 2): D-E Slope = 25 mm × 5 × 1.30 = 163 mm/sec

D. E-F Slope (Normal adult range = 80–150 mm/sec)[1, 2, 70]

This slope is obtained by constructing a triangle with the following three steps:
(1) Draw a diagonal line through the steepest *initial* part of the E-F portion of the anterior mitral leaflet.

(2) Draw a horizontal line near the bottom of the tracing leftward, beginning at a point where line 1 intersects one of the time lines on the tracing.

(3) Construct a vertical line perpendicular to line 2 at a point along line 2 that is exactly 1 sec from the intersection of lines 1 and 2. (Note the distance between time lines on the tracing.) The length of this line 3, measured in mm, from where it intersects lines 1 and 2 multiplied by the calibration factor is the E-F slope of the anterior mitral leaflet in mm/sec.

Example (Position 2): E-F Slope = 82 mm/sec × 1.30 = 107 mm/sec

RIGHT VENTRICULAR (RV) DIMENSION (Position 3—Figure D)

(Normal adult range—supine   = 0.8–2.3 cm)[1, 2, 4, 146, 296]
         —left lateral   = 0.9–2.6 cm)[4, 296]
(Right Ventricular Index   = 0.4–1.3 cm/m²)[4, 296]

Measure the vertical distance from the internal side of the anterior right ventricular wall to the right ventricular side of the septum in end-diastole at a point corresponding to the R wave of the electrocardiogram on tracings that include properly recorded left ventricle posteriorly. Note that recordings made with the patient in the left lateral position may show larger right ventricular dimensions.

Example (Position 3): 8.0 cm × 1.29 = 1.0 cm

The right ventricular index is obtained by dividing the right ventricular dimension by the patient's body surface area.

INTERVENTRICULAR SEPTUM (IVS) (Position 3—Figure D)

All measurements should be made on tracings that include a properly recorded left ventricle posteriorly.

POSITION 3

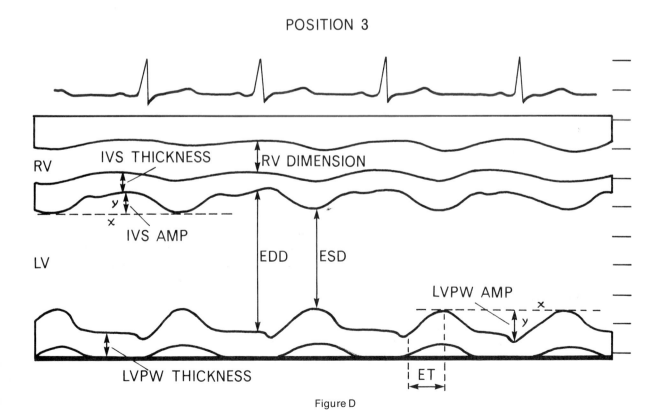

Figure D

A. IVS Thickness (Normal adult range = 7–11 mm)[1]

Measure the vertical distance from the right ventricular side of the IVS to the left ventricular side of the IVS in end-diastole at a point corresponding to the R wave of the electrocardiogram.

Example (Position 3): IVS Thickness = 5.5 mm × 1.30 = 7 mm

B. IVS Amplitude (Normal adult range = 5–10 mm)[137]

Measure the posterior motion of the LV side of the IVS. This measurement is made by first drawing a horizontal line between the most posterior points of the left ventricular side of the septum during systole (line x), and then measuring the maximal vertical distance from this line to the IVS just before the septum begins to move posteriorly in systole (line y).

Example (Position 3): IVS Amplitude = 5.5 mm × 1.30 = 7 mm

C. Percentage Systolic Septal Thickening (% IVS Thickening) (Normal adult range = 30–64%)[137]

Measure the systolic thickness of the IVS as the maximal vertical distance that occurs between the right ventricular and left ventricular sides of the IVS during systole. Measure the diastolic septal thickness in a similar manner at end-diastole, as described under A above. The percentage systolic septal thickening is calculated by the following formula:

$$\% \text{ IVS Thickening} = \frac{\text{Systolic Thickness} - \text{Diastolic Thickness}}{\text{Diastolic Thickness}} \times 100$$

Example (Position 3):

$$\% \text{ IVS Thickening} = \frac{(9 \text{ mm})(1.30 - (5.5 \text{ mm})(1.30)}{5.5 \text{ mm } (1.30)} \times 100 = 64\%$$

LEFT VENTRICLE (Position 3 — Figure D)

These measurements should be made on a tracing that was recorded just inferior to the tip of the anterior mitral leaflet and that includes portions of the mitral apparatus (i.e., chordae tendineae). The septal and left ventricular posterior wall (LVPW) endocardium should be distinct, continuous lines throughout the cardiac cycle. Popp et al.[147] have demonstrated that, for the most accurate reproducibility, the left ventricle should be recorded from the "standard interspace." This interspace is defined as the one from which the mitral valve is recorded with the transducer perpendicular to the chest wall, with only slight medial, but no superior or inferior angulation.

A. End-Diastolic Diameter (EDD) (Normal adult range = 3.8–5.6 cm)*

Measure the vertical distance from the endocardium of the LVPW to the endocardium of the IVS in end-diastole at a point corresponding to the R wave of the electrocardiogram.

Example (Position 3): EDD = 3.7 cm × 1.29 = 4.8 cm

B. End-Systolic Diameter (ESD) (Normal adult range = 2.2–4.0 cm)*

Measure the vertical distance from the endocardium of the LVPW at the peak of its anterior motion during systole to the endocardium of the IVS. This measurement may or may not correspond with the peak of posterior motion of the IVS in systole.

Example (Position 3): ESD = 2.6 cm × 1.29 = 3.4 cm

C. LVPW Amplitude (Normal adult range = 5–12 mm)*

Measure the anterior motion of the LVPW during systole. This measurement is made by first drawing a horizontal line between the most anterior points of the left ventricular endocardium in systole (line x) and then measuring the maximal vertical distance from this line to the endocardium of the LVPW at a point just before the left ventricular free wall begins to move anteriorly in systole (line y).

Example (Position 3): LVPW Amplitude = 8.0 mm × 1.29 = 10 mm

D. LVPW Thickness (Normal adult range = 7–11 mm)[1]

Measure the vertical distance from the epicardium of the LVPW to the endocardium in end-diastole at a point just prior to the presystolic "thinning" of the LVPW.

Example (Position 3): LVPW Thickness = 7 mm × 1.29 = 9 mm

E. LV Volume

An estimate of LV end-diastolic volume (EDV) and end-systolic volume (ESV) can be obtained by using the appropriate dimension (EDD or ESD) for the value of D in the following equation as published by Teichholtz.[148]

$$\text{Volume} = \frac{7}{2.4 + D} \times D^3$$

*Based on 53 normals, ages 22–72, studied at Presbyterian Hospital, Pacific Medical Center, San Francisco.

Example (Position 3): $\text{EDV} = \dfrac{7}{(2.4 + 4.8)} \times (4.8 \text{ cm})^3 = 107 \text{ cc}$

$$\text{ESV} = \dfrac{7}{(2.4 + 3.4)} \times (3.4 \text{ cm})^3 = 47 \text{ cc}$$

This method of estimating ventricular volumes for calculation of left ventricular ejection fraction has been used in this workbook. A table showing the volumes obtained through this formula for different ventricular dimensions (EDD and ESD) is included at the end of this section.

Two alternative methods of calculating LV volume have been proposed using the appropriate dimension (EDD and ESD) described above. First, Pombo has proposed that the appropriate dimension (EDD and ESD) can be cubed to obtain an estimate of the diastolic and systolic LV volumes (EDV and ESV):

$$\text{Volume} = D^3$$

Second, Fortuin has proposed two regression formulae for calculation of these volume measurements (L7):

$$\text{EDV} = 59 \text{ EDD} - 153$$

$$\text{ESV} = 47 \text{ ESD} - 120$$

INDICES OF LV FUNCTION[151-161]

A. Ejection Fraction (Ej.Fr.) $= \dfrac{\text{EDV} - \text{ESV}}{\text{EDV}} \times 100$
(Normal adult range = 53–77%)*

Example (Position 3): $\text{Ej.Fr.} = \dfrac{107 \text{ cc} - 47 \text{ cc}}{107 \text{ cc}} = 56\%$

B. Percentage Change of Minor Diameter (% Change)
(Normal adult range = 24–46%)*

$$\% \text{ Change} = \dfrac{(\text{EDD} - \text{ESD})}{\text{EDD}} \times 100$$

Example (Position 3): $\% \text{ Change} = \dfrac{4.8 \text{ cm} - 3.4 \text{ cm}}{4.8 \text{ cm}} = 29\%$

---

*Based on 53 normals, ages 22–72, studied at Presbyterian Hospital, Pacific Medical Center, San Francisco, California.

C. Velocity of Circumferential Fiber Shortening (Vcf)
(Normal adult range = 0.88–1.55 circumferences/sec)*

$$Vcf = \frac{(EDD - ESD)/EDD}{ET}$$

Example (Position 3): $Vcf = \dfrac{(4.8 \text{ cm} - 3.4 \text{ cm})/4.8 \text{ cm}}{0.240 \text{ sec}} = 1.22 \text{ circ/sec}$

ET = left ventricular ejection time and is the time in seconds from the point the LVPW endocardium first begins to move anteriorly in systole until it reaches the peak of its anterior motion. When the motion of the LVPW is gradual, the exact point at which it begins to move anteriorly often is indistinct. On such an echo, estimation of the ET from the LVPW is inaccurate.

There are two alternative methods for measuring left ventricular ejection time (ET), both of which are more accurate than obtaining it from the LVPW echo. On a simultaneously recorded carotid pulse tracing, the left ventricular ejection time is the time from the beginning of the upstroke to the dicrotic notch. The ejection time also can be accurately measured from an echo of the aortic valve cusps and is the time from the point where the aortic valve opens to the point where it closes (Position 1). Care must be taken to define clearly these opening and closing points by recording both the anterior and posterior aortic cusps and to use cycle lengths equivalent to those where the left ventricular dimensions are taken.

Because of variations in paper speed with strip chart recorders, the distance between time lines often varies slightly. To correct for this variation, all measurements of time should be related to a proportion of a known distance and time on that particular echo tracing. For example, suppose we wish to determine how many milliseconds (msec) a distance of 13 mm represents on a certain tracing. First, we measure and find that on that tracing 48 mm represents a time of 1 second (1000 msec). Then, by the proportion:

$$\frac{48 \text{ mm}}{1000 \text{ msec}} = \frac{13 \text{ mm}}{x}$$

$$x = 270 \text{ msec}$$

---

*Based on 53 normals, ages 22–72, studied at Presbyterian Hospital, Pacific Medical Center, San Francisco, California.

Normal Adult Values of Echocardiographic Measurements

	Range
Aortic Diameter (AO)[1]	20–37 mm
Aortic Amplitude[11]	5–16 mm
Aortic Valve Opening[4]	1.5–2.6 cm
Left Atrium (LA)[182]	1.9–4.0 cm
Left Atrial Index[182]	1.2–2.1 cm/m²
LA/Ao Ratio[183]	0.87–1.11
Mitral Valve (MV)	
C-E Amplitude[45, 70]	20–32 mm
D-E Amplitude[70]	17–30 mm
D-E Slope[70]	240–380 mm/sec
E-F Slope[1, 2]	80–150 mm/sec

Right Ventricular Dimension (RV)[1, 2, 4, 146, 296] — supine = 0.7–2.3 cm

— left lateral = 0.9–2.6 cm

Right Ventricular Index[4, 296] = 0.4–1.3 cm/m²

Interventricular Septal Thickness[1]	7–11 mm
Interventricular Septal Amplitude[137]	5–10 mm
Percentage Septal Thickening[137]	30–64%
Left Ventricular Posterior Wall Thickness[1]	7–11 mm
Left Ventricular Posterior Wall Amplitude*	5–12 mm

Left Ventricular Minor Diameter: *

	Mean ± S.D.	*Range*
EDD	4.8 ± 0.4 cm (4.4–5.2)	3.8–5.6 cm
ESD	3.1 ± 0.5 cm (2.6–3.6)	2.2–4.0 cm

Indices of Left Ventricular Function: *

Ejection Fraction	66 ± 7% (59–73%)	53–77%
Percentage Change of Minor Diameter	36 ± 5% (31–41%)	24–46%
Velocity of Circumferential Fiber Shortening	1.23 ± 0.18 circ/sec (1.05–1.41)	0.88–1.55 circ/sec
LV Ejection Time (From the LVPW)	295 ± 20 msec (275–315)	250–352 msec

*Based on 53 normals, ages 22–72, studied at Presbyterian Hospital, Pacific Medical Center, San Francisco, California.

Table of Ventricular Volumes

Ventricular volumes (EDV and ESV) calculated from ventricular dimensions (EDD and ESD) according to the formula of Teichholtz:[148] $Volume = \frac{7}{2.4 + D} \times D^3$

Dim.	Vol.	Dim.	Vol.	Dim.	Vol.
2.0	13	4.0	70	7.0	254
2.1	14	4.1	74	7.1	265
2.2	16	4.2	79	7.2	272
2.3	18	4.3	83	7.3	280
2.4	20	4.4	88	7.4	288
2.5	22	4.5	92	7.5	300
2.6	25	4.6	97	7.6	307
2.7	27	4.7	103	7.7	315
2.8	30	4.8	107	7.8	327
2.9	31	4.9	113	7.9	336
3.0	35	5.0	118	8.0	343
3.1	38	5.1	123	8.1	356
3.2	41	5.2	129	8.2	364
3.3	44	5.3	135	8.3	372
3.4	47	5.4	142	8.4	385
3.5	51	5.5	148	8.5	393
3.6	55	5.6	155	8.6	407
3.7	59	5.7	159	8.7	415
3.8	62	5.8	166	8.8	429
3.9	66	5.9	174	8.9	439
		6.0	180		
		6.1	187		
		6.2	194		
		6.3	202		
		6.4	209		
		6.5	216		
		6.6	224		
		6.7	232		
		6.8	240		
		6.9	246		

CASE 1

This 61-year-old printer with a 25-year history of a heart murmur noted dyspnea while carrying a large stack of paper across his shop one month ago. Since then his symptoms have progressed to the point of dyspnea on climbing one flight of stairs. He denies syncope, palpitation, or chest pain. Physical examination shows a prominent LV impulse, no thrill, normal S1, single S2, and a Grade III/VI systolic murmur at the base. Another Grade 2/6 "musical" systolic murmur is also described at the left sternal border and axilla. The carotid pulses are quick-rising but of low amplitude. Chest x-ray reveals mild cardiomegaly. An echocardiogram is ordered to delineate the etiology of his murmurs.

MEASUREMENTS (Echo tracings A-C)   **Time lines = 200 msec**

cf	=	Ejection fraction	=
Ao dimension	=	Percentage change	=
Ao valve opening	=	Ejection time	=
LA	=	Vcf	=
E-F slope	=	IVS amplitude	=
D-E amplitude	=	LVPW amplitude	=
EDD	=	LVPW thickness	=
ESD	=		

QUESTIONS

1. Using the above measurements, what two observations can be made from the echo to confirm the etiology of this patient's murmur? What is this diagnosis?

2. Is there echo evidence of disease of more than one valve? What is this evidence?

3. From the echo, what is the best estimate of the severity of this patient's valvular disease?
   (A) Mild
   (B) Moderate
   (C) Severe
   (D) None of the above

4. What anatomic diagnosis can be made in reference to the left ventricle to explain the patient's cardiomegaly on x-ray?

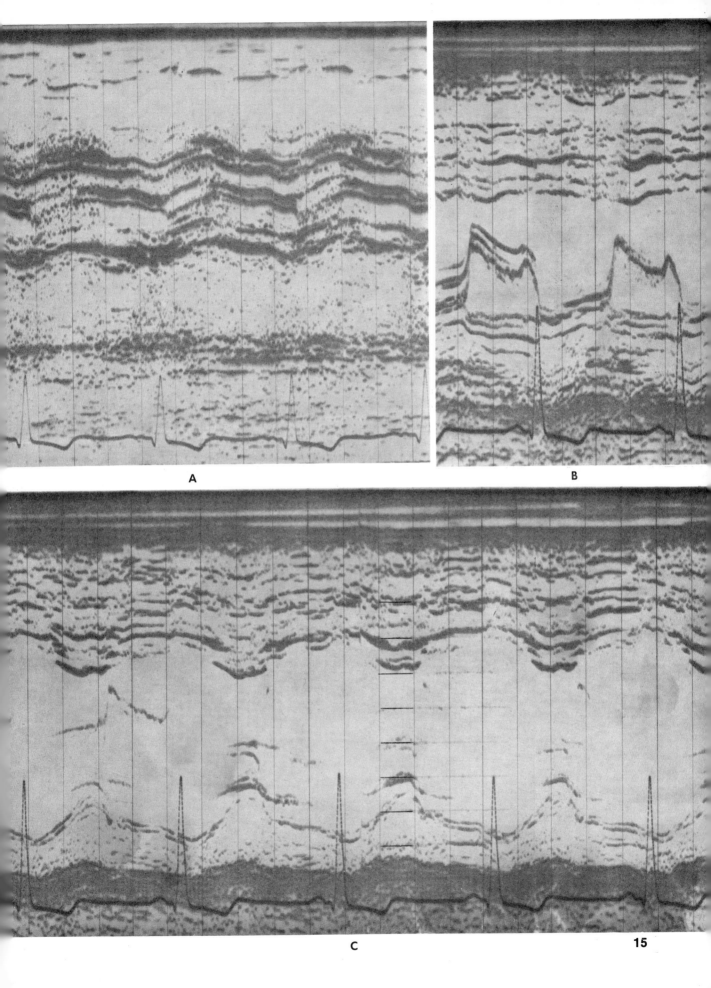

A

B

C

ANSWERS TO CASE 1
Calcific Aortic Stenosis
Left Ventricular Hypertrophy

MEASUREMENTS

cf	= 1.08	Ejection fraction	= 63%
Ao dimension	= 30 mm	Percentage change	= 35%
Ao valve opening	= 0.4 cm	Ejection time	= 310 msec
LA	= 2.9 cm	Vcf	= 1.12 circ/sec
E-F slope	= 50 mm/sec	IVS amplitude	= 12 mm
D-E amplitude	= 19 mm	LVPW amplitude	= 14 mm
EDD	= 5.8 cm	LVPW thickness	= 13 mm
ESD	= 3.8 cm		

ANSWERS

1. The observation of multiple, dense aortic root echoes combined with decreased opening of the aortic cusps (less than 1.5 cm) makes the echo diagnosis of valvular aortic stenosis (Table 1–1).[1, 11, 12] As illustrated in Figure 1–1, the aortic cusps *(open arrow)* are seen to have a markedly reduced opening during systole. Aortic valve opening is properly measured as the maximal opening obtained using the *internal* borders of the echoes from these cusps. Maximal opening almost always occurs in early systole just as the valve opens.

   Technical Hints. The following points will improve one's ability to record the often elusive aortic valve:

   (1) Make multiple, slow sweeps from the base of the aorta to the anterior mitral leaflet.

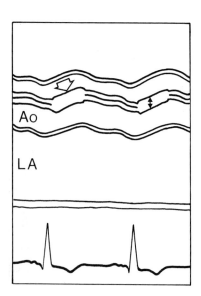

Figure 1–1 (Echo tracing *A*). Calcific aortic stenosis with reduced opening of the aortic cusps in systole *(open arrow)*. Note that the opening of the aortic valve is measured as the maximal opening obtained using the internal borders of the aortic cusp echoes *(double-headed arrow)*.

TABLE 1–1.   Calcific Aortic Stenosis

Diagnostic Criteria
1. Aortic valves opening less than 1.5 cm.
2. Echo-dense aorta.

Possible Associated Findings
1. Left ventricular hypertrophy and/or left ventricular dilatation.
2. Decreased E-F slope of the anterior mitral leaflet.
3. Fine diastolic shuddering of the anterior mitral leaflet.
4. Decreased aortic amplitude.
5. Dilated aortic root.
6. Echo-dense mitral annulus.

---

(2) Try different adjustments of the gain and damping controls as well as the depth compensation. It often is useful to have the depth compensation fully anterior and to have a slowly increasing slope of the time gain control. However, excessive gain can create the false impression of a dense aortic root. For this reason, the aortic root is best recorded with gain settings that optimize the mitral valve and right anterior ventricular wall.

(3) Use slightly different transducer angles and several different transducer positions; one interspace above the optimal position for the anterior mitral leaflet is often useful.

(4) Try recording the leaflets with the patient in a 30° left lateral position.

2. There is no evidence for intrinsic disease of the mitral valve shown in echo tracing *B*. The thin mitral leaflets with an appropriately moving posterior mitral leaflet (Fig. 1–2) exclude concomitant rheumatic mitral disease, despite the slightly reduced E-F slope of the anterior mitral leaflet. It is common to have a slight reduction in the E-F slope of the anterior mitral leaflet with loss of left ventricular compliance as in left ventricular hypertrophy (Table 1–1).[55, 59]

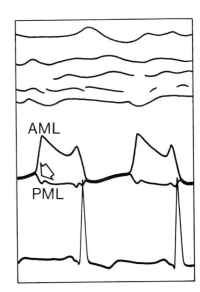

Figure 1–2 (Echo tracing *B*). Normal posterior motion of the posterior mitral leaflet in diastole *(open arrow)* and the thin mitral valve echo exclude concomitant rheumatic mitral disease despite the slightly reduced E-F slope.

The systolic murmur heard at the apex in this patient, therefore, most likely does not represent associated mitral regurgitation, but rather is transmitted from the aortic area. Note that there is no suggestion of associated aortic insufficiency in this case, as the thin anterior mitral leaflet does not show the fine shuddering in diastole characteristic of aortic regurgitation.[19-21]

Clinical Application. This case illustrates that echocardiography can be useful in determining if there is multiple valvular involvement. For example, when disease of one valve is evident and it is difficult to determine clinically if there is also involvement of another valve, an echocardiogram will often resolve this dilemma.

3. (D) None of the above.

Clinical Application. The severity of valvular aortic stenosis is poorly estimated by single element echocardiography.[13, 14] Not only may minimal degrees of aortic stenosis be overlooked, but severe stenosis cannot be distinguished reliably from moderate or even mild disease.

However, echocardiography remains useful in evaluating the presence of aortic stenosis. If thin, normally opening aortic cusps are recorded, the diagnosis of calcific valvular aortic stenosis is excluded. On the other hand, the finding of an echo-dense aortic root with reduced leaflet opening strongly suggests aortic stenosis. Congenital aortic stenosis, however, has different echocardiographic findings and is discussed elsewhere.

4. Symmetric left ventricular hypertrophy and slight dilatation of the left ventricular cavity are diagnosed by the thickened interventricular septum and left posterior ventricular wall and by the increased end-diastolic dimension of the left ventricle (Table 1-1). It should be noted that in symmetric left ventricular hypertrophy, both the left ventricular posterior wall and the interventricular septum are thickened approximately to the same extent.

Technical Hints. There are several technical points necessary to ensure accurate and reproducible left ventricular measurements.

(1) In adults, the end-diastolic and end-systolic diameters should be measured just inferior to the tip of the anterior mitral leaflet with fragments of the mitral apparatus visible. In children, the mitral valve lies relatively lower in the left ventricle, and measurements should be made at the level of the posterior mitral leaflet with this structure visible in the echo.[2, 144, 145]

(2) The transducer position and the damping and gain controls should be adjusted to identify positively and record continuous endocardial echoes simultaneously from both the interventricular septum and the left ventricular posterior wall, as well as the epicardial and pericardial interfaces.[1, 220]

(3) Popp, et al.,[147] found that for the most reproducible results, the left ventricle should be recorded from a "standard interspace." This interspace will vary from patient to patient, but is defined as the interspace from which the anterior mitral leaflet is recorded while the transducer is perpendicular to the chest wall, with only slight medial but no superior or inferior angulation.

(4) To make reliable serial measurements in a patient being followed longitudinally, the echo should always be obtained with the patient in the same position and from the same place on the chest wall. This is particularly important in patients with an enlarged left ventricle, which can be recorded from several different interspaces with conflicting dimensions. Noting the actual interspace and transducer position used in the echo report and making LV measurements on recordings that

show very similar landmarks will help minimize these sources of error in following patients longitudinally.

Cardiac catheterization in this patient showed an integrated aortic gradient of 53 mm Hg with a calculated aortic valve area of 0.8 cm². There was no pressure gradient across the mitral valve, and the contour of the LA pressure was normal. The LV cineangiogram showed no mitral regurgitation and normal LV contractility, with an ejection fraction of 82 per cent, change of the minor axis of 37 per cent, and Vcf of 1.3 circ/sec (right anterior oblique projection). At surgery, the aortic valve was stenotic and heavily calcified, with fusion of the commissures. The left ventricle was markedly hypertrophied.

CASE 2

A 50-year-old realtor, previously in good health, is hospitalized with a three-week history of increasing dyspnea on exertion, fatigue, and fever. Three times during the week prior to admission, he awoke short of breath at night. Physical examination reveals a temperature of 39° C, normal S1 and S2, a systolic ejection murmur at the base, an early diastolic blowing murmur along the left sternal border, and an apical mid-diastolic rumble. Bibasilar rales are present on chest examination. The chest x-ray shows moderate cardiomegaly. An echocardiogram is ordered to delineate the etiology of his valvular disease.

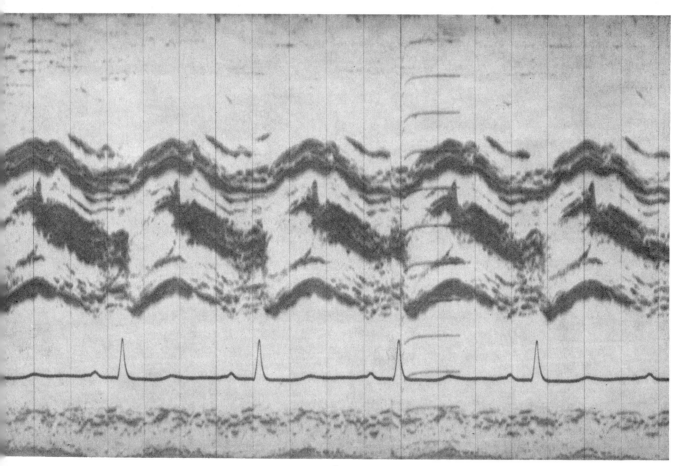

A

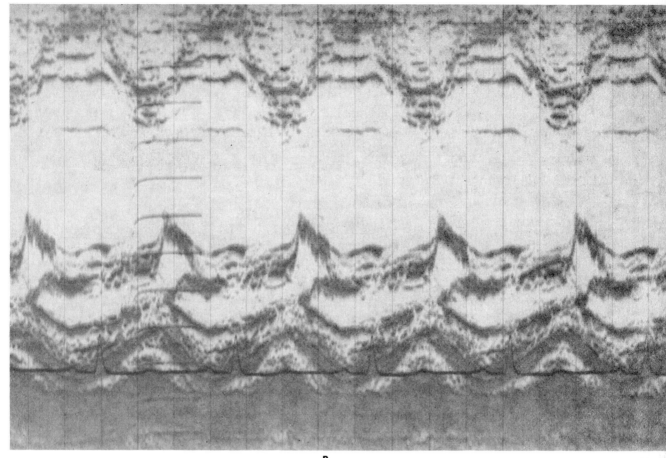

B

MEASUREMENTS (Echo tracings A-C)   **Time lines = 200 msec**

cf	=	Percentage change	=
Ao dimension	=	Ejection time	=
Ao valve opening	=	Vcf	=
EDD	=	IVS amplitude	=
ESD	=	LVPW amplitude	=
Ejection fraction	=	IVS thickness	=
		LVPW thickness	=

QUESTIONS

1. For each of the three diagnoses listed in the chart below, check the appropriate space to indicate whether the echo confirms or excludes this diagnosis; then supply the echo findings that allow this differentiation.

	Echo		
	Confirms	*Excludes*	*Findings that Allow this Differentiation*
A. Aortic stenosis			
B. Aortic insufficiency			
C. Mitral stenosis			

2. What observations from the echo suggest an etiology of this patient's valvular disease? What diagnosis is suggested?

3. What echo observation is *best* for judging this patient's valvular disease to be hemodynamically severe?
   (A) Left ventricular dilatation
   (B) Fine shuddering of the anterior mitral leaflet (AML)
   (C) Left ventricular hypertrophy
   (D) Early closure of the mitral valve
   (E) The ejection fraction and Vcf

4. What is the *best* description of this patient's left ventricle?
   (A) Normal left ventricular size and contractility
   (B) Hyperdynamic left ventricle with increased ejection fraction and increased Vcf
   (C) Decompensated left ventricle with decreased ejection fraction and decreased Vcf
   (D) Left ventricular volume overload with ejection fraction and Vcf that are within normal limits

5. Name two causes of this patient's cardiomegaly observed on x-ray.

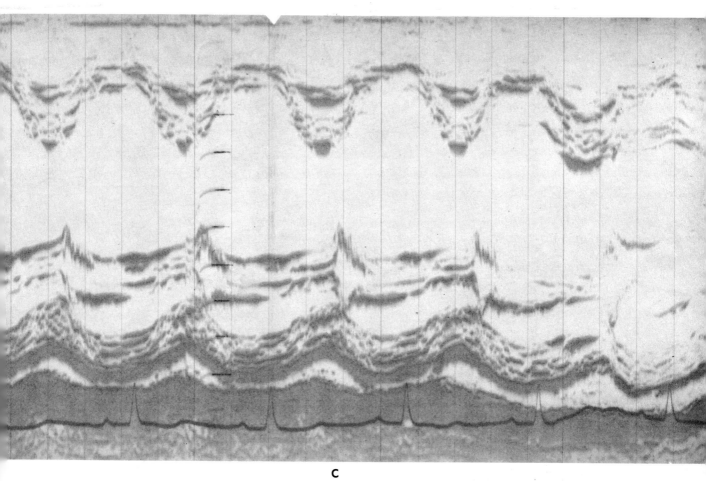

C

ANSWERS TO CASE 2
Aortic Insufficiency with Aortic Vegetations
Early Mitral Closure
Left Ventricular Volume Overload

MEASUREMENTS

cf	= 1.02	Percentage change	= 39%
Ao dimension	= 38 mm	Ejection time	= 300 msec
Ao valve opening	= 1.5 cm	Vcf	= 1.30 circ/sec
EDD	= 6.7 cm	IVS amplitude	= 16 mm
ESD	= 4.1 cm	LVPW amplitude	= 8 mm
Ejection fraction	= 68%	IVS thickness	= 7 mm
		LVPW thickness	= 12 mm

ANSWERS

1. (A) Aortic stenosis: Normal opening of the aortic leaflets excludes the diagnosis of calcific aortic stenosis (Fig. 2–1).
   (B) Aortic insufficiency: Fine, high frequency diastolic shuddering of the anterior mitral leaflet confirms the diagnosis of aortic insufficiency (Fig. 2–2).[19-21] The increased amplitude of the interventricular septum also supports this diagnosis.
   (C) Mitral stenosis: The thin anterior mitral leaflet with an appropriately moving posterior mitral leaflet excludes the diagnosis of mitral stenosis (Fig. 2–2).

   Technical hints. When there is fine diastolic shuddering of the anterior mitral leaflet, as seen in aortic insufficiency, care must be taken to record the mitral valve

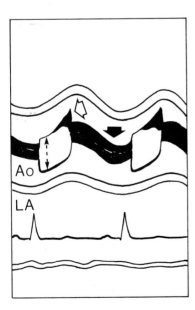

Figure 2–1 (Echo tracing *A*). Aortic vegetations are suggested by the nonuniform thickening of the anterior aortic cusp *(open arrow)* and by echo densities that occur primarily during diastole *(closed arrow)*. Note that calcific aortic stenosis is excluded by the normal opening of the aortic valve *(dashed, double-headed arrow)*.

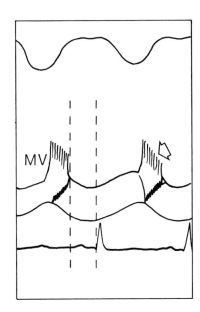

Figure 2–2 (Echo tracing *B*). Aortic insufficiency is indicated by the fine, high frequency shuddering of the anterior mitral leaflet in diastole *(open arrow)*. Early closure of the mitral valve prior to the QRS is also illustrated. Note too that the posterior mitral leaflet moves posteriorly at the beginning of diastole.

with the *minimal* amount of gain necessary to record the valve clearly. If too much gain is used, the fine diastolic shuddering will be obscured and, instead, a false impression of mitral thickness might be obtained. In this case, notice how much clearer the fine diastolic shuddering of the anterior mitral leaflet is when the gain is lower, as on echo tracing *C*. Likewise, one must be careful not to over-read minor degrees of equivocal diastolic shuddering as indicating aortic insufficiency.

2. On echo tracing *A*, prominent echo densities are observed within the aorta, primarily during diastole. The aortic valve opens normally but appears to be nonuniformly thickened in that the anterior cusp is unusually echo-dense in the latter part of systole, whereas the rest of both cusps are of normal echo density (Fig. 2–1). This nonuniform thickening of an aortic cusp that exhibits normal opening and the prominent echo densities within the aorta, primarily during one part of

TABLE 2–1. Valvular Vegetations
(In the Appropriate Clinical Setting)

Aortic Valve
1. Nonuniform thickening of the aortic cusps.
2. Normal opening of the aortic cusps.
3. Multiple linear or coalescent echo densities within the aorta in different parts of the cardiac cycle with different angles of the transducer. Rarely may persist throughout cardiac cycle.
4. Irregular, chaotic vibrating echo densities prolapsing into the left ventricular outflow tract during diastole.

Mitral and Tricuspid Valve
1. Nonuniform thickening of the leaflet.
2. Normal leaflet opening.
3. Possible signs of prolapse or ruptured chordae tendineae.

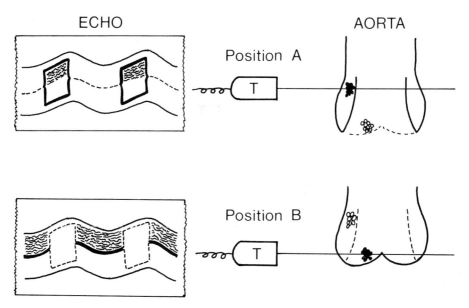

ECHO   AORTA

Position A

Position B

Figure 2–3. Illustration of how aortic vegetations may be recorded in different parts of the cardiac cycle. In position *A*, the vegetation is in the path of the echo beam only when the valve opens, and thus appears on the recorded echo during systole. However, in position *B*, only when the valve is closed is the vegetation in the path of the echo beam. Consequently, in this position the echo densities are recorded only during diastole.

the cardiac cycle, suggest the presence of aortic valvular vegetations and endocarditis as an etiology of this patient's valvular disease (Table 2–1).[26-31] Vegetations may have a variable appearance on the echo. They may appear as an irregular or "shaggy" thickening of normally opening valves or as multiple linear or coalescent echoes in one part of the cardiac cycle. Other appearances will be discussed in subsequent cases. When aortic vegetations are present, it often is possible to record these prominent echo densities either primarily in systole or primarily in diastole with slightly different angles of the transducer, as explained in Figures 2–3 and 2–4.

Clinical Applications. In the clinical setting of fever of unknown etiology or in the presence of a cardiac murmur and fever, echo evidence of vegetations should suggest the diagnosis of endocarditis. However, it should be realized that a normal echo does not exclude endocarditis, because vegetations may not be large enough to be seen and because they may be present on a part of the valve that is not recorded. But, when present, echo evidence of vegetations does support a clinical diagnosis of endocarditis and may localize the infection to one or more valves. In addition, the echo cannot distinguish between sterile and infected vegetations.[29] Evidence of vegetations may be detected echocardiographically even after complete recovery from endocarditis.

Because false-positive echo findings for vegetations occur, the diagnosis of valvular vegetations should not be made from the echo alone in the absence of a clinical suspicion of endocarditis. The causes of these false-positive echoes for aortic vegetations include: (1) nonspecific thickening of the aortic leaflets or root; (2) congenital aortic stenosis; and (3) too high a gain setting on the echo machine.

3. (D) Early closure of the mitral valve prior to the QRS is the best echo indicator of severity in acute aortic insufficiency (Fig. 2–2).[19, 21, 22, 30] This observation reflects the precarious hemodynamic finding of the left ventricular pressure

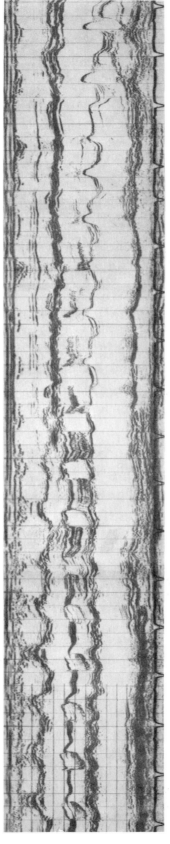

Figure 2–4. Echocardiogram from another patient with bacterial endocarditis (anaerobic streptococcus) and a large vegetation on the noncoronary cusp that was found almost destroyed at surgery. Notice how, with slightly different angles of the transducer, the echo densities are recorded primarily during systole on the left, where the leaflets appear nonuniformly thickened, or during diastole in the center of the tracing.

exceeding the left atrial pressure early in diastole, secondary to a large volume of blood acutely regurgitating across the aortic valve into a chamber that has not had a chance to dilate and is relatively noncompliant. As a consequence, the mitral valve closes early and the ability to increase the cardiac output is limited. Pharmacologic interventions that alter the left ventricular filling pressure or the afterload, or both, or changes in the left ventricular compliance with time, may alter this finding of early closure of the mitral valve. For example, amyl nitrite, by lowering systemic resistance and reducing left ventricular end-diastolic pressure, would tend to abolish early closure. In chronic aortic insufficiency the left ventricle dilates and is able to handle a large regurgitant volume without developing a high enough end-diastolic pressure to close the mitral valve early in systole.[30] On the other hand, early closure of the mitral valve may be seen without aortic insufficiency in the presence of first-degree heart block, slow junctional rhythms, or intermittently with other irregular arrhythmias.

Fine, high frequency diastolic shuddering of the anterior mitral leaflet as seen in aortic insufficiency is a poor indicator of the severity of the aortic regurgitation.[23] Prominent shuddering may be associated with either mild or severe aortic insufficiency. In acute, severe aortic insufficiency associated with early closure of the mitral valve, diastolic shuddering may be minimal or even absent.

Technical Hint. Before diagnosing early closure of the mitral valve, one must positively identify that coaptation of the anterior and posterior mitral leaflets (C point) occurs prior to the QRS (Fig. 2–2). Relying solely on the rapid closing descent of the anterior mitral leaflet without identification of the point at which the anterior and posterior leaflets coapt may give a false impression of early closure of the mitral valve.

Clinical Application. Assessment of the severity and rate of progression of acute aortic regurgitation secondary to endocarditis is critical to the proper timing of aortic valve replacement in patients with significant aortic insufficiency and congestive heart failure. The echo finding of closure of the mitral valve prior to the QRS in these patients has proved to be indicative of significant aortic regurgitation and to suggest a precarious hemodynamic situation. Consequently, it is recommended[19, 22] that these patients be considered for urgent surgical correction of the aortic regurgitation.

4. (D) Left ventricular volume overload, as may occur in aortic insufficiency, mitral regurgitation, and patent ductus arteriosus, is suggested by (1) increased EDD of the left ventricle and (2) increased amplitude, but appropriately timed motion, of the interventricular septum (Table 2–2). In compensated states of left ventricular volume overload, the calculated left ventricular ejection fraction and Vcf usually are within the normal range, although the amplitude of the septum and posterior wall is high. Consequently, echocardiography can be used to follow serially patients with aortic insufficiency in order to detect signs of decompensation that might be reflected in falling ejection indices.[24, 169a, 295]

5. The two causes of this patient's cardiomegaly are: (1) dilatation of the left ventricular cavity, as indicated by the increased end-diastolic and end-systolic measurements; and (2) small pericardial effusion, as shown by the presence of an echo-free space posterior to the left ventricular wall throughout both systole and diastole.[220]

TABLE 2–2. Ventricular Volume Overload

---

*Right Ventricular Volume Overload**
1. Right ventricular dilatation.
2. Abnormally timed motion of interventricular septum.

Left Ventricular Volume Overload†
1. Dilatation of left ventricular cavity.
2. Increased amplitude, but appropriately timed motion,
   of interventricular septum.

---

*May occur in atrial septal defect, tricuspid insufficiency, anomalous pulmonary venous drainage, pulmonic insufficiency, and aorta-to-right heart shunts.

†May occur in aortic or mitral regurgitation, patent ductus arteriosus, and ventricular septal defect.

At cardiac catheterization, this patient had severe aortic insufficiency and evidence of biventricular failure (right ventricle = 61/17 and pulmonary artery wedge = 34 mm Hg). Significant pulmonary hypertension with a pulmonary artery pressure of 62/42 mm Hg also was present. At surgery for aortic valve replacement, the aortic cusps were found to be mobile, but there was a large vegetation on the right coronary cusp, which itself was almost totally sloughed away. Blood cultures prior to surgery were positive for Pneumococcus.

CASE 3

A 21-year-old lumberjack with a murmur known since an Army discharge physical examination four years previously is referred for evaluation after beginning to experience dizziness and increasing fatigue while working. There is no history of fever, weight loss, or night sweats. Physical examination reveals a blood pressure of 130/85, a temperature of 38° C, and a systolic ejection murmur at the base. No diastolic murmur is appreciated. Chest x-ray shows minimal cardiomegaly. An echocardiogram is ordered to help define the etiology of this murmur.

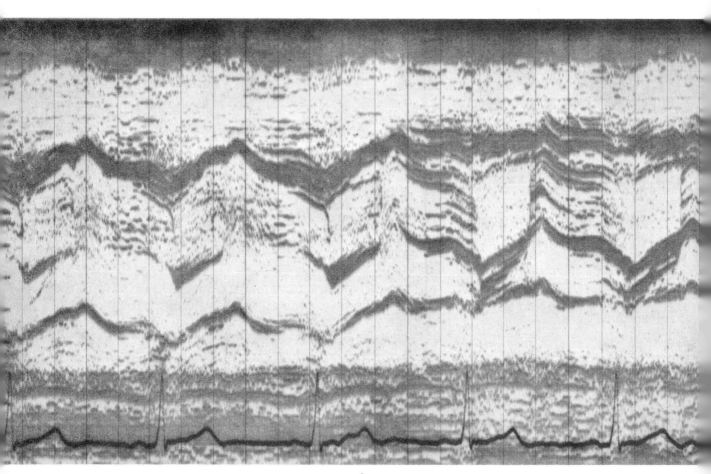

A

QUESTION

(Echo tracings *A* and *B*)   Time lines = 200 msec

With which diagnosis is the echo most compatible?
(A) Calcific aortic stenosis
(B) Congenital aortic stenosis
(C) Endocarditis of aortic valve
(D) Mitral stenosis with regurgitation
(E) Heart tumor

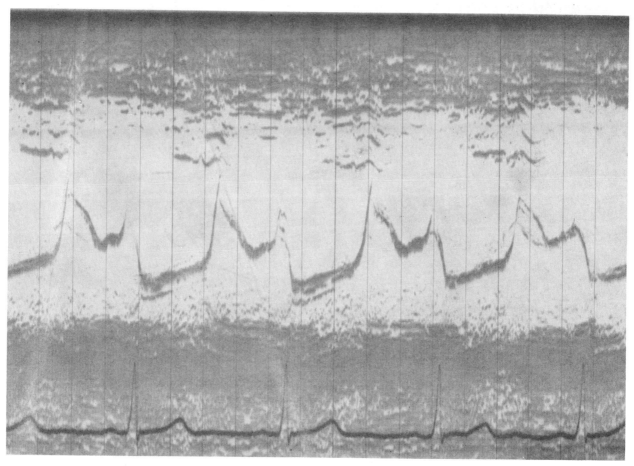

B

ANSWER TO CASE 3
Congenital Aortic Stenosis

ANSWER

(B) This echocardiogram shows the aortic cusps to open normally (Fig. 3–1), and, of the choices given, congenital aortic stenosis is the most likely answer in this clinical setting.

In congenital aortic stenosis, the aortic valve often opens normally, even in the presence of severe stenosis. As illustrated in Figure 3–2, this results from the echo beam passing through the base of a mobile, doming aortic valve, which during ventricular systole comes in close proximity to the aortic walls. The echo only detects the base of the valve and thus shows the cusps to open normally. It fails to detect the narrow opening at the top of the dome where the cusps are not perpendicular to the transducer and do not reflect echoes well. In addition, one often detects multiple linear echoes during diastole in congenital aortic stenosis, as illustrated on this echo.[2, 16] These linear densities probably result from nonspecific thickening of the valve or from nodular excrescences present in the cusps,[17] but are not specific for congenital aortic stenosis, as they may also be seen in calcific aortic stenosis. Note that these dense diastolic echoes associated with a normally opening aortic valve closely resemble the echo pattern often seen with aortic valvular vegetations (Case 2).

This echo also suggests a bicuspid aortic valve, as reported by Nanda, et al.[15] Recognizing that in bicuspid aortic valves one of the cusps usually predominates in size and the aortic orifice is thus eccentrically located, these authors noted an eccentricity of the aortic cusps within the aorta on echoes from patients with surgically or angiographically proved bicuspid aortic valves. From these patients, they calculated an Eccentricity Index (Fig. 3–1) and found that it was always greater than 1.5 in patients with bicuspid aortic valves.

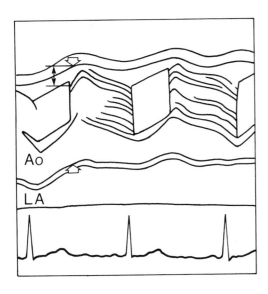

Figure 3–1 (Echo tracing *A*). Congenital aortic stenosis of a bicuspid aortic valve. Note that the aortic valve opens normally and that there is eccentricity of the point where the valve opens and closes. In calculation of the Eccentricity Index, the internal aortic root diameter (open arrows) and the minimal distance between the closing point of the aortic cusps (double-headed arrow) are measured at the onset of diastole.

CONGENITAL AORTIC STENOSIS

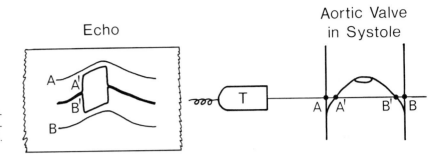

Figure 3–2. Illustration of how normally opening aortic leaflets are recorded in congenital aortic stenosis. See text for discussion.

$$\text{Eccentricity Index} = \frac{\frac{1}{2}\ \text{internal aortic diameter at beginning diastole}}{\text{minimal distance between cusp and aortic wall in diastole}}$$

This Eccentricity Index[15] for a bicuspid aortic valve is calculated by dividing one-half of the *internal* aortic diameter measured at the onset of diastole by the *minimal distance* between the closing point of aortic cusps and the inside of the closest aortic wall (Fig. 3–1). In a bicuspid aortic valve this Eccentricity Index is greater than 1.5 according to Nanda[15] and greater than 1.3 according to Radford.[16]

Radford and colleagues[16] have reported that 74 per cent of patients with surgically or angiographically proved bicuspid aortic valves have an Eccentricity Index equal to or greater than 1.3. However, a normal Eccentricity Index did not exclude the presence of a bicuspid aortic valve, since central aortic leaflet closing occurred in 26 per cent of cases with a bicuspid valve. However, all tricuspid aortic valves had central aortic cusp echoes. They also found that approximately one-third of patients with a high membranous ventricular septal defect had an Eccentricity Index of greater than 1.3. In making this measurement, care must be taken to identify where the aortic cusp echoes merge into a line in diastole. Sometimes this can be difficult if there are multiple linear echoes in diastole.

In the patient shown in this case, the Eccentricity Index is calculated to be 2.2. At cardiac catheterization, the integrated aortic gradient was 45 mm Hg, and the calculated aortic valve area was 1.2 cm². The aortic valve was seen to be stenotic with mobile, doming cusps on left ventricular cineangiography. At surgery when an aortic commissurotomy was done, the valve was stenotic and bicuspid with thickened, mobile aortic cusps.

CASE 4

This 35-year-old former intravenous amphetamine user presents with a two-week history of fever, chills, and malaise. He is hospitalized and found to have systolic and diastolic murmurs and to have multiple pulmonary infiltrates on chest x-ray. An echocardiogram is ordered.

QUESTIONS

(Echo tracings A-C)   **Time lines = 200 msec**

1. Which two of the following diagnoses does the echo suggest as an explanation for this patient's murmurs?
   (A) Aortic stenosis
   (B) Aortic insufficiency
   (C) Mitral stenosis
   (D) Mitral regurgitation
   (E) Tricuspid stenosis
   (F) Tricuspid regurgitation

2. What etiology for the above diagnosis(es) does the echo suggest?

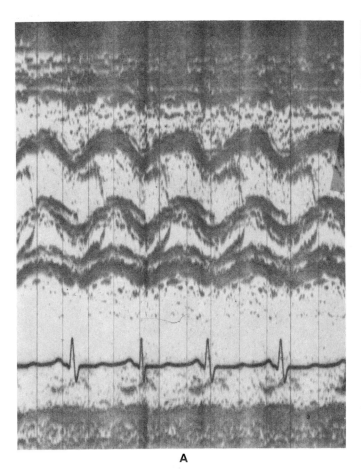

A

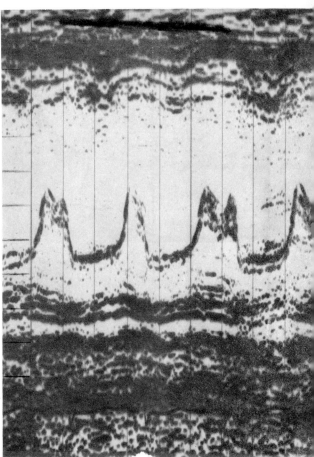

B

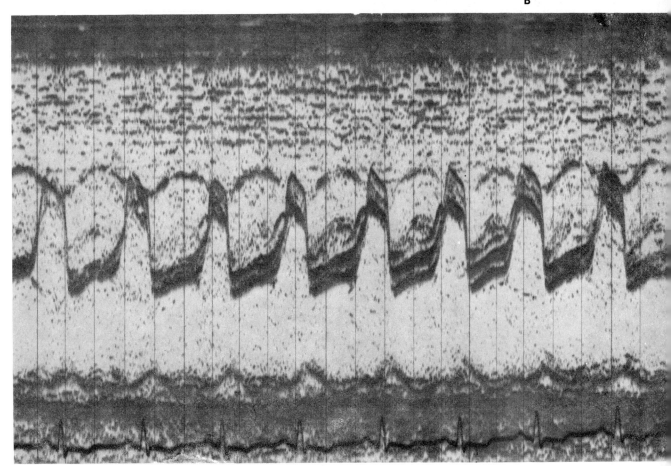

C

35

ANSWERS TO CASE 4
Tricuspid and Aortic Vegetations

ANSWERS

1. (B), (F).

2. The aortic, mitral, and tricuspid valves are shown. The tricuspid valve seen in echo tracing *C* has a normal amplitude of motion and, although in places it appears thin, in others there is nonuniform thickening with abnormal echo densities recorded both in systole and diastole (Fig. 4–1, *open arrows*). In the clinical setting of this patient, these findings are most consistent with a vegetation on the tricuspid valve (Table 2–1). In the absence of an intrinsic echo abnormality of the mitral valve, these findings suggest that the cause of this patient's pansystolic murmur is tricuspid regurgitation secondary to endocarditis. The aortic valve is seen and opens normally, excluding aortic stenosis. However, the prominent echo densities seen within the aortic walls throughout the cardiac cycle are abnormal (Fig. 4–2). In this clinical setting, with tricuspid vegetations and the possibility of fine, high frequency diastolic shuddering of the anterior mitral leaflet, these aortic densities suggest that endocarditic vegetations also involve the aortic valve, with accompanying aortic regurgitation.

   Blood cultures in this man were positive for *Staphylococcus aureus*, coagulase positive. After prolonged antibiotic therapy, the documentation of gross (4+) aortic insufficiency on cardiac catheterization and continuing congestive heart failure, the patient underwent aortic and tricuspid valve replacement. At operation, there was a strong systolic thrill palpated in the right atrium consistent with tricuspid regurgita-

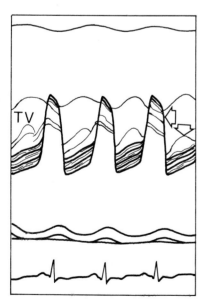

Figure 4–1 (Echo tracing C). Vegetations on the tricuspid valve. Note the increased echo densities *(open arrows)* during systole and diastole of the tricuspid valve that shows a normal amplitude of motion.

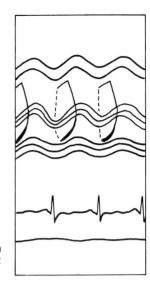

Figure 4–2 (Echo tracing *A*).   Vegetation of the aortic valve located on the commissure between the right and left cusps at the time of surgery. Note echo densities within the aortic root that persist throughout the cardiac cycle and normal opening of the aortic leaflets.

tion. A large, grape-sized vegetation was found in the area of the septal leaflet of the tricuspid valve, and this leaflet had almost disappeared. The aortic valve was thin and tricuspid, but had one vegetation involving the commissure between the right and the left coronary cusps and another vegetation on the noncoronary cusp. A moderate-sized hole was present in the noncoronary cusp. There was no recurrence of infection postoperatively after more than one year of follow-up.

The degree of high frequency vibrations of the anterior mitral leaflet recorded in aortic insufficiency is dependent more on the direction of the regurgitant jet than on the severity of the insufficiency. If the regurgitation is directed away from the anterior leaflet, mitral vibrations may be minimal even though the degree of aortic insufficiency is significant. Apparently, this is the explanation for the slight degree of mitral shuttering in this patient who had a hole in the posterior, noncoronary aortic cusp and gross aortic insufficiency.

CASE 5

This 25-year-old bricklayer experienced the acute onset of left upper quadrant abdominal pain one month ago, and, after obtaining a diagnosis of splenic infarct, underwent splenectomy in another city. Since discharge, he has experienced several transient episodes of difficulty in seeing and attacks of numbness in his right fingers and in his toes. Because of increasing malaise and weight loss associated with fever and chills at night, he consults a local physician, who orders an echocardiogram to rule out a left atrial myxoma. Both systolic and diastolic murmurs are also described.

QUESTIONS

(Echo tracings *A-C*. Tracings *B* and *C* are continuous.)

1. What etiology for this patient's apparent peripheral emboli does the echo suggest?

2. Where should the difficulty be localized?

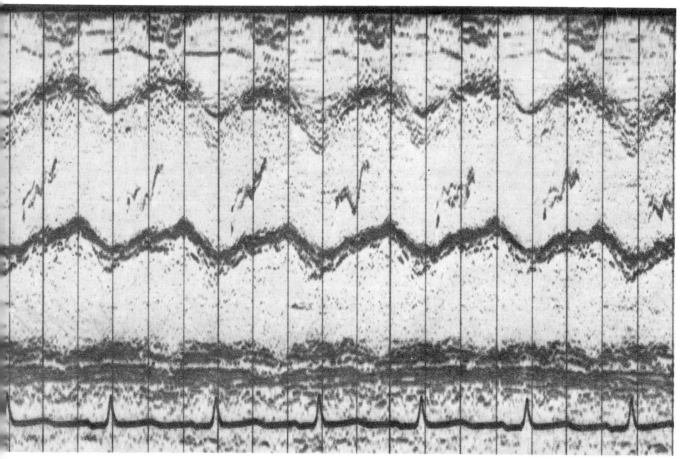

A

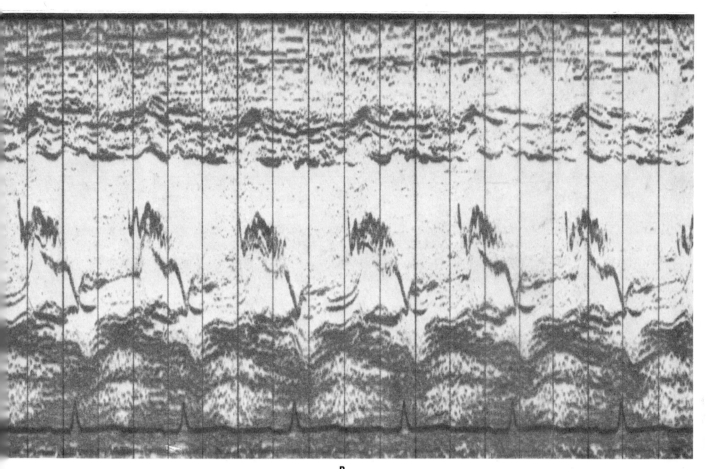

B

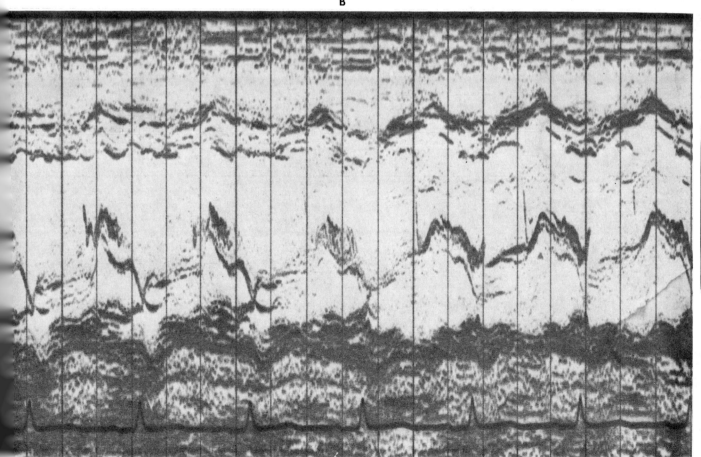

C

39

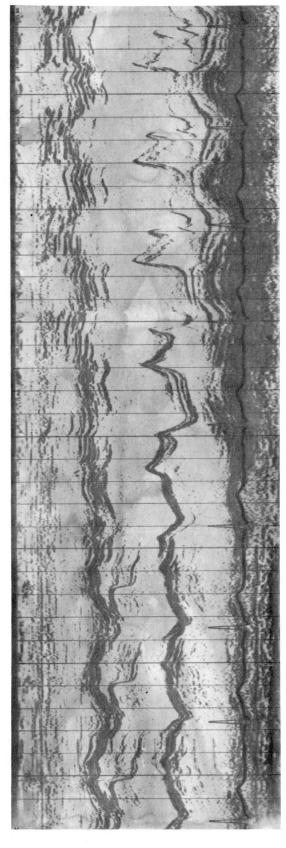

Figure 5–1. M-mode scan of the aorta and mitral valve in the patient shown in this case after three weeks of penicillin therapy, showing the absence of the previously demonstrated aortic vegetation within the left ventricular outflow tract. Note the evidence of aortic regurgitation with diastolic shuddering of the anterior mitral leaflet. Evidence of peripheral emboli was not recognized clinically after initiation of antibiotic therapy.

ANSWERS TO CASE 5
Prolapsing Aortic Valvular Vegetation

ANSWERS

1 and 2. The aortic root echo shows an unusual structure within the aorta in systole in the region of the posterior noncoronary aortic cusp. This structure is thin, moves erratically, and does not have the characteristic motion of a posterior aortic cusp. On an M-mode scan, an irregularly vibrating echo-dense structure is seen within the left ventricular outflow tract during diastole between the septum and the anterior leaflet of the mitral valve. Posterior to this structure, both the anterior and posterior mitral leaflets appear normal.

Note that this structure is present in the left ventricular outflow tract *prior to* the time when the anterior mitral leaflet comes forward in diastole and that it appears to be separate from the mitral valve. In the clinical setting of fever and apparent peripheral emboli of undetermined etiology associated with cardiac murmurs, these findings are suggestive of an endocarditic vegetation of the aortic valve, with prolapse of the vegetation into the left ventricular outflow tract in diastole (Table 2–1). A similar echo pattern has been described as indicating a flail aortic valve in bacterial endocarditis.[32-35, 35a] However, such a finding would not seem to be specific for a flail aortic leaflet, but rather to be another manifestation of aortic endocarditis in which the vegetation prolapses into the left ventricular outflow tract in diastole and is recorded as an irregular vibrating structure. Abnormal echoes may or may not be recorded within the aortic root during systole. One might speculate that this is

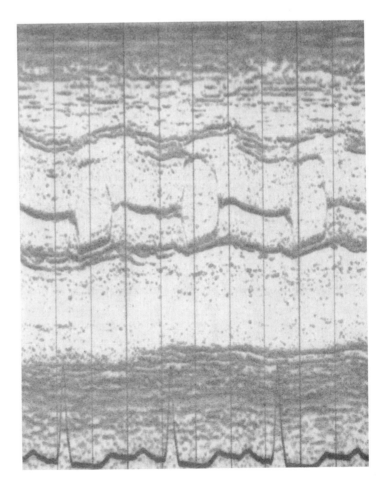

Figure 5–2. Echocardiogram of the posterior aortic cusp obtained after three weeks of antibiotic therapy at the same time as Figure 5–1.

the mechanism of the "kissing lesions" of the mitral valve described in aortic valvular endocarditis.

It is of interest that, after three weeks of penicillin therapy following blood cultures positive for alpha Streptococcus, the patient in this case no longer showed evidence of vegetations within the left ventricular outflow tract nor of the unusual structures in the region of the posterior aortic cusp (Fig. 5–1). In fact, a normal-appearing echo was obtained from the posterior aortic cusp on the later echocardiogram (Fig. 5–2). This supports the idea that the mass prolapsing into the left ventricular outflow tract was primarily an aortic vegetation. Aortic insufficiency was evident from the anterior mitral leaflet, but the mitral valve otherwise remained normal. Because the patient has remained relatively asymptomatic, he has not undergone cardiac catheterization or surgery, but does have clinically evident aortic regurgitation without evidence of mitral disease.

CASE 6

A 45-year-old delicatessen owner with hypertension, congestive heart failure, and stable exertional angina since her "heart attack" eight years ago experienced the abrupt onset of severe substernal pain and dyspnea while restocking the shelves of her store. On the way to the hospital, she became increasingly dyspneic as the pain increased in severity and spread through to her back. On admission to the Coronary Care Unit, she is hypertensive (200/120) and diaphoretic, with peripheral vasoconstriction. Diffuse inspiratory rales are present in the lungs. A Grade II/VI systolic ejection murmur at the base and a Grade II/VI diastolic murmur at the left sternal border are associated with a gallop rhythm. Peripheral pulses are intact. ECG shows loss of precordial R waves and diffuse ST-T wave abnormalities. The chest x-ray reveals marked cardiomegaly.

MEASUREMENTS (Echo tracings A-C)   **Time lines = 100 msec**

cf	=	EDD	=
Ao dimension	=	ESD	=
		Ejection fraction	=
LA	=	Percentage	
		change	=
E-F slope	=	IVS thickness	=
RV	=	LVPW thickness	=

QUESTIONS

1. What etiology for this patient's chest pain does the echo suggest?

2. Name one entity that may cause a false-positive echocardiographic pattern for this diagnosis.

3. What two complications that occur with this entity might the echo reliably detect? Is there evidence of either of these on this patient's echo?

4. From the echo, should this patient's left ventricular function be judged compensated or decompensated? What evidence can be cited to support this judgment?

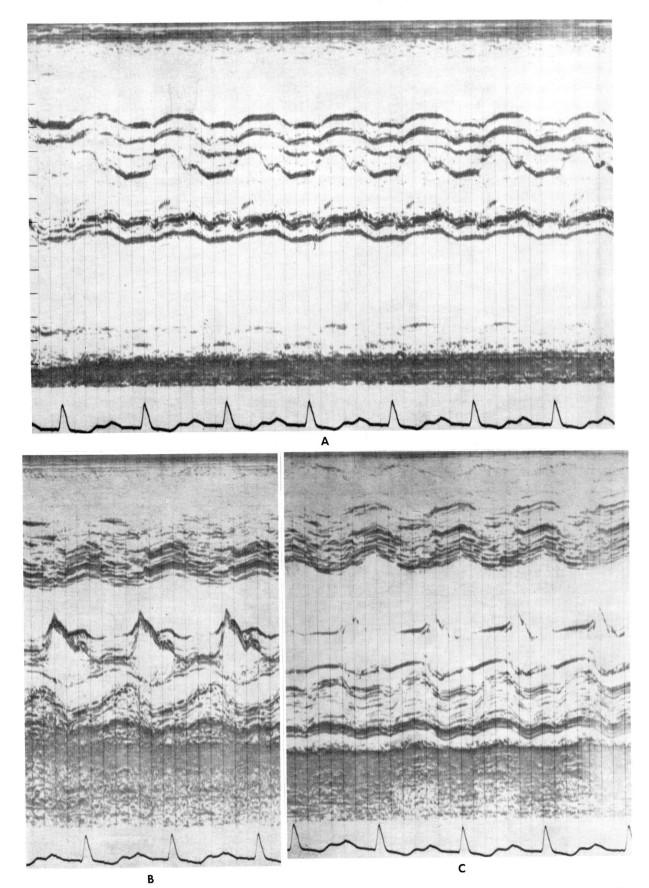

A

B

C

43

ANSWERS TO CASE 6
Aortic Root Dissection
Aortic Insufficiency
Pericardial Effusion

MEASUREMENTS

cf	= 1.59	EDD	= 5.4 cm
Ao dimension	= 49 mm	ESD	= 4.5 cm
		Ejection fraction	= 35%
LA	= 5.8 cm	Percentage	
		change	= 17%
E-F slope	= 70 mm/sec	IVS thickness	= 21 mm
RV	= 1.3 cm	LVPW thickness	= 18 mm

ANSWERS

1. Dissecting aneurysm of the ascending aorta is suggested by the following echo findings, as reported by Nanda (Table 6–1):[37] (1) enlargement of the aortic root (42 mm or more); (2) separation and marked widening of the anterior aortic wall (16 to 21 mm) and posterior aortic wall (10 to 13 mm); (3) maintenance of parallel motion of the separated aortic walls throughout the cardiac cycle; and (4) preservation of normal opening of the aortic valve. In this study, aortic root width was determined as the external measurement from the most anterior echo of the anterior aortic wall to the most posterior echo from the posterior aortic wall during systole (Fig. 6–1, *open arrows*). Wall thickness was measured from the outer limit of each wall to the inner limit of the more central, lesser component of that wall during systole (Fig. 6–1, *solid, double-headed arrows*).

In the echo from this case (Fig. 6–1), the aortic root is widened (51 mm), and double anterior and posterior aortic walls are seen which remain parallel throughout the cardiac cycle. But the thicknesses of the anterior wall (13 to 14 mm) and the posterior wall (7 to 8 mm) are less than those previously reported in this entity. Care should be taken in diagnosing aortic dissection from an echo when all the criteria listed below are not rigidly met. However, angiography performed just after

TABLE 6–1. Aortic Root Dissection

Echo Findings (All) (In the Appropriate Clinical Setting)[37]
1. Dilatation of the aortic root (greater than 42 mm).
2. Separation and widening of the anterior aortic wall
   (16 to 21 mm) and the posterior wall (10 to 13 mm).
3. Maintenance of parallel motion of the separated
   aortic walls.
4. Normal opening of the aortic valve.

Possible Associated Conditions
1. Aortic insufficiency.
2. Pericardial effusion.

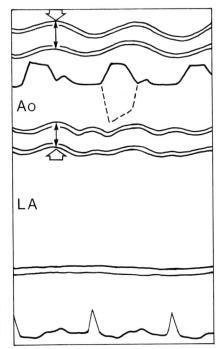

Figure 6–1 (Echo tracing *A*). Dissection of aortic root showing a dilated aortic root *(open arrows)* and thickened, double anterior and posterior aortic walls *(solid, double-headed arrows)* that maintain parallel motion throughout the cardiac cycle. See text for details of measurement.

this echocardiogram revealed that the patient did have a dissecting aneurysm of the ascending aorta.

2. The most common cause of false-positive echoes for aortic dissection is *dilatation of the ascending aorta,* as may occur in aortic insufficiency, cystic medial necrosis, Marfan's syndrome, hypertension, or bulging aortic aneurysm. In these cases, a widened aortic root, double aortic walls that remain parallel, and normally opening aortic leaflets may be recorded. One possible explanation for the double echo recorded from the aortic walls in dilatation of the aortic root is that echoes may be obtained from the curved aortic walls at different levels from the transducer. Such echoes might then be recorded as thick aortic walls that remain parallel throughout the cardiac cycle (Fig. 6–2).

   Calcific aortic stenosis also may produce multiple parallel lines within the aortic lumen and thus simulate aortic dissection. However, identifying a normally opening aortic valve should exclude this cause of false-positives.

Figure 6–2. Illustration of how "double aortic walls" might occur in dilatation of the aortic root. If echoes are obtained within the width of the echo beam from each curved aortic wall at different levels from the transducer, thickened or "double aortic walls" that move parallel will be recorded. In this manner, aortic dilatation may exactly simulate dissection of the aortic root (Table 6–1).

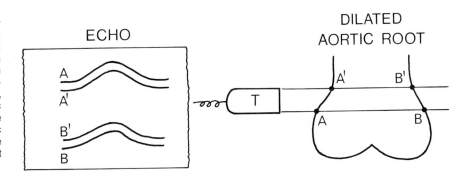

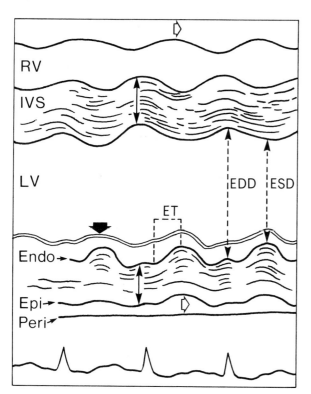

Figure 6–3 (Echo tracing C). Symmetric left ventricular hypertrophy and pericardial effusion posteriorly and anteriorly *(open, single-headed arrows)*. The endocardium *(Endo)*, epicardium *(Epi)*, and pericardium *(Peri)* of the left ventricle are identified. Just above the LVPW, echoes from the mitral apparatus, i.e., chordae tendineae, are seen *(closed, single-headed arrow)*. A scan to the mitral valve would show these echoes to be continuous with that valve. The proper places for measurement of septal and LVPW thickness at mid-diastole *(solid, double-headed arrows)*, LV cavity dimensions *(dashed, double-headed arrows)*, and ejection time *(ET)* also are illustrated.

Nonspecific thickening or calcium in the ascending aortic root could also closely simulate the echo picture of aortic root dissection.[38]

Pericardial fluid in the transverse sinus between the posterior aortic wall and the left atrium may give a double contour to the posterior aortic wall.[37] In such cases, the other criteria for the diagnosis of aortic dissection would not be present.

The echocardiographic pattern of aortic dissection may be seen in some patients without clinical or angiographic evidence of any disease of the aorta. Brown, et al.,[39] reported a series of 10 patients without clinical indications of aortic root dissection or aortic valve disease, of whom five patients had all the necessary echo criteria for dissection of the aorta, and five patients had at least two of the criteria. Because none of these patients had the extreme degree of thickening of the anterior aortic wall previously reported by Nanda[37] (16 to 21 mm), the authors thought that this finding was the most specific in this entity and that the echo criteria for aortic root dissection were most reliable when clinical indications of the abnormality are present.

On the other hand, false-negative echocardiograms may be obtained if the dissection occurs in the aortic wall asymmetrically[40] or in the interstitial space around the aorta, as we recently observed in one patient.

3. Aortic insufficiency and pericardial effusion, two entities associated with dissecting aneurysm of the ascending aorta, are more reliably detected by the echocardiogram than the dissection itself. There is evidence for both of these complications on this echo. A moderate pericardial effusion is indicated by the relatively echo-free space posterior to the left ventricular posterior wall, as well as anterior to the heart (Fig. 6–3, *open single-headed arrows*). Aortic insufficiency is also indicated by the fine, high frequency vibrations of the anterior mitral leaflet during

diastole. Early closure of the mitral valve is not present. Both of these complications were confirmed at operation in this patient.

In addition, there is evidence of symmetric left ventricular hypertrophy in this patient, who had long-standing systemic hypertension.

Clinical Application.   Considering all the causes of false-positive echo criteria for dissection of the aortic root, one should be extremely wary of making this diagnosis on the basis of the echo unless (1) the clinical setting is suggestive of dissection, and (2) all four echo criteria listed above are rigidly met. Echocardiography may be useful in detecting the aortic insufficiency and pericardial effusion that may be associated with dissection of the ascending aorta.

4. Although the left ventricle is symmetrically hypertrophied, the calculated left ventricular ejection fraction and percentage change of the minor axis are significantly reduced and indicate some left ventricular decompensation. Figure 6–3 illustrates the proper locations for making these left ventricular measurements.

After the diagnosis of a dissecting aneurysm of the ascending aorta and moderately severe aortic insufficiency had been established by angiography, the patient underwent surgery, at which a nearly complete circumferential dissection of the ascending aorta was confirmed. It began just above the noncoronary aortic leaflet and extended to the aortic arch. The noncoronary leaflet was found to prolapse through a widely dilated aortic annulus. Approximately 900 ml straw-colored pericardial fluid was present, and the heart was markedly enlarged, owing principally to massive hypertrophy.

CASE 7

This 73-year-old former commercial fisherman with a history of exertional angina for several years began to develop severe, increasingly disabling dyspnea despite diuretics and digitalis. One year ago, he began to notice peripheral edema and was hospitalized for congestive heart failure. At present, his physician notes a Grade III/VI harsh systolic ejection murmur at the base with radiation to the neck, a Grade II/VI early diastolic blow along the left sternal border, and a Grade II/VI high-pitched systolic murmur at the apex. S1 is normal and S2 decreased. The venous pressure is elevated. The liver is enlarged and slightly tender; peripheral edema (2+) is present around the ankles. An echo is ordered to delineate the etiology of his murmurs and to assess his left ventricular function.

MEASUREMENTS   (Echo tracings A–E)   **Time lines = 200 msec**

cf	=	Ejection fraction	=
Ao dimension	=	Percentage change	=
Ao valve opening	=	Ejection time	=
LA	=	Vcf	=
RV	=	IVS amplitude	=
EDD	=	LVPW amplitude	=
ESD	=	IVS thickness	=
		LVPW thickness	=

QUESTIONS

1. Which diagnosis(es) is(are) the most appropriate interpretation of this echocardiogram? More than one answer may apply.
   (A) Calcific aortic stenosis
   (B) Echo-dense aortic root
   (C) Aortic insufficiency
   (D) Dissection of the aortic root

2. Considering this patient's symptoms of right-sided failure, is there echo evidence of tricuspid insufficiency or pulmonary hypertension? If so, what is this evidence?

3. What is the *best* description of this patient's left ventricle?
   (A) Hyperdynamic, consistent with aortic insufficiency
   (B) Slightly dilated, with normal ejection indices
   (C) Hypertrophic, with segmental abnormalities
   (D) Decompensated

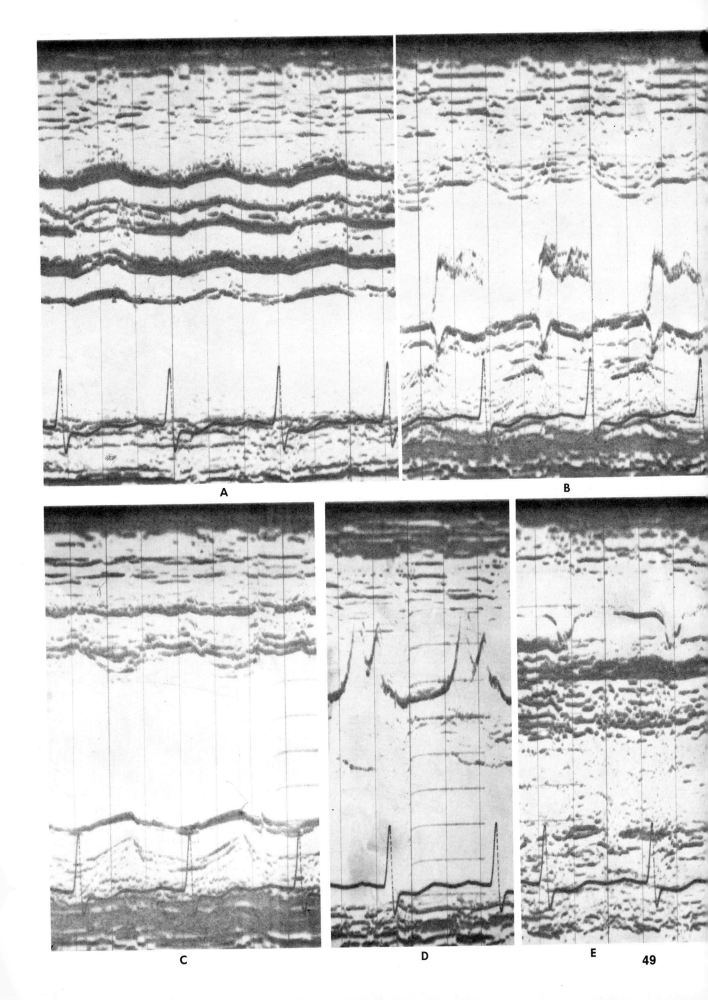

A

B

C

D

E

ANSWERS TO CASE 7
Echo-Dense Aortic Root (Aortic Stenosis)
Aortic Insufficiency
Pulmonary Hypertension

MEASUREMENTS

cf	= 1.05	Ejection fraction	= 42%
Ao dimension	= 36 mm	Percentage	
		change	= 20%
Ao valve opening	= not seen	Ejection time	= 270 msec
LA	= 3.7 cm	Vcf	= 0.69 circ/sec
RV	= 2.1 cm	IVS amplitude	= 7 mm
EDD	= 5.8 cm	LVPW amplitude	= 7 mm
ESD	= 4.6 cm	IVS thickness	= 12 mm
		LVPW thickness	= 14 mm

ANSWERS

1. (B), (C) Aortic insufficiency is indicated by the fine, high frequency diastolic shuddering of the anterior mitral leaflet (Fig. 7–1)[19-21] (see Case 2). It should be noted that early closure of the anterior mitral leaflet is not seen, and that this sign is not expected in chronic aortic regurgitation. Increased echo densities of the aortic root certainly are evident. However, to make the diagnosis of calcific aortic stenosis from the echo, definite aortic cusps with decreased opening must be identified (Table 1–1).[1] It is not rare for calcium in the aortic walls and/or annulus

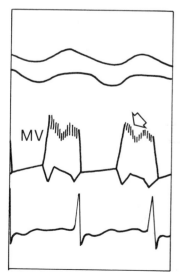

Figure 7–1 (Echo tracing *B*). Aortic insufficiency is indicated by the fine, high frequency diastolic shuddering of the anterior mitral leaflet *(open arrow)*. The lack of mitral rheumatic involvement is also established by the thin mitral echo and the normal motion of the posterior leaflet.

to produce increased echo densities on the echogram of the aortic root very similar to that shown in this patient in the absence of aortic valvular stenosis.[2] The degree of echo density alone does not correspond with the presence or severity of aortic stenosis. For this reason, increased echo densities of the aortic root without definitely identifiable aortic cusps that have a decreased opening should not be read as diagnostic of aortic stenosis. Under such circumstances it is more appropriate to read that there are increased echo densities of the aortic root, but, because the aortic cusps are not identified, a definite diagnosis of aortic stenosis cannot be made. It is true in this patient that the index of suspicion of aortic stenosis is increased with echo evidence of aortic insufficiency and left ventricular hypertrophy.

Dissection of the aortic root is not suggested from this echo, even though multiple parallel lines are recorded throughout the cardiac cycle. The aortic root is not dilated, the walls are not sufficiently thickened, aortic cusps are not identified, and the clinical setting is not suggestive of dissection (Table 6–1).[37]

2. The right ventricle is normal in size, and the motion of the interventricular septum is appropriately timed with reference to the left ventricular posterior wall. Thus, there is no echo evidence of tricuspid insufficiency, i.e., right ventricular volume overload (Table 2–2). However, the echogram of the pulmonary valve seen in echo tracing *E* is consistent with pulmonary hypertension. In this panel, one leaflet of the pulmonary valve is seen to move posteriorly as it opens following the QRS and to have a horizontal slope during diastole. It is this horizontal slope during diastole, with the absence of an "A wave" in the presence of sinus rhythm, which suggests pulmonary hypertension. The echo findings in pulmonary hypertension will be discussed in subsequent cases.

3. (B) Measurement of the left ventricle shows that it is symmetrically hypertrophied and slightly dilated, but calculation of the ejection indices, i.e., ejection fraction, percentage change of the minor diameter, and Vcf, shows that all these measurements are significantly decreased below normal, indicating some degree of left ventricular decompensation. There is no evidence of segmental abnormalities, and with normal amplitudes of the septum and left ventricular posterior wall, no evidence of a hyperdynamic left ventricle.

This elderly gentleman refused cardiac catheterization and surgery, stating he had "lived long enough." At necropsy, done soon after the echo, very severe calcific aortic stenosis was found, with a dilated left ventricle that showed hypertrophy and extensive fibrosis on microscopic examination.

CASE 8

A 46-year-old airline executive has episodic palpitations associated with shortness of breath and fatigue. These occur once or twice per week and last from two minutes to four hours. In addition, his exercise tolerance has decreased over the last year. Physical examination shows a loud S1, a normal S2, a Grade II/VI apical systolic murmur, and a Grade II/IV low-pitched diastolic murmur at the apex. An S3 is described. ECG shows atrial fibrillation. An echocardiogram is ordered to define the etiology of his presumed valvular disease.

MEASUREMENTS   (Echo tracings *A-D*)   **Time lines = 200 msec**

cf	=		Percentage change	=
LA	=		Ejection fraction	=
E-F slope	=		IVS amplitude	=
D-E amplitude	=		LVPW amplitude	=
EDD	=		LVPW thickness	=
ESD	=			

QUESTIONS

1. What two abnormalities of this echo allow a definitive diagnosis? What is this diagnosis?

2. Should this lesion be judged of a mild, moderate, or severe nature from the echo?

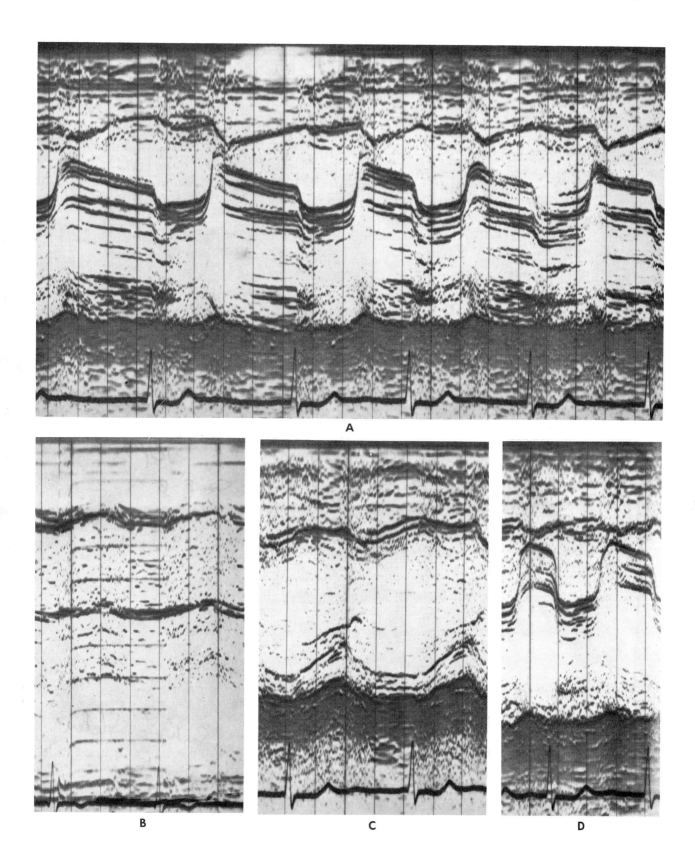

A

B

C

D

ANSWERS TO CASE 8
Mitral Stenosis, Moderate

MEASUREMENTS

cf	= 1.16	Percentage change	= 33%
LA	= 5.5 cm	Ejection fraction	= 62%
E-F slope	= 18 mm/sec	IVS amplitude	= 5 mm
D-E amplitude	= 17 mm	LVPW amplitude	= 10 mm
EDD	= 4.2 cm	LVPW thickness	= 10 mm
ESD	= 2.8 cm		

ANSWERS

1. Mitral stenosis is substantiated by the thickened, echo-dense mitral valve, by the reduced E-F slope of the anterior mitral leaflet, and by the abnormal anterior motion of the posterior mitral leaflet in diastole (Table 8–1).[42-47] The left atrium also is enlarged, a finding consistent with this diagnosis. Although the valve is moderately thickened, its mobility (D-E amplitude) remains within normal limits. The absent A wave is expected in atrial fibrillation.

   The reduced E-F slope in mitral stenosis results primarily from a decreased rate of flow across a narrowed mitral orifice. Because it takes longer for blood to flow from the left atrium to the left ventricle, the duration of the pressure gradient across the valve is increased, and thus the anterior mitral leaflet stays in an open position for a longer period.[46] In addition, with decreased rate of flow across the mitral valve, there will be less motion of the mitral annulus and, consequently, less motion of the anterior mitral leaflet, both in systole and diastole.[46, 48] For both of these reasons, the diastolic slope of the anterior mitral leaflet is reduced in mitral stenosis. As the rheumatic process progresses and the mitral leaflets and chordae tendineae become thickened, fused, and calcified, the mitral echo will exhibit diminishing mobility (D-E amplitude), progressive reduction in the A wave, even in the presence of sinus rhythm, and increasing echo densities.

TABLE 8–1.   Mitral Stenosis

Echo Findings
1. Increased echo density of mitral leaflets.
2. Low E-F slope.
2. Abnormal motion of posterior mitral leaflet.

Possible Associated Findings
1. Reduced C-E and D-E amplitudes.
2. Diminished or absent A wave.
3. Left atrial enlargement.
4. Right ventricular dilatation.
5. Pulmonary hypertension.

---

2. Moderate mitral stenosis is indicated by the E-F slope of 19 mm/sec, by the moderate amount of thickening of the mitral valve that has retained a normal mobility, and by the enlarged left atrium. The right ventricle, however, appears normal in size although it is not well illustrated.

Considerable variation of opinion exists in the literature as to what range of E-F slope corresponds to a given severity of mitral stenosis.[1, 49-51, 53] However, we have found that the values shown in Table 8–2 provide the most accurate guide to a rough judgment of the severity of mitral stenosis. It should be recognized clearly, however, that overlap definitely occurs among these categories. Severe mitral stenosis usually is associated with a very reduced E-F slope (less than 8 mm/sec). However, all patients with markedly reduced diastolic slopes do not have severe mitral stenosis. Although in mild mitral stenosis the E-F slope usually is in the range of 20 to 40 mm/sec, it may be higher or sometimes lower. Other causes of a low E-F slope besides mitral stenosis usually have only minimal reduction in this slope, although they may be associated with a very low value.

Although the E-F slope is one of the best indicators of the severity of mitral stenosis, it may be misleading if considered alone.[48, 53] The degree of mitral stenosis can be judged more accurately using a composite of: (1) the E-F slope; (2) the amount of mitral thickness or calcification as judged by the relative density of the mitral echo; (3) any reduction in mobility (D-E amplitude) of the anterior mitral leaflet; (4) an absent or diminished A wave in the presence of sinus rhythm; (5) the degree of left atrial and right ventricular enlargement; and (6) any evidence of pulmonary hypertension from the echo of the pulmonary valve (Table 8–2). However, even considering all these factors, the echo provides only a rough qualitative estimate of the severity of mitral stenosis and cannot reliably be used to predict the mitral valve area.[53]

Henry and colleagues[54] recently reported a high correlation between the mitral valve orifice measured at surgery in 20 patients with mitral stenosis and the orifice size estimated from real time, cross-sectional echocardiography.

Cardiac catheterization showed that this patient had an integrated mitral gradient of 12 mm Hg and a calculated mitral valve area of 0.6 cm², although there was

TABLE 8–2. Qualitative Assessment of Severity of Mitral Stenosis

Based on E-F Slope of Anterior Mitral Leaflet (mm/sec)*	
Severe	0 to 8
Moderate	8 to 20
Mild	20 to 40
Consider another cause of low E-F slope	40 to 60

Severity Must be Based on a Composite of:
1. Low E-F slope.
2. Degree of mitral thickening or calcification.
3. Amplitude of motion of the anterior mitral leaflet.
4. Absent or diminished A wave in the presence of sinus rhythm.
5. Left atrial size.
6. Right ventricular size.
7. Evidence of pulmonary hypertension from the pulmonary valve.

*Significant overlap may occur

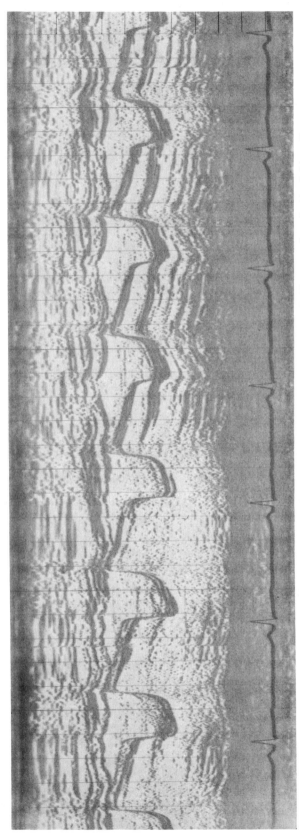

Figure 8–1. M-mode scan of the mitral valve in another patient with mitral stenosis. The posterior mitral leaflet is well recorded with the transducer aiming toward the base of the valve (right), but maximal mitral amplitude is detected more distally on the valve (left). Cardiac catheterization in this patient revealed moderate mitral stenosis (calculated mitral valve area = 0.9 cm², integrated mitral gradient = 13 mm Hg with cardiac index = 2.2 L/min).

mild mitral regurgitation on the left ventricular cineangiogram. The cardiac index determined by the Fick method was 1.6 L/min. At the time of mitral valve replacement, the mitral valve was stenotic and moderately calcified.

Technical Hints. As the position of the transducer may greatly influence the recording of the mitral valve, it is very important to scan the entire valve to record both the greatest mitral amplitude, as well as the posterior mitral leaflet. As shown in Figure 8–1, the mitral amplitude is greatest on the left, with the transducer aimed more distally on the mitral valve than on the right with the transducer aimed more toward the base of the valve. In the latter case, mitral mobility falsely appears to be reduced but, as is often the case, the posterior mitral leaflet is more easily recorded toward the base of the valve. When recording or measuring the C-E or D-E amplitudes, however, the mitral amplitude should always be measured at the place showing maximal amplitude.

In addition, because the mitral leaflets in mitral stenosis may be relatively thin in places, with eccentric thickening, the entire valve should be scanned in order to assess accurately the degree of mitral thickening.

CASE 9

A 36-year-old asymptomatic nurse is returning to work after her youngest child entered school. Pre-employment physical examination reveals a "heart murmur." Work-up includes a normal-sized heart on x-ray, normal ECG, and normal blood pressure. The patient is referred to you for an echo.

MEASUREMENTS (Echo tracings *A* and *B*)   **Time lines = 40 msec**

cf	=	E-F slope	=
Ao valve opening	=	D-E amplitude	=
LA	=		
RV	=		

QUESTIONS

1. What diagnosis does this echo suggest? Of what severity should it be judged?

2. What is the single most important observation in making this diagnosis?

3. Should a cardiac catheterization be done to complete her evaluation?

4. Which condition(s) can cause a low E-F slope of the anterior mitral leaflet?

   (A) Hypertension
   (B) Rheumatic heart disease
   (C) Recurrent pulmonary emboli
   (D) Hypertrophic subaortic stenosis
   (E) Aortic stenosis
   (F) Coronary artery disease
   (G) Cardiomyopathy
   (H) Heart tumors
   (I) Chronic obstructive pulmonary disease

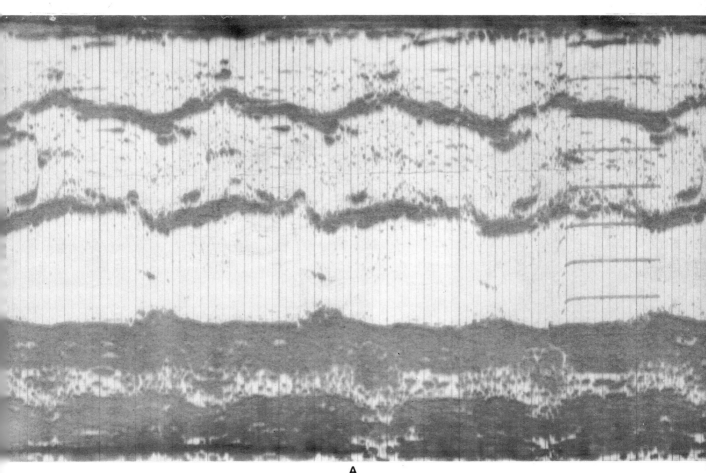

A

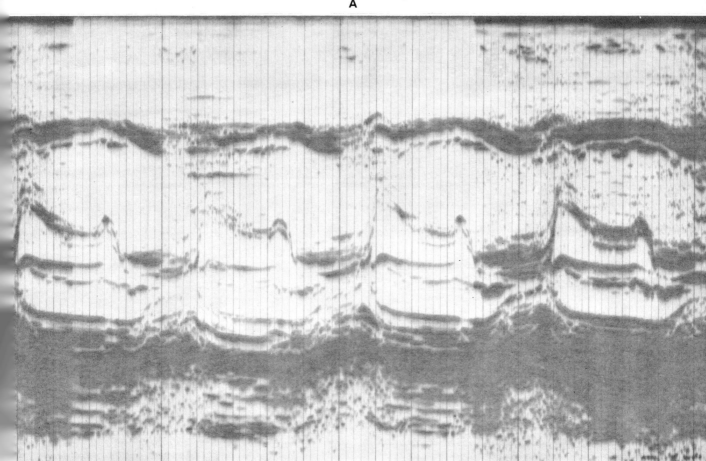

B

59

ANSWERS TO CASE 9
Mitral Stenosis, Mild

MEASUREMENTS

cf	= 1.03	E-F slope	= 36 mm/sec
Ao valve opening	= 1.5 cm	D-E amplitude	= 23 mm
LA	=.3.4 cm		
RV	= 1.9 cm		

ANSWERS

1. The slight reduction in the E-F slope of the anterior mitral leaflet, the mild degree of mitral thickening, and the anterior motion of the posterior mitral leaflet during diastole establish the diagnosis of mild mitral stenosis (Tables 8–1 and 8–2).[55] The normal-sized left atrium and right ventricle and the normal A wave are also consistent with this diagnosis.

   Actually, soon after this echo was recorded, the patient developed significant symptoms of exertional chest discomfort that threatened her ability to continue working. She then underwent cardiac catheterization and was found to have an integrated mitral gradient of 8 mm Hg and a calculated mitral valve area of 2.0 cm². With exercise, the mean pulmonary artery wedge pressure rose from 18 to 27 mm Hg and the cardiac index increased from 3.2 to 5.9 L/min. The coronary arteriograms were normal.

2. When different causes of a reduction in the E-F slope of the anterior mitral leaflet are being considered or when the degree of thickening of the mitral valve is minimal, demonstration that the posterior mitral leaflet moves anteriorly from the D point during diastole is the most important abnormality in establishing the diagnosis of mitral stenosis (Fig. 9–1, A).[55] In all other causes of a low E-F slope, the diastolic motion of the posterior mitral leaflet is posterior, beginning at the D point. However, it should be noted that in mitral stenosis the posterior mitral leaflet may not always move anteriorly in diastole. It may move horizontally (Fig. 9–1, B), although in this case it must be distinguished from the mitral annulus, which may have a similar motion. It may even move slightly posteriorly from the D point for about 50 msec, or at the A point, even though its predominant motion is anterior with the anterior mitral leaflet (Fig. 9–1, C).[56] In fact, recently several cases of catheterization-proved significant mitral stenosis have been reported in which the posterior mitral leaflet moved posteriorly throughout all of diastole (Fig. 9–1, D).[56-58] However, these cases were still recognizable as mitral stenosis because of the increased density of the mitral echo and the reduced diastolic slope.

   Cross-sectional multi-element echocardiography has confirmed that in some cases of mitral stenosis in which the posterior mitral leaflet remains relatively mobile the mitral valve may dome into the left ventricle in diastole, with some parts of the posterior mitral leaflet moving away from the anterior mitral leaflet. A single-element echo beam aimed across the base of such a doming valve might record the posterior leaflet as moving away from the anterior leaflet in diastole. For these reasons, a diagnosis of mitral stenosis should not necessarily be excluded just because the posterior leaflet moves opposite to the anterior leaflet in diastole. However, in such cases the diagnosis should be evident from the increased echo densities of the mitral valve and the decreased diastolic slope.

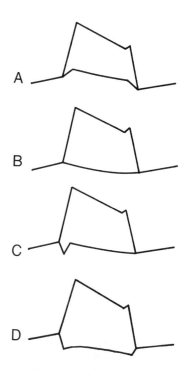

Figure 9–1.　Patterns of motion of the posterior mitral leaflet in mitral stenosis. See text for discussion.

Why the posterior mitral leaflet moves anteriorly with the anterior mitral leaflet during diastole in mitral stenosis is not completely understood. A basic principle of echocardiography is that the motion of any cardiac structure as displayed by echo is the algebraic sum of the motion of that structure *plus* the motion of the heart as a whole with reference to the transducer at a fixed point on the chest wall. In mitral stenosis, fusion of the mitral commissure restricts the actual motion of the posterior leaflet. In this case, if the anterior motion of the entire mitral apparatus exceeds the posterior motion of the posterior leaflet, the echo will record the posterior leaflet as moving anteriorly in diastole, even though it actually may move slightly posteriorly.[1, 56] As commissural fusion and thickening of the posterior leaflet progress in mitral stenosis, one would expect to record a spectrum of motion of the posterior mitral leaflet from posterior to anterior in diastole (Fig. 9–1, *A-D*). When posterior motion of the posterior leaflet is seen in mitral stenosis, it may mean that the posterior leaflet is still flexible and that its total posterior motion is relatively greater than usual in this condition.[57] But when the mobility of the posterior leaflet is considerably restricted it may be recorded as moving anteriorly in diastole with the anterior leaflet.

3. In the asymptomatic or minimally symptomatic patient, echocardiography can establish the diagnosis of mitral stenosis and, provided there are no complicating factors, obviate the need for cardiac catheterization at that time.

4. All the conditions listed may be associated with a low E-F slope of the anterior mitral leaflet and should be considered in the differential diagnosis of this abnormality.

Reduction in the E-F slope of the anterior mitral leaflet is primarily a reflection of decreased rate of left ventricular filling. The resultant reduction in the motion of the mitral annulus is also a contributor to this lower diastolic slope.[46] In mitral stenosis[46] and left atrial myxoma,[90, 91] obstruction at the mitral orifice results in a decreased rate of left ventricular filling, and this contributes at least in part to the reduced E-F slope. In aortic stenosis, systemic hypertension with left ventricular hypertrophy, in hypertrophic and congestive cardiomyopathies, and in some patients with coronary artery disease, a reduction in left ventricular compliance causing a slower rate of left ventricular filling may be associated with a low E-F slope.[48, 49, 59, 66, 125, 126, 162, 163] In pulmonary hypertension, a reduced E-F slope may also be found,[60, 220] and it has been theorized that this finding results from decreased left ventricular filling either from a disturbance of left ventricular geometry secondary to right ventricular dilatation or from changes in the actual diastolic compliance of the left ventricular myocardium.[60]

CASE 10

This 50-year-old liquor store manager with a heart murmur known since his college years was well until he suddenly became very dyspneic while playing golf three years ago and was found for the first time to have atrial fibrillation. Since then, his exercise tolerance has steadily decreased, and occasional paroxysmal nocturnal dyspnea leads him to consult his physician. Physical examination reveals normal carotid pulses and a blood pressure of 150/90. A normal S1 and S2, a Grade I/VI systolic ejection murmur at the left sternal border without radiation to the neck, a Grade I/VI early diastolic blow at the sternal edge, and a Grade III/VI diastolic rumble at the apex are heard. No gallops or opening snap are present. ECG: first degree AV block, borderline left ventricular hypertrophy.

MEASUREMENTS   (Echo tracings A-C)   **Time lines = 200 msec**

cf	=	EDD	=
Ao valve opening	=	ESD	=
LA	=	Ejection fraction	=
RV	=	Percentage change	=
E-F slope	=	LVPW thickness	=
C-E amplitude	=	IVS amplitude	=
		LVPW amplitude	=

QUESTIONS

1. What diagnosis does the echo suggest? Of what severity should this lesion be judged?

2. In a patient with mitral stenosis, what observations from the echo are helpful in making a decision about whether the patient is a candidate for mitral commissurotomy?

3. From this echo, should aortic stenosis or aortic regurgitation be predicted?

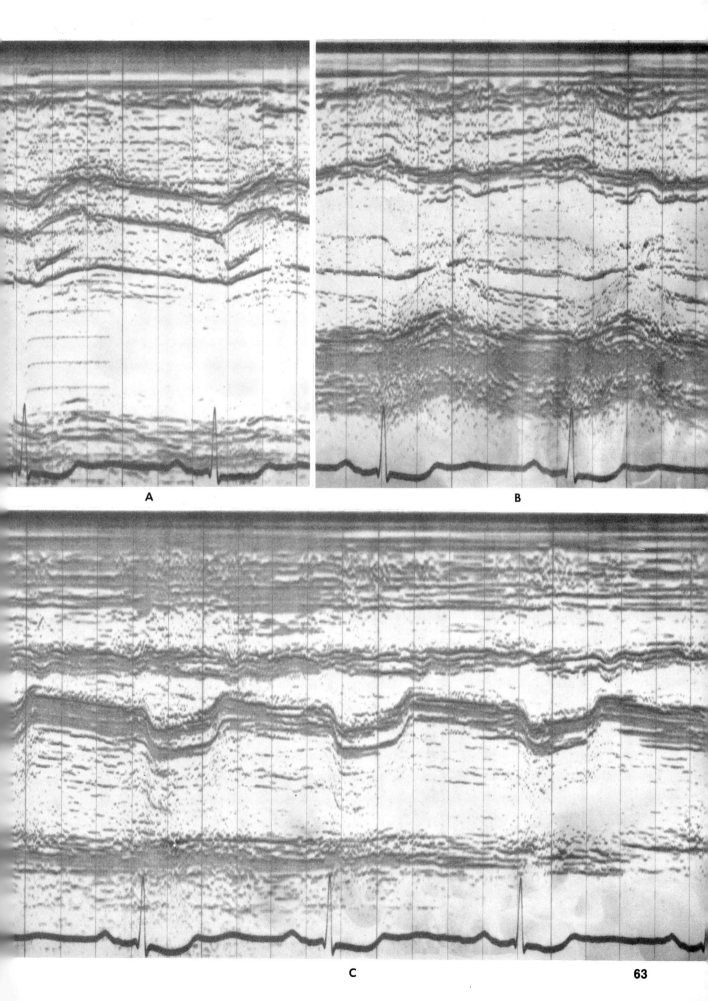

A

B

C

ANSWERS TO CASE 10
Mitral Stenosis, Severe

MEASUREMENTS

cf	= 1.46	EDD	= 4.5 cm
Ao valve opening	= 1.3 cm	ESD	= 2.7 cm
LA	= 5.7 cm	Ejection fraction	= 71%
RV	= 2.0 cm	Percentage change	= 40%
E-F slope	= 7 mm/sec	LVPW thickness	= 16 mm
C-E amplitude	= 15 mm	IVS amplitude	= 8 mm
		LVPW amplitude	= 12 mm

ANSWERS

1. Severe mitral stenosis is suggested both by the markedly reduced E-F slope of the anterior mitral leaflet that has decreased mobility, moderately heavy thickening, and an absent A wave in the presence of sinus rhythm, as well as by the left atrial enlargement (Table 8–2).

   At cardiac catheterization, this patient had an integrated mitral gradient of 18 mm Hg and a calculated mitral area of 0.8 cm². There was significant passive pulmonary hypertension, with a pulmonary artery pressure equal to 63/26. With moderate exercise, the mean pulmonary artery wedge rose from 23 to 45 mm Hg, and the cardiac index increased only from 2.1 to 2.8 L/min. Only slight mitral regurgitation was present on the left ventricular cineangiogram. No aortic gradient was present.

   At the time of mitral valve replacement, there was very heavy calcification of the mitral leaflets, commissures, and annulus, and severe stenosis of the mitral orifice. Only very mild aortic regurgitation was present. Postoperatively, an aortic systolic ejection murmur was present.

2. In patients with pure or predominant mitral stenosis, echocardiography can be helpful in selecting those suitable for mitral commissurotomy by assessing mitral mobility and the degree of mitral thickening or calcification.[44, 45, 49, 51, 52, 61] Nanda and associates[61] evaluated these two factors in 57 patients with pure or predominant mitral stenosis with reference to commissurotomy or valve replacement. These authors proposed that mitral calcification be judged as (1) heavy (thick conglomerate mitral echoes), (2) light (multiple, discrete linear echoes), or (3) none (thin, single or double echoes). In making this semiqualitative judgment, the sensitivity of the instrument was adjusted to record only the left side of the septum. Neither the timed-varied gain nor the reject knobs were used. Nanda and his coworkers found that absence of mitral calcification was the most useful echo indicator for commissurotomy (18 of 19 cases) and that heavy mitral calcification was the most reliable criterion for valve replacement (11 of 11 cases). Reduced

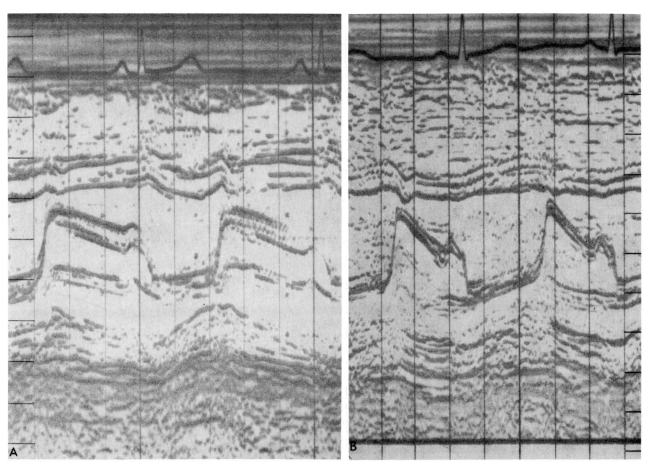

Figure 10–1. Mitral echo before (*A*) and after (*B*) a successful mitral commissurotomy for moderate mitral stenosis. Note that the E-F slope of the anterior leaflet increases from 15 to 60 mm/sec.

leaflet mobility (C-E amplitude less than 20 mm) was a less reliable sign, although C-E amplitudes of less than 15 mm were regularly associated with valve replacement. These findings are in agreement with others,[50] but some workers have found the echo less reliable in predicting which patients will receive mitral valve replacement.[53]

The effects on the mitral valve echo of a successful commissurotomy are well illustrated in Figure 10–1 from another patient who had symptomatic moderate mitral stenosis (calculated mitral valve area of 1.0 cm² with an integrated mitral gradient of 11 mm Hg at rest and 30 mm Hg with exercise). After the mitral commissurotomy, the E-F slope of the anterior leaflet increased from 15 to 60 mm/sec, probably as a result of increased mitral flow. There was only a slight increase in the C-E amplitude from 18 mm to 21 mm. Postoperatively, the posterior leaflet appeared to be moving horizontally during diastole rather than anteriorly, a finding that probably reflects increased mobility of the posterior leaflet secondary to commissurotomy.

3. Although the opening of the aortic valve is slightly decreased (1.3 cm) below normal and the leaflets appear slightly prominent, there are no multiple echo densities from the aortic root and thus no reliable echo evidence of aortic stenosis. In our experience, in severe mitral stenosis it is not unusual to observe a slight reduction in the opening of the aortic valve (1.3 to 1.4 cm) and slightly prominent aortic cusps in the absence of any aortic gradient measured at cardiac catheterization or clinically evident aortic stenosis even after mitral surgery. Such findings probably indicate some rheumatic involvement of the aortic valve, but usually are not associated with an aortic gradient. In this patient, no gradient was recorded on pullback across the aortic valve at the time of catheterization, although he undoubtedly had aortic valve disease with aortic regurgitation present on physical examination and thickening of quite mobile aortic cusps seen on left ventricular cineangiogram.

The mitral thickening of mitral stenosis usually prevents echo detection of associated aortic insufficiency, as is the case in this patient. This represents a limitation of echo in the assessment of multivalvular disease.

Clinical Applications in the Area of Mitral Stenosis. 1. To confirm or exclude mitral stenosis in a patient with suggestive clinical findings or in a patient with recurrent atrial fibrillation or peripheral emboli.

2. To judge the severity of mitral stenosis roughly as mild, moderate, or severe (Table 8–2).[44, 45, 49, 50-52]

3. To rule out mitral stenosis in a patient presenting with pulmonary hypertension, especially in a patient severely ill with a low cardiac output and pulmonary hypertension in whom auscultation may be difficult or the mitral stenosis "silent."

4. To aid in the selection of patients suitable for mitral commissurotomy by assessing mitral valve mobility and the degree of mitral thickening or calcification.[44, 45, 49, 50-52, 61]

5. To follow longitudinally any progression in patients with mild mitral stenosis or in patients after mitral commissurotomy.[44, 45, 49, 61, 62]

6. To judge whether the small size of the left ventricular outflow tract warrants consideration of a low profile prosthesis when planning mitral valve replacement.

Nanda[63] found a higher mortality rate in patients in whom there was less than 20 mm between the C point of the mitral valve and the interventricular septum when a Starr-Edwards prosthesis was used for mitral replacement than in patients with a similar reduction in this measurement in whom a low profile valve was employed.

7. To exclude the diagnosis of left atrial myxoma, an entity that may exactly masquerade as mitral stenosis.

8. To determine in patients with aortic insufficiency whether an apical diastolic murmur represents associated mitral stenosis or is an Austin-Flint murmur.

CASE 11

A 48-year-old school teacher with a history of rheumatic fever presents with slowly progressive dyspnea on exertion, palpitations, and easy fatigability. Physical examination reveals a normal S1, a systolic ejection murmur at the base, an early diastolic blowing murmur along the left sternal border and a mid-diastolic rumble at the apex with presystolic accentuation. A cardiac series shows left ventricular and left atrial enlargement. Clinical impression is aortic insufficiency and mitral stenosis.

MEASUREMENTS (Echo tracings A-C)   **Time lines = 200 msec**

cf	=	Percentage change =	
D-E amplitude	=	Ejection time	=
EDD	=	Vcf	=
ESD	=	IVS amplitude	=
Ejection fraction	=	LVPW amplitude	=

QUESTIONS

1. Does the echo substantiate the clinical impression? Explain.

2. What is the best description of this left ventricle?

   (A) Left ventricular dilatation with increased ejection fraction and Vcf
   (B) Left ventricular dilatation with decreased measurements of LV function
   (C) Left ventricular dilatation with evidence of volume overload
   (D) Hyperdynamic left ventricle with segmental abnormality

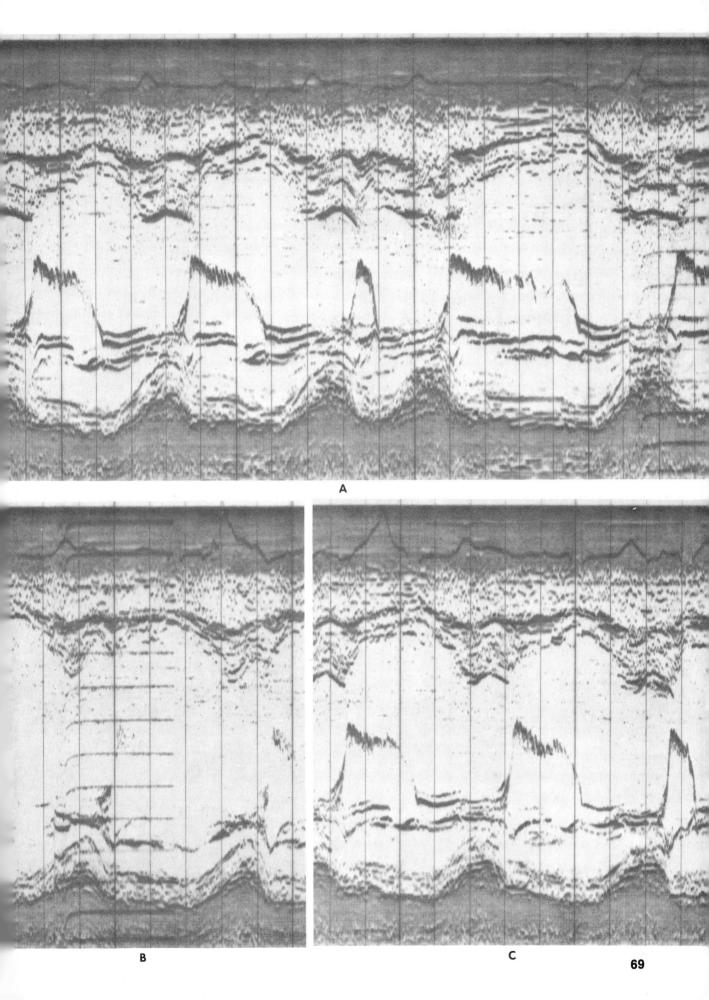

A

B

C

69

ANSWERS TO CASE 11
Aortic Insufficiency with Austin-Flint Murmur

MEASUREMENTS

cf	= 1.14	Percentage change	= 35%
D-E amplitude	= 24 mm	Ejection time	= 290 msec
EDD	= 7.9 cm	Vcf	= 1.20 circ/sec
ESD	= 5.1 cm	IVS amplitude	= 17 mm
Ejection fraction	= 63%	LVPW amplitude	= 13 mm

ANSWERS

1. No. As suspected clinically, aortic insufficiency is substantiated by the fine, high frequency diastolic shuddering of the anterior mitral leaflet (Fig. 11–1, *open arrow*). However, mitral stenosis is excluded by the thin anterior mitral leaflet and the normally moving posterior mitral leaflet. Hence, the mid-diastolic rumble heard in this patient represents an Austin-Flint murmur, not mitral stenosis.

   Clinical Application. In a patient with known aortic insufficiency in whom a diastolic rumble is present, it often is clinically difficult to decide whether there is associated mitral stenosis or if this murmur represents an Austin-Flint murmur. However, echocardiography can easily settle this difficult question by letting us see the mitral thickness and the motion of the posterior mitral leaflet.[21, 23] If the mitral valve is thin and the posterior mitral leaflet moves appropriately, mitral stenosis is excluded. It should be noted that if mitral stenosis *is* present, the thickening of the anterior mitral leaflet will most likely prevent mitral shuddering, even in the presence of significant aortic regurgitation. Therefore, if mitral stenosis is known to be present, the echo will not reliably detect associated aortic insufficiency. Of course, fine diastolic shuddering is not specific for an Austin-Flint murmur and is present in aortic insufficiency without this auscultatory sign.[21]

   The timing of aortic valve replacement in patients with chronic aortic insufficiency often is very difficult. Although many patients can tolerate significant aortic insufficiency for years without myocardial deterioration and do not require surgery, one would like to operate before significant irreversible myocardial damage has occurred. By allowing serial noninvasive evaluation of left ventricular performance, echocardiography may permit early detection of left ventricular decompensation and thus aid in the timing of surgery for aortic insufficiency.[24, 25, 169a, 295]

   In chronic aortic insufficiency, premature closure of the mitral valve is not seen, even though the aortic regurgitation may be severe and the hemodynamics significantly abnormal.[30]

2. (C) The increased end-diastolic diameter (EDD) of the left ventricle is associated with an increased amplitude of the septum and the left ventricular posterior wall. Such a pattern is most consistent with left ventricular volume overload (Table 2–2). In compensated states of aortic insufficiency, the ejection fraction, the percentage change of the minor axis, and Vcf are within normal limits, as in this case. If one wall of the left ventricle is segmentally involved and has a decreased ampli-

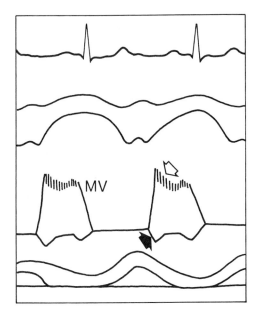

Figure 11–1 (Echo tracing *C*).   Mitral valve in Austin-Flint murmur. Aortic insufficiency is indicated by the fine, high frequency diastolic shuddering of the anterior mitral leaflet (*open arrow*). Mitral stenosis is excluded by the thin, normally opening mitral leaflets and by the posterior motion of the posterior leaflet in diastole (*closed arrow*).

tude of motion, it is common for a compensatory increase to occur in the motion of the other walls. Therefore, if there is clinical or echocardiographic evidence for segmental wall dyskinesia, one should be cautious in reading increased amplitude of the left ventricular wall as evidence of left ventricular volume overload. On the echo of this patient, there is no evidence of a segmental abnormality of the septum or left ventricular posterior wall, and thus (D) would not be the best answer.

Cardiac catheterization in this patient revealed moderate (2+) aortic insufficiency with an enlarged left ventricle that had good contractility. There is no diastolic gradient across the mitral valve.

CASE 12

This 55-year-old doctor's secretary who had rheumatic fever as a child and a known murmur was treated for congestive heart failure for 10 years. Her symptoms increased progressively until over the past six months she could barely walk across a room, could never lie flat, and was dyspneic at rest. Physical examination showed small carotid pulses, a right ventricular lift, a loud S1, a prominent and widely split S2, and a Grade II/VI apical pansystolic murmur. Chest x-ray showed moderate cardiomegaly unchanged for five years. ECG showed right ventricular hypertrophy. Her physician orders an echocardiogram to evaluate the severity of her rheumatic heart disease.

QUESTIONS

(Echo tracing A)   **Time lines = 100 msec**

1. What echo abnormalities allow a definitive diagnosis in this case?

2. What is this diagnosis?

3. After cardiac surgery, in what range would the E-F slope probably fall?

    (A) 10 to 20
    (B) 20 to 40
    (C) 40 to 80
    (D) 80 to 150
    (E) None of these

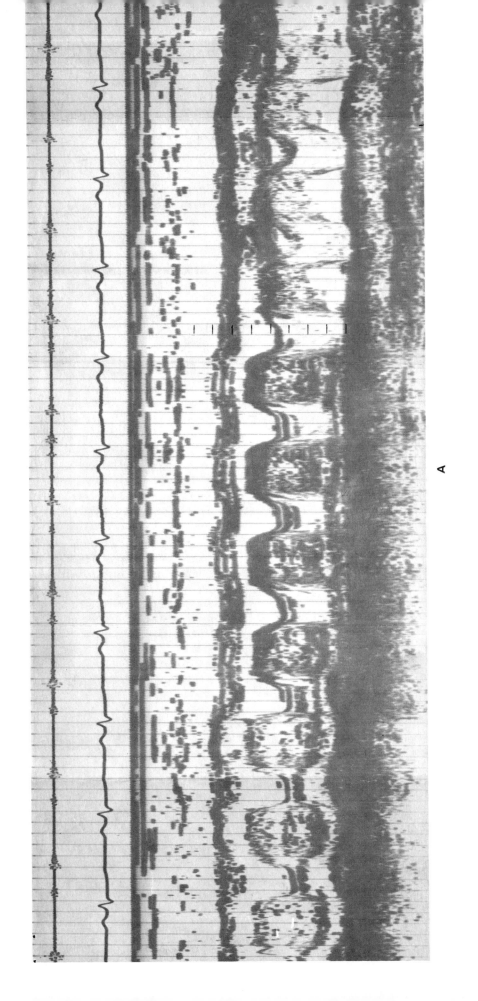

A

ANSWERS TO CASE 12
Left Atrial Myxoma

MEASUREMENTS

cf   = 1.94
LA   = 4.7 cm
E–F slope   = 0–2 mm/sec
C–E amplitude = 22 mm

ANSWERS

1. and 2. A left atrial space-occupying mass (most likely a left atrial myxoma) is indicated by the following observations from this echo (Fig. 12–1):[90-97, 109, 111]

(1) A collection of echo densities which appears in the left atrium during ventricular systole and is absent or less obvious during ventricular diastole (Fig. 12–1, *closed arrow*).

(2) Dense echoes posterior to the anterior mitral leaflet during ventricular diastole, but not during systole.

(3) The thin edge of the anterior mitral leaflet in diastole (D-E segment) being seen prior to and separate from the edge of the prolapsing echo-dense mass (Fig. 12–1, *open arrow*).

On a pulmonary artery cineangiogram in this patient, a large lobulated left atrial mass was seen prolapsing through the mitral valve. There was a 20 mm Hg gradient between the mean pulmonary artery wedge and left ventricular end-diastolic pressure, with a cardiac index of 1.0 L/min, severe active and passive pulmonary hypertension and significant (2+ to 3+) mitral regurgitation. At surgery, a large gelatinous left atrial myxoma was found that measured $10 \times 6 \times 3$ cm; the mitral valve was normal. Postoperatively there was no murmur.

3. (D) Left atrial myxomas that prolapse into the mitral orifice obstruct and prolong the flow of blood from the left atrium to the left ventricle. Consequently, a low E-F slope of the anterior mitral leaflet occurs. The mitral leaflet is intrinsically normal and, after removal of this obstruction, would be expected to have a normal E-F slope—i.e., 80 to 150 mm/sec.

Technical Hints. For the diagnosis of left atrial myxoma: 1. *Find the edge of the mass that moves "appropriately" in the left atrium* (Fig. 12–1, *closed arrow*). On an echo tracing of the left atrium, a left atrial myxoma moves posteriorly within the left atrium during ventricular systole and anteriorly during ventricular diastole as it prolapses into the left ventricle. If the myxoma is very large and almost fills the infe-

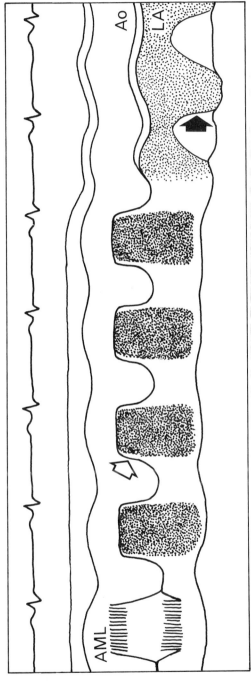

Figure 12-1 (Echo tracing A). Left atrial myxoma. Note (1) the thin edge of the mitral leaflet (*open arrow*) preceding the echo densities seen behind the mitral valve; (2) the densities, primarily in the left atrium, during ventricular systole (*closed arrow*) being less obvious during ventricular diastole; and (3) the fine diastolic shuddering of the anterior mitral leaflet distal to where the myxoma prolapses into the left ventricle.

rior portion of the left atrium, the transducer may have to be aimed very superiorly in the left atrium in order to identify the appropriately moving edge of the mass.

2. *Look for the thin, leading edge of the anterior mitral leaflet* (D-E segment) (Fig. 12–1, *open arrow*) Fig. 12–2 to precede by a small distance the beginning of the echo density seen behind the mitral valve.[91, 93] This difference in timing probably results from the inertia of the left atrial myxoma, causing it to lag behind the flow of blood and the opening of the anterior mitral leaflet.[98] In mitral stenosis, there is no such space preceding the dense mitral echoes, and thus this sign becomes helpful in making the diagnostic distinction between these two entities.

3. *Observe that the echo densities are primarily behind the mitral valve only in diastole* and not in systole.[90, 92, 96, 99] In mitral stenosis[91] or calcified mitral annulus, the echo densities persist throughout the cardiac cycle.

4. *Make several slow, careful sweeps* between the aorta and the mitral valve in all cases of suspected left atrial myxoma. This maneuver will more likely record those large myxomas that only partially prolapse into the left ventricle. Case 12 shows that the myxoma is recorded behind the basilar portion of the anterior mitral leaflet but disappears on scanning toward the tip of the valve. Too rapid a sweep may fail to detect densities behind the mitral valve, recording only the valve more distally.

5. *Use adequate gain.* Care should be taken not to have the gain setting too low, or the dampening control too high, as one will fail to detect the left atrial mass and dial out the proper diagnosis. It often is useful to make a short recording of the left atrium with excessive gain to assure that a mass is not missed. Of course, too much gain will create echo densities, but these echoes tend to occur throughout the tracing rather than being confined behind the mitral valve during diastole.[91]

6. *Do not be misled by fine diastolic shuddering of the anterior mitral leaflet seen distal to the prolapsing myxoma* (Fig. 12–1). This finding, though not previously reported, often is seen in prolapsing left atrial myxomas and may result from turbulent flow of blood around the obstructing myxoma in the presence of a thin mitral valve.

It should be recognized that, even with adequate technique, echocardiography may fail to detect a left atrial myxoma if it is too small, if it fails to prolapse through the mitral orifice because of excessive size or lack of mobility, or if the acoustical impedance of the tumor is not sufficiently different from blood. Because such left atrial tumors produce a reduced E-F slope and dense mitral echoes, one must always be on guard to exclude them in all cases of suspected mitral stenosis.[96] However, it should be recognized that myxomas may not necessarily produce a low E-F slope if they do not prolapse behind the mitral valve[97, 100] or reduce mitral flow.

Clinical Applications.   Since a left atrial myxoma often exactly simulates mitral stenosis in its clinical presentation[93] and may even masquerade as mitral stenosis during cardiac catheterization,[90, 93, 96] echocardiography should be used to aid in this difficult differential diagnosis. Echo examination for a left atrial myxoma also may be useful in patients with syncope, systemic emboli, or suspected endocarditis.

In a patient with suspected mitral stenosis in whom only a left ventricular angiogram and not a pulmonary artery injection is planned, a left atrial myxoma should *always* be excluded by echo. Failure to do this has resulted in missing a left atrial myxoma at cardiac catheterization.[90, 96] Likewise, a left atrial myxoma should be excluded prior to a trans-septal catheterization, as this procedure has caused systemic embolization of undiagnosed left atrial myxomas.[101] Because left atrial myx-

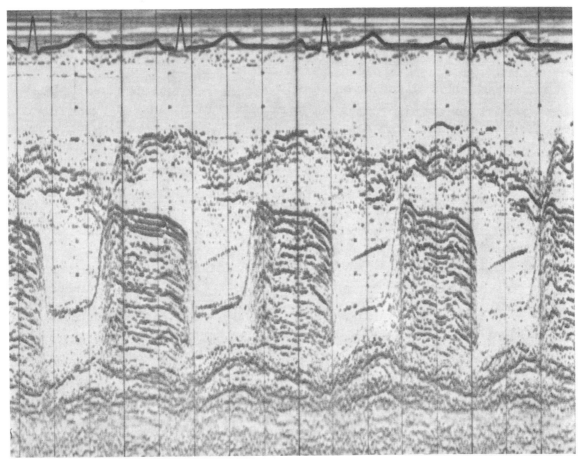

Figure 12–2. Echocardiogram in another patient with a left atrial myxoma. Note the thin leading edge of the mitral valve preceding the echo densities at the beginning of diastole and that these increased echoes are recorded primarily behind the mitral valve during diastole.

omas have been reported to recur,[102] echocardiograms should be performed periodically in patients who have had these tumors removed. Current surgical techniques make their recurrence less likely.

Echocardiography also has been reported to be helpful in diagnosing right atrial,[91, 103-106] right ventricular,[107-109] and left ventricular tumors.[110]

CASE 13

This 60-year-old former dancer and teacher consults her physician because, despite digitalis and diuretics, she is experiencing increasing dyspnea, even while walking on flat ground. Recently, she has even noticed disturbing palpitations associated with substernal tightness and dyspnea at night. On examination an irregular pulse is detected and a Grade II/VI midsystolic apical murmur and a diastolic rumble are heard. An echocardiogram is ordered to help delineate the cause of her disability.

MEASUREMENTS (Echo tracings *A-D*)   **Time lines = 200 msec**

cf	=	D-E slope =	
Ao valve opening	=	RV	=
E-F slope	=	LA	=
C-E amplitude	=	EDD	=
D-E amplitude	=	ESD	=

QUESTIONS

1. Which of the following observations are present on this echo? More than one may apply.
   (A) Increased density of mitral echoes
   (B) Decreased E-F slope of the anterior mitral leaflet
   (C) Thin leading edge of the anterior leaflet separate from the increased mitral densities
   (D) Increased mitral echoes primarily behind the mitral valve in diastole
   (E) Multiple mitral echoes primarily in systole
   (F) Anterior motion of the posterior mitral leaflet in diastole
   (G) Posterior motion of the posterior mitral leaflet in diastole
   (H) Enlarged left atrium with mobile space-occupying mass

2. Which one of the following diagnoses explains this patient's increased disability?
   (A) Aortic stenosis   (C) Left atrial myxoma
   (B) Mitral stenosis   (D) Mitral valve prolapse

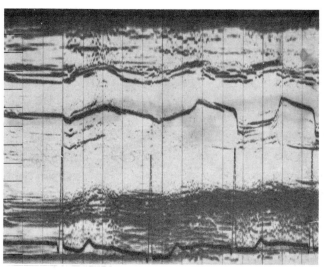

A

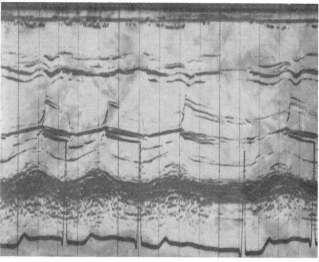

B

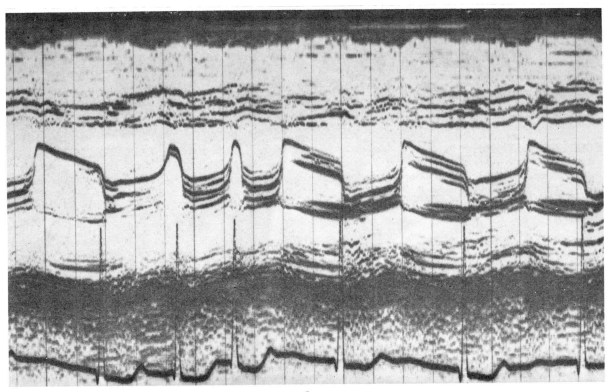

C

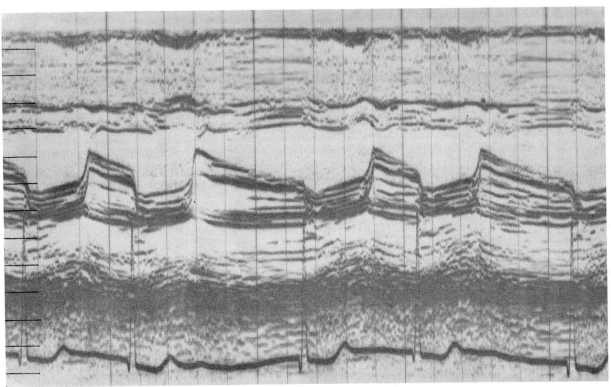

D

ANSWERS TO CASE 13
Mitral Stenosis with Posterior Motion of the Posterior Leaflet During Diastole

MEASUREMENTS

cf (echo *A* and *B*)	= 2.06
cf (echo *C* and *D*)	= 1.40
Ao valve opening	= 1.6 cm
E-F slope	= 25 mm/sec
C-E amplitude	= 25 mm
D-E amplitude	= 20 mm

D-E slope	= 400–470 mm/sec
RV	= 2.0 cm
LA	= 4.7 cm
EDD	= 4.6 cm
ESD	= 3.7 cm

ANSWERS

1. (A), (B), and (G)

2. (B)

On these tracings, increased density of mitral echoes is seen as multiple, discrete, linear echoes throughout the entire cardiac cycle. As was discussed in Case 10, these multiple linear echoes are consistent with the light mitral thickening or calcification described by Nanda.[61] Such mitral thickening in combination with a decreased E-F slope of the anterior leaflet points to mitral stenosis as the explanation for this patient's disability (Table 8–1). Considering the mitral echo and the left atrial enlargement, the mitral stenosis appears to be of moderate severity (Table 8–2).

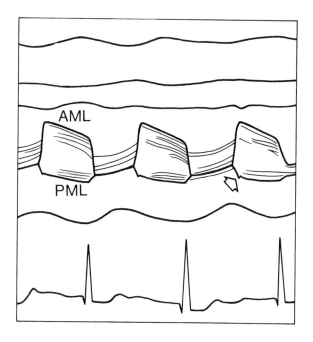

Figure 13–1 (Echo tracing *C*). Mitral stenosis with posterior motion of the posterior mitral leaflet (*PML*) throughout diastole (*open arrow*).

The posterior mitral leaflet is observed in echo tracing *C* to move posteriorly with the onset of diastole and to remain in a posterior position throughout all of diastole (Fig. 13–1). Such normal motion of the posterior leaflet does not exclude the diagnosis of mitral stenosis. As was discussed in Case 9, significant mitral stenosis may exist even in the presence of posterior motion of the posterior leaflet in diastole (Fig. 9–1).[56-58] This may result from the echo beam traversing the base of a doming, mobile mitral valve where the posterior leaflet is actually moving away from the anterior leaflet during diastole. In these cases, the diagnosis of mitral stenosis is still apparent on the basis of increased mitral thickening and a decreased diastolic slope.

At cardiac catheterization, moderate mitral stenosis was substantiated with a resting mitral gradient of 12 mm Hg and a calculated mitral valve area of 1.0 cm^2. With exercise, the pulmonary artery wedge pressure rose from 18 to 38 mm Hg. On a pulmonary artery cineangiogram, the mitral valve was seen to be mildly thickened and to dome prominently into the left ventricle with good mobility.

This echo does not show the abnormalities necessary for the diagnosis of a left atrial myxoma (see Case 12).[90-93, 96, 97] Increased mitral echoes extend throughout the cardiac cycle and are not seen behind the anterior leaflet primarily during diastole; the anterior leaflet is not seen as a thin line moving anteriorly before the increased mitral echoes; and there is no mobile, space-occupying left atrial mass. Although there are multiple lines seen in systole, their motion does not meet the criteria for mitral prolapse, as will be discussed in subsequent cases.

CASE 14

This 55-year-old policeman with the history of a cardiac murmur for years consulted his physician because of progressive dyspnea and effort intolerance. He denies chest discomfort or syncope. The physician detects both systolic and diastolic murmurs and orders an echocardiogram to help delineate their etiology.

MEASUREMENTS (Echo tracings *A-D*)   **Time lines = 200 msec**

cf	=	Ejection fraction	=	
Ao valve opening	=	Percentage change	=	
LA	=	Ejection time	=	
E-F slope	=	Vcf	=	
C-E amplitude	=	IVS thickness	=	
D-E amplitude	=	LVPW thickness	=	
RV	=	IVS amplitude	=	
EDD	=	LVPW amplitude	=	
ESD	=			

QUESTIONS

1. What cause(s) of this man's disability does the echo suggest? Of what severity should the lesion(s) be judged?

2. What is the best description of this man's left ventricle?

   (A) Normal left ventricle and measurements of function
   (B) Borderline compensated with ejection indices slightly below normal
   (C) Decompensated with ejection indices markedly depressed
   (D) Consistent with left ventricular volume overload

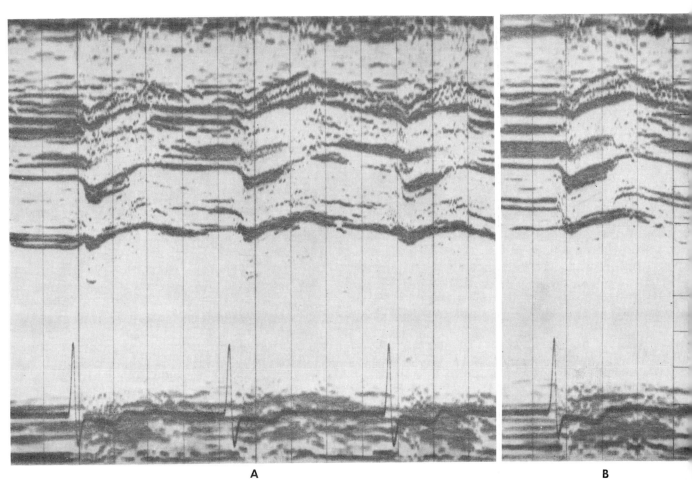

A   B

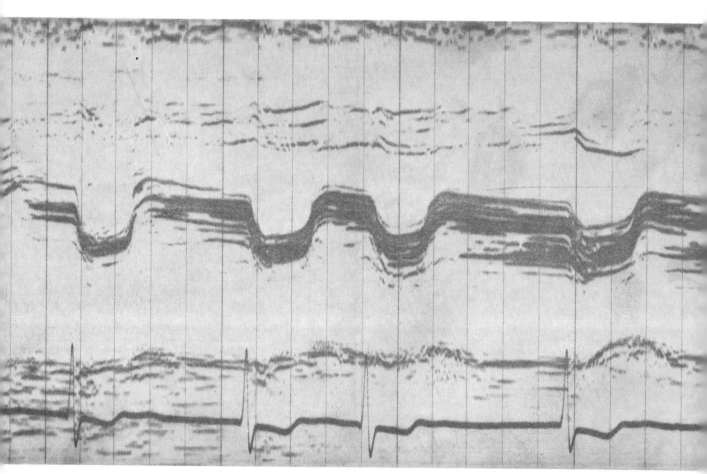

C

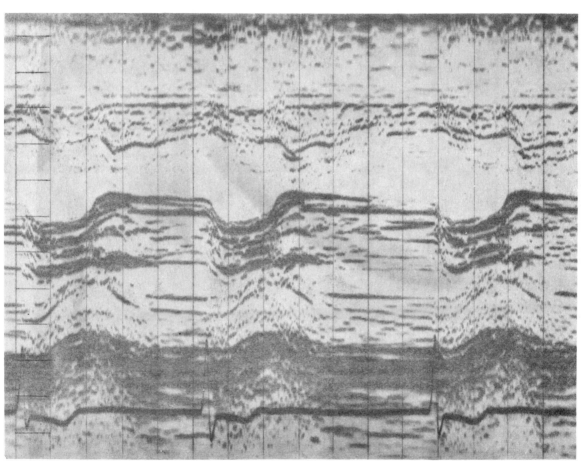

D

ANSWERS TO CASE 14
Aortic Stenosis and Mitral Stenosis

MEASUREMENTS

cf	= 1.05	Ejection fraction	= 43%
Ao valve opening	= 0.5 cm	Percentage	
LA	= 5.0 cm	change	= 22%
E-F slope	= 3 mm/sec	Ejection time	= 310 msec
C-E amplitude	= 18 mm	Vcf	= 0.71 circ/sec
D-E amplitude	= 17 mm	IVS thickness	= 10 mm
RV	= 2.0 cm	LVPW thickness	= 11 mm
EDD	= 5.1 cm	IVS amplitude	= 3 mm
ESD	= 4.0 cm	LVPW amplitude	= 9 mm

ANSWERS

1. Aortic stenosis is suggested by the marked reduction in the opening of the echo-dense aortic valves and by the increased echo densities recorded in the aortic root (Fig. 14–1) (Table 1–1).[1, 11] As previously stated in Case 1, the severity of aortic stenosis cannot be detected reliably by single-element echocardiography.[13]

   Severe mitral stenosis is also suggested by the extreme reduction in the E-F slope, by the very dense mitral echoes—even with the gain adjusted to record only the septum—and by the reduced amplitude of the mitral valve. The enlarged left atrium also supports this diagnosis (Tables 8–1 and 8–2).[42-46]

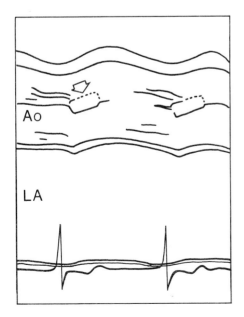

Figure 14–1 (Echo tracing *A*). Calcific aortic stenosis showing decreased opening of thickened aortic cusps in systole (*open arrow*) and increased echo densities in the aortic root.

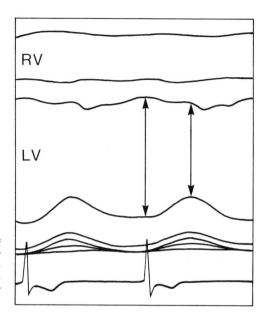

Figure 14–2 (Echo tracing *D*).   Left ventricle showing the proper place of measurement of EDD at end-diastole and ESD at the peak of the anterior motion of the left ventricular free wall. The endocardium of the left ventricular posterior wall is chosen as the line that tends to be the most continuous throughout the cardiac cycle and that has the steepest anterior motion during systole.

Technical Hint.   Measuring mitral C-E and D-E amplitudes in significant mitral stenosis often can be difficult because of the multiple lines that are recorded from these thickened and calcified valves. Echo tracing *C* in this case illustrates that sometimes this difficulty can be resolved by slight changes in the angle of the transducer. To the left of this echo tracing, the maximal mitral amplitude is recorded and the multiple diastolic lines that are seen to the right are resolved so that a reasonable amplitude can be measured. In these cases, this measurement should be taken from the top of the echoes forming the C-D portion to the top of the mitral valve in diastole (E point).

2. (B) The left ventricular cavity is normal in size (Fig. 14–2), but all three of the calculated ejection indices—i.e., ejection fraction, percentage change in the minor axis, and velocity of circumferential fiber shortening—are slightly reduced below the normal range. Of the choices given, then, "borderline compensated" is the best description of this left ventricle.

Cardiac catheterization revealed that this patient had moderately severe aortic stenosis (integrated gradient = 22 mm Hg, aortic valve area = 0.8 cm²), mild aortic insufficiency (1+), moderately severe mitral stenosis (integrated gradient = 15 mm Hg, mitral valve area = 0.9 cm²), and mild mitral regurgitation (1+). Cardiac index was 1.8 L/min. The left ventricle was slightly enlarged, with a calculated ejection fraction of 40 per cent.

CASE 15

This 57-year-old insurance broker, who had acute rheumatic fever at age seven and a murmur first heard five years ago when he emigrated from Egypt, is admitted to the hospital with dyspnea on exertion and orthopnea progressive over the last six months. Within the last week, be began noticing periodic fever, pleuritic chest pain, and dyspnea, even with mild exertion. On physical examination, the temperature is 39°C and the blood pressure is 150/80; the venous pressure is not elevated. The carotid pulses, the left ventricular impulse, S1, and S2 are normal. A Grade III/VI holosystolic murmur at the apex and a Grade II/VI harsh systolic ejection murmur at the base without radiation to the neck are described. Likewise, an apical low-pitched diastolic rumble is present, but no opening snap is heard. Chest x-ray reveals moderate cardiomegaly with pulmonary vascular congestion and a right pleural effusion. On thoracocentesis, straw-colored fluid with an increased eosinophil count is withdrawn. A tuberculin skin test is positive. An echocardiogram is ordered to delineate the etiology of the patient's valvular disease.

MEASUREMENTS (Echo tracings A-C)   **Time lines = 200 msec**

cf	=	IVS thickness	=	
Ao valve opening	=	LVPW thickness	=	
LA	=	IVS amplitude	=	
RV	=	LVPW amplitude	=	
E-F slope	=	Ejection fraction	=	
D-E amplitude	=	Percentage change	=	
EDD	=	Ejection time	=	
ESD	=	Vcf	=	

QUESTIONS

1. What maneuver is illustrated on echo tracing *B*, and what does it establish?

2. Check the diagnosis(es) that should be made from this echo. Opposite *each* of the lettered diagnoses below (A to F), list either the findings present on this echo that allow the diagnosis to be suggested or those that prevent the diagnosis from being made.

Diagnoses	Check If Echo Suggests	List Appropriate Findings that Establish or Prevent Diagnosis from Being Made
A. Aortic stenosis		
B. Aortic insufficiency		
C. Mitral stenosis		
D. Tricuspid stenosis		
E. Tricuspid insufficiency		
F. Valvular vegetations		

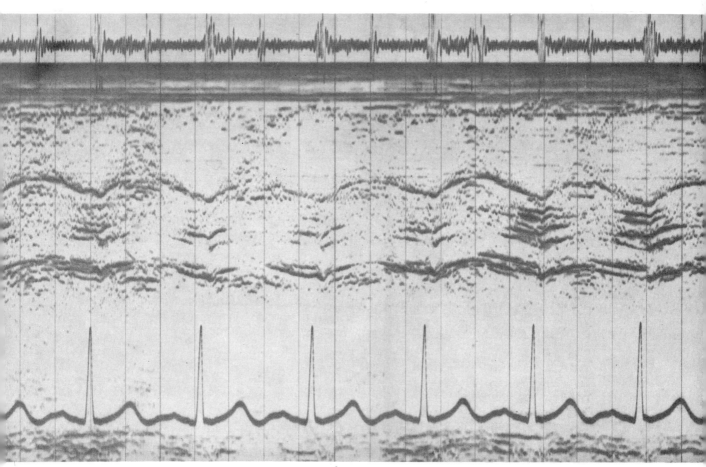

A

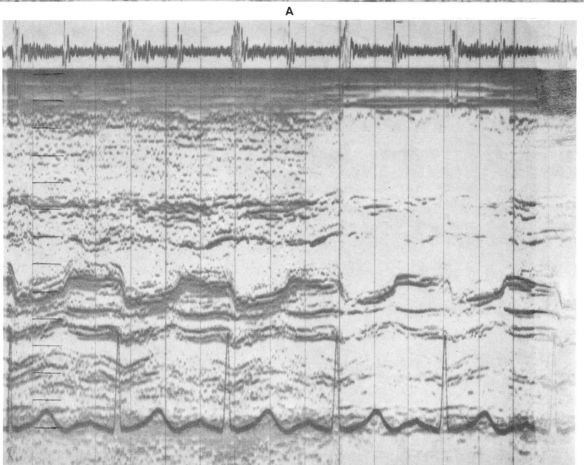

B

89

3. What cause(s) of this patient's "moderate cardiomegaly" described on the chest x-ray does this echo suggest?

   (A) Left ventricular cavity dilatation
   (B) Left ventricular hypertrophy
   (C) Hypertrophic subaortic stenosis
   (D) Right ventricular cavity dilatation
   (E) Left atrial enlargement
   (F) Pericardial effusion

4. Name three independent abnormalities present on this echo that may contribute to the reduced E-F slope of this patient's anterior mitral leaflet.

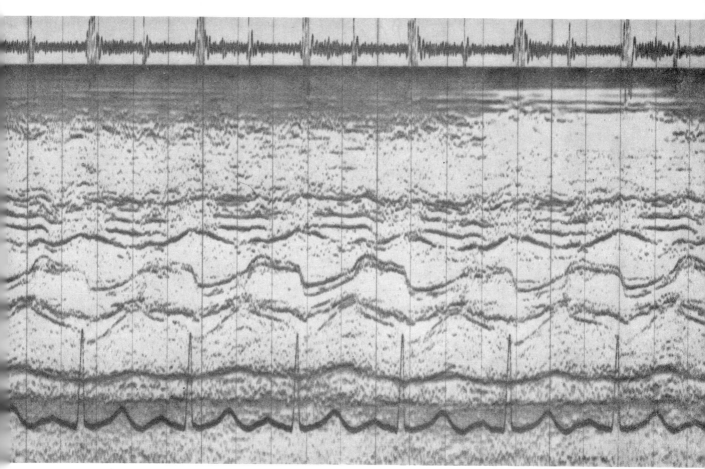

C

ANSWERS TO CASE 15
Aortic Stenosis, Mitral Stenosis and Left Ventricular Hypertrophy

MEASUREMENTS

cf	= 1.39	IVS thickness	= 14 mm
Ao valve opening	= 0.3 cm	LVPW thickness	= 18 mm
LA	= 6.3 cm	IVS amplitude	= 5 mm
RV	= 2.5 cm	LVPW amplitude	= 12 mm
E-F slope	= 3 mm/sec	Ejection fraction	= 74%
D-E amplitude	= 12 mm	Percentage change	= 42%
EDD	= 3.8 cm	Ejection time	= 270 msec
ESD	= 2.2 cm	Vcf	= 1.5 circ/sec

ANSWERS

1. On the right-hand side of echo tracing *B*, the total gain has been reduced to the point of almost obliterating the interventricular septum and posterior left ventricular wall. We observe that there is persistence of the mitral echo during this maneuver and can thus establish that there is mitral thickening and therefore rheumatic involvement of the mitral valve.

2. The echo suggests A and C. Aortic stenosis is established by the increased echo densities in the aortic root and by the decreased opening of the aortic valve (Fig. 15–1) (Table 1–1)[1, 11] (See Case 1). Likewise, concomitant mitral stenosis is strongly suggested by the markedly reduced E-F slope of the anterior mitral leaflet, by the mitral thickening recorded as conglomerate dense echoes when the left ventricular side of the septum is properly recorded, and by the reduced mobility and absent A wave of the mitral valve (Table 8–1)[42–46] (See Cases 4 and 9). The posterior mitral leaflet appears to have a predominantly horizontal motion in diastole.

   Aortic insufficiency could not be diagnosed from this echo because thickening of the mitral valve would prevent appreciation of the findings associated with this diagnosis. Tricuspid stenosis could not be diagnosed because the tricuspid valve is not recorded. Although the right ventricle is enlarged, the motion of the interventricular septum is appropriately timed, and therefore there is no echo evidence for right ventricular overload, i.e., tricuspid insufficiency (Table 2–2). Valvular vegetations could not be diagnosed from this echo because of the presence of aortic and mitral stenosis. Because valvular thickening and calcification in rheumatic involvement of a valve can closely emulate the echo picture of vegetations, a normally opening valve should be identified before endocarditic vegetations are diagnosed from the echo (Table 2–1).[26, 30]

3. (B), (D), (E), (F). Symmetric left ventricular hypertrophy, right ventricular cavity dilatation, and left atrial enlargement contribute to this patient's cardiomegaly, appreciated on x-ray. In addition, the patient has a small pericardial effusion, as evidenced by a small, relatively echo-free space posterior to the left ventricular posterior wall (Fig. 15–2). The size of the left ventricular cavity is below the limits of normal, but there is no evidence of hypertrophic subaortic stenosis from the mitral valve or septum.

Figure 15–1 (Echo tracing *A*). Calcific aortic stenosis showing decreased opening of the aortic cusps in systole (*open arrow*).

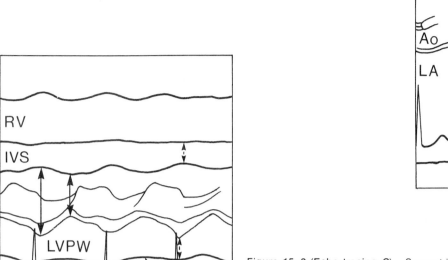

Figure 15–2 (Echo tracing *C*). Symmetric hypertrophy of the left ventricular posterior wall and septum (*dashed, double-headed arrows*) with small left ventricular end-diastolic and systolic minor diameters (*solid, double-headed arrows*). A small pericardial effusion (*open arrow*) is also seen posterior to the left ventricular posterior wall.

4. Three independent abnormalities present on this echo that contribute to the reduced E-F slope of the anterior mitral leaflets are (1) mitral stenosis, (2) left ventricular hypertrophy associated with aortic stenosis, and (3) a small pericardial effusion. Each of these entities may retard the velocity of flow from the left atrium to the left ventricle and thus contribute to the reduced diastolic slope of the mitral valve.[46, 55, 59] With these multiple causes of a reduced E-F slope of the anterior mitral leaflet, it is difficult to judge the severity of the associated mitral stenosis, especially if only the E-F slope is considered in making this assessment. However, if the significant mitral thickening and reduced mobility are considered with the marked left atrial and right ventricular enlargement, the mitral stenosis would be roughly judged as moderately severe to severe.

Although aortic stenosis tends to reduce the mitral E-F slope, significant mitral stenosis usually can be excluded in these patients: (1) if high frequency, diastolic shuddering of the anterior mitral leaflet seen with associated aortic insufficiency indicates that the mitral valve is not significantly thickened; (2) if a prominent A wave is seen in the mitral valve; (3) if the posterior mitral leaflet moves normally in diastole;[13] and (4) if the E-F slope is not greatly reduced. Aortic stenosis alone *tends* to be associated with diastolic slopes above 30 mm/sec, but this is not invariably the case. However, despite these points it may be very difficult to always exclude absolutely associated mitral stenosis in the presence of aortic stenosis.

Cardiac catheterization in this patient revealed that he had severe aortic stenosis (integrated gradient of 51 mm Hg and aortic valve area of 0.4 to 0.5 cm²) and moderate mitral stenosis (integrated gradient of 24 mm Hg and mitral valve area of 1.0 to 1.3 cm²). There was severe active and passive pulmonary hypertension with a PA pressure of 113/46 mm Hg. A left ventricular cineangiogram showed good contractility. At the time of surgery, the aortic valve was stenotic, with calcium involving the leaflets, commissures, and annulus and extending down to the anterior mitral leaflet. The mitral valve was very stenotic and calcified. The left ventricle was also very hypertrophied.

Clinical Application.   This case and several previous ones (Cases 1, 7, 11, 13, and 14) illustrate that echocardiography can be beneficial in multivalvular disease when clinical assessment of several valves may be difficult. For example, when there is obvious aortic disease, is the mitral valve also involved? When rheumatic mitral disease is present, is there associated aortic disease? However, the presence of significant mitral stenosis usually prevents echo detection of associated aortic insufficiency, and thus this represents a limitation of the echo assessment of multivalvular involvement.

In addition, Cases 14 and 15 illustrate that the degree of left ventricular compensation or decompensation in significant valvular disease can be assessed by echocardiography. Despite very significant multivalvular disease in both these cases, the left ventricle was relatively compensated, as judged by analysis of the echo and as later confirmed by angiography. One would then predict that significant symptomatic improvement could be obtained by surgical correction of the valvular defects.

CASE 16

This 57-year-old gasoline station owner with the history of a heart murmur heard three years ago now has symptoms of dyspnea and cough with exertion. On physical examination, the patient has a normal S1 and a Grade III/VI pansystolic apical murmur. No opening snap or S3 is heard. An echo is requested to determine the etiology of his murmur.

MEASUREMENTS   (Echo tracings *A* and *B*)   Time lines = **200 msec**

cf =	E-F slope =
Ao =	D-E amplitude =
LA =	D-E slope =

QUESTIONS

1. What maneuver is demonstrated in echo tracing *A*, and what does it establish?

2. Which of the following causes of a murmur of mitral regurgitation does this echo suggest?
   (A) Nonrheumatic disease with ruptured chordae tendineae
   (B) Systolic mitral prolapse
   (C) Rheumatic heart disease
   (D) Papillary muscle dysfunction

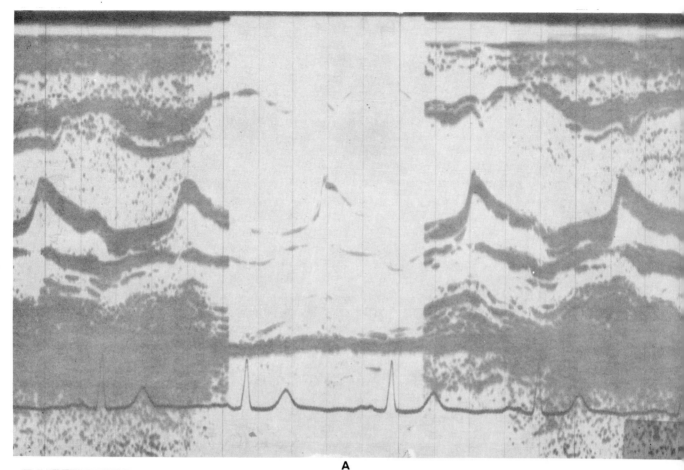

A

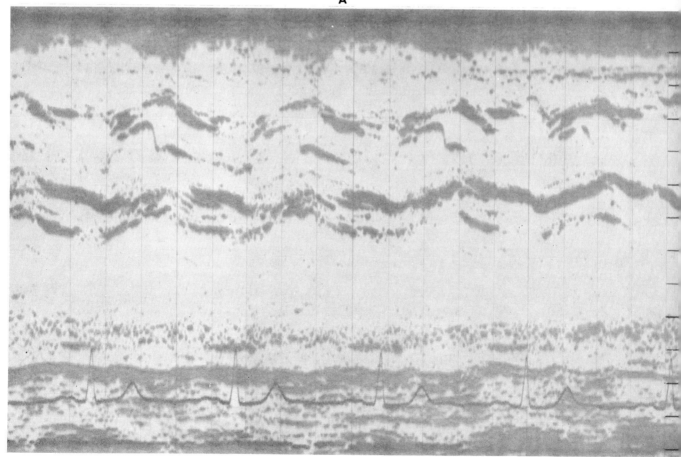

B

95

ANSWERS TO CASE 16
Rheumatic Mitral Regurgitation

MEASUREMENTS

cf $= 1.14$

Ao $= 34$ mm

LA $= 5.0$ cm

E-F slope $= 75$ mm/sec

D-E amplitude $= 22$ mm

D-E slope $= 240$–260 mm/sec

ANSWERS

1. Even after the dampening control in echo tracing A is increased until the septum and left ventricular free wall are nearly obliterated, the anterior mitral leaflet is still recorded. This maneuver establishes that the mitral valve is echo-dense; it is no longer thin and filamentous, but rather thickened and probably partially calcified. Such increased echo density or thickening is the basic abnormality seen with rheumatic mitral involvement and can be used to distinguish rheumatic from nonrheumatic causes of mitral regurgitation. The density of the mitral valve can also be compared with that of the septum and left ventricular wall by decreasing the total gain. However, the anterior gain should not be used for this maneuver because if it affects only the septum, a false impression of mitral thickening will be obtained.

2. (C) Increased echo density or thickness of the mitral valve establishes the diagnosis of rheumatic mitral disease, and a reduced E-F slope of the anterior leaflet is usually an accompanying finding. When evidence for rheumatic mitral thickening occurs in combination with a relatively normal E-F slope, especially when the anterior leaflet has a "ski slope" appearance, as in this case, it has been suggested that this indicates rheumatic mitral regurgitation.[44, 45, 50] Certainly, an E-F slope with an initial rapid motion and then a slower descent is seen in some cases of rheumatic mitral regurgitation. However, the mitral echo alone cannot reliably separate those patients with predominant mitral stenosis from those with predominant or even pure rheumatic mitral regurgitation.[1, 64, 70] Even in pure mitral regurgitation, the mitral echo may be indistinguishable from mitral stenosis. In fact, unless the degree of rheumatic mitral regurgitation is very severe, the mitral echo usually reflects mitral stenosis. Such variability probably results because the E-F slope reflects a variety of factors—i.e., mitral flow secondary to both right ventricular stroke volume and mitral regurgitant volume,[48, 65, 66] leaflet fibrosis or calcification, chordal fusion and shortening, and left ventricular compliance.[59] Thus, the configuration of the anterior mitral leaflet may suggest rheumatic mitral regurgitation, but its diagnostic sensitivity is low. Sometimes an enlarged left ventricular cavity that shows evidence of left ventricular volume overload may offer additional support for the diagnosis of mitral regurgitation.

   Echocardiography has been suggested as helpful in detecting left atrial thrombi, especially when there are scattered echoes anterior to the left atrial wall, as seen in tracing B of this case. However, because the left atrial posterior wall often is hazy, even in normal individuals, and because the echo examines only a limited part of

TABLE 16–1. Echocardiographic Patterns of Mitral Regurgitation

1. Rheumatic mitral disease
2. Mitral prolapse
   a. Late systolic prolapse
   b. Pansystolic prolapse
3. Flail mitral valve
   a. Ruptured chordae tendineae to the anterior mitral leaflet
   b. Ruptured chordae tendineae to the posterior mitral leaflet
4. Mitral regurgitation secondary to left ventricular dilatation and dysfunction, "double-diamond" mitral valve
5. Hypertrophic subaortic stenosis
6. Calcified mitral annulus

the left atrium, echocardiography is not a reliable method for detecting left atrial clots. It is our opinion that this diagnosis should not be made from the echo on the basis of such scattered left atrial echoes.

Table 16–1 lists the varied echocardiographic patterns seen in different kinds of mitral regurgitation. These patterns will be thoroughly discussed in subsequent cases and are extremely useful in establishing the etiology of a murmur of mitral regurgitation.[70]

Cardiac catheterization and left ventricular cineangiography in this patient documented severe mitral regurgitation with a pulmonary artery wedge pressure of 22 mm Hg, a mitral valve gradient of 7 mm Hg, and a cardiac index of 2.0 L/min. Contracted, thickened mitral leaflets with predominant regurgitation were found at surgery for mitral valve replacement. Pathologic examination of the surgical specimen was consistent with chronic rheumatic valvulitis.

CASE 17

A 37-year-old pediatrician is referred for an echocardiogram because of increasingly frequent palpitations and because her heart murmur has recently increased in intensity. She was first told of a murmur 15 years ago during a pre-employment physical examination and remembers irregular heartbeats since she was a teenager. Physical examination is normal except for a grade III/VI late systolic murmur. No clicks are audible. Electrocardiogram demonstrates frequent premature ventricular contractions.

QUESTIONS

(Echo tracings *A* and *B*)   Time lines = 200 msec

1. This patient's mitral echocardiogram demonstrates:

   (A) Hypertrophic subaortic stenosis
   (B) Ruptured chordae tendineae to the posterior leaflet
   (C) Late systolic prolapse
   (D) Pansystolic prolapse
   (E) Rheumatic mitral regurgitation

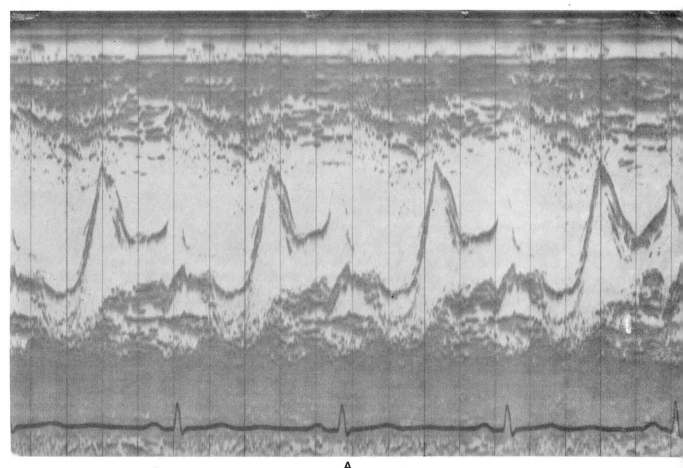

A

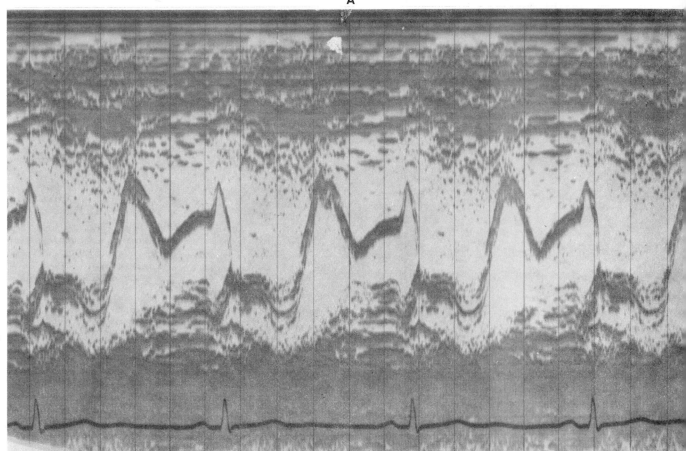

B

99

ANSWERS TO CASE 17
Late Systolic Prolapse of the Mitral Valve

ANSWERS

1. (C) Late systolic prolapse is demonstrated by the abnormal motion of the C-D portion of the mitral valve in systole (Fig. 17–1). Instead of the normal continuous anterior motion of the mitral valve throughout systole, the mitral valve abruptly moves posteriorly in midsystole toward the left atrium. It then returns anteriorly to the D point just prior to mitral diastolic opening. This type of abnormal motion of the mitral valve has been described as an abrupt sagging, bulging, or buckling of the mitral valve in mid- to late systole and as a "question mark lying on its side."[68-74] As is illustrated in Figure 17–2, with the echo pattern of late systolic prolapse the initial portion of the C-D segment of the mitral valve may move slowly anteriorly, horizontally, or even slowly posteriorly prior to its abrupt posterior motion in mid- to late systole. It is the abrupt onset in mid- to late systole of bowing posterior to the D point of the mitral valve that characterizes the echo pattern of late systolic prolapse.

Markiewicz, et al.,[74] have attempted to define this pattern of late systolic prolapse more precisely. They found that when the abrupt, posterior motion of the mitral valve bowed more than 2 mm posterior to an imaginary line connecting the C and D points, this pattern had a high correlation with phonocardiographic evidence of mid- to late systolic click and/or mid- to late systolic murmurs (Fig. 17–1). In this study, if the D point could not be clearly defined by recording the separation of the anterior and posterior leaflets in diastole, the point where the anterior leaflet

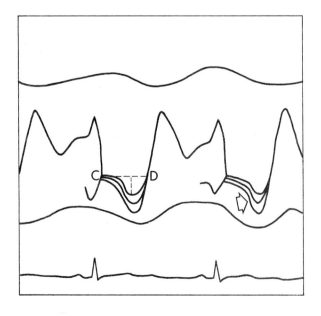

Figure 17–1 (Echo tracing *B*). Late systolic prolapse of the mitral valve (*open arrow*). As per Markiewicz,[74] and as discussed in the text, the construction of an imaginary *C–D* line with measurement of the degree of prolapse is also illustrated.

MITRAL PROLAPSE

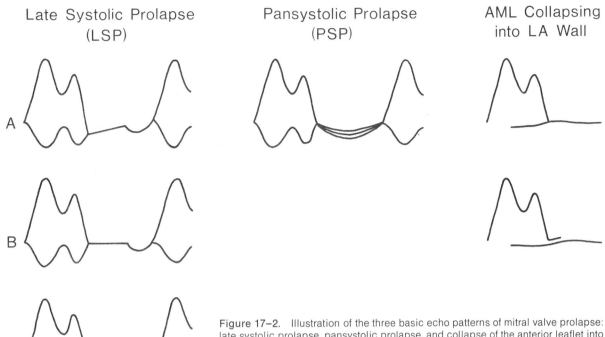

Late Systolic Prolapse (LSP)   Pansystolic Prolapse (PSP)   AML Collapsing into LA Wall

Figure 17–2. Illustration of the three basic echo patterns of mitral valve prolapse: late systolic prolapse, pansystolic prolapse, and collapse of the anterior leaflet into the left atrial wall.

moved sharply anteriorly or the posterior leaflet moved sharply posteriorly was taken as the D point in order to construct the imaginary C-D line.

Such a pattern of late systolic prolapse is only one of the three echo patterns that have been described in patients with angiographically documented mitral prolapse and in patients with late systolic murmurs with or without systolic clicks (Fig. 17–2).[68-74] The other two echo patterns of pansystolic prolapse and collapse of the mitral valve into the left atrial wall will be discussed in subsequent cases. It should be emphasized that these different patterns of late systolic prolapse or pansystolic prolapse may be recorded in the same patient with slightly different angula-

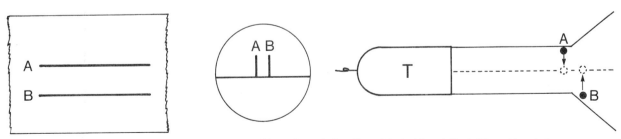

Figure 17–3. Illustration of the problem of lateral resolution. Two objects (A and B) at different levels from the transducer are seen within the width of the echo beam, electronically "verticalized" as if they were in a straight line and recorded on the echo tracing as if point B was directly behind point A.

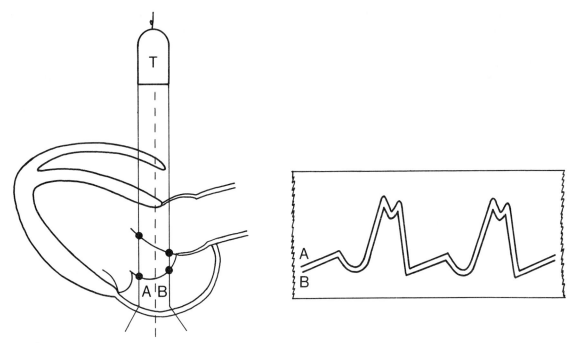

Figure 17–4. Illustration of how recording *only* the anterior leaflet at different places can result in multiple mitral echoes.

tion of the transducer. With cross-sectional echocardiography, the entire spectrum of M-mode patterns from late systolic to pansystolic prolapse may be recorded simultaneously in the same patient at the same time.[75] Thus, the pattern recorded by single crystal technique depends in part on the portion of the mitral valve transversed by the echo beam and does not represent different types of mitral prolapse.

In mitral prolapse, multiple systolic mitral echoes are characteristically recorded, as illustrated in this case (Fig. 17–1). The explanation for these multiple systolic echoes lies in a consideration of the inherent width of the echo beam[76] and the resulting problems of lateral resolution.[2, 76] All surfaces that are "seen" within the echo beam are recorded as if they were all in a straight line. This electronic "verticalization" occurs with objects within the finite width of the beam and is a particular problem when the beam begins to disperse laterally, as even beams from focused transducers do. Figure 17–3 illustrates that because the echo machine electronically "verticalizes" the echoes from points A and B along the broken line, they will be recorded as if they were directly behind each other. In point of fact, they are primarily at different levels from the transducer, and point B is not directly behind point A. In this manner, an object may be displaced on the echo recording as if it were present in a cardiac chamber where it does not exist. This "verticalization" of objects seen within the echo beam forms the problems of lateral resolution of echoes and is one of the most serious limitations of currently used echo systems. An understanding of these problems of lateral resolution is essential to the proper interpretation of many echocardiograms.

When these problems of lateral resolution and the inherent width of the echo beam are applied to the mitral valve, they provide an explanation for the multiple systolic lines that can be recorded in normal subjects and that are characteristically recorded in patients with mitral prolapse (Fig. 17–4). If several different places on the anterior mitral leaflet are recorded at different distances from the transducer within the width of the echo beam, they will be electronically "verticalized," and multiple systolic echoes, each behind another, will be recorded. As a result, multiple parallel systolic echoes of the mitral valve do not imply separation of the mitral leaflets. Since such echoes may be recorded in normal subjects, multiple systolic echoes of the mitral valve alone are not an echo pattern suggestive of mitral regurgitation. Because of similar considerations in late systolic prolapse, it usually is not possible from the echo to say which leaflet is prolapsing. Just because an echo is recorded posterior to another does not necessarily mean that the anterior echo is from the anterior leaflet and the posterior one from the posterior leaflet. Both echoes may be from two different areas on the anterior leaflet, with one prolapsing and the other remaining stable. If both these areas are "seen" within the echo beam, one area may be recorded as if it were posterior to the other, even though it originates from the anterior leaflet.

Thus, echo readings specifying which leaflet is prolapsing—i.e. "late systolic prolapse of the posterior mitral leaflet"—are misleading and probably inaccurate. Actually, both leaflets usually show myxomatous degeneration, and with cross-sectional echocardiography both leaflets have abnormal posterior and superior motion into the left atrium during systole.[75]

CASE 18

This 31-year-old television news commentator consults his physician because of palpitations with exertion and the recent onset of episodic chest pains unrelated to activity. Despite the diagnosis of "congenital heart disease" at age 17, he has remained active, skiing and swimming without difficulty. On physical examination, the left ventricular impulse is active, a systolic thrill is present, and a grade IV/VI holosystolic murmur is heard at the apex, as well as along the left sternal border and in the carotids. An electrocardiogram shows prominent QRS voltage and nonspecific T abnormalities. An echocardiogram is ordered.

QUESTIONS

(Echo tracings A-C)   Time lines = 200 msec

1. What etiology of this patient's pansystolic murmur does the echo suggest?

2. What effect would amyl nitrite be expected to produce on the abnormality demonstrated in this patient's echocardiogram?

3. Match the following auscultatory findings (1–4) with the lettered echo patterns with which they may be associated. More than one auscultatory finding may be appropriate for each echo pattern.

   (1) Late systolic murmur
   (2) Pansystolic murmur
   (3) Systolic clicks only
   (4) No abnormal auscultatory findings
   _____ (A) Echo pattern of late systolic mitral prolapse
   _____ (B) Echo pattern of pansystolic mitral prolapse
   _____ (C) Normal mitral echocardiogram

4. Which of the following drawings (A-D) represent echocardiographic features consistent with mitral valve prolapse?

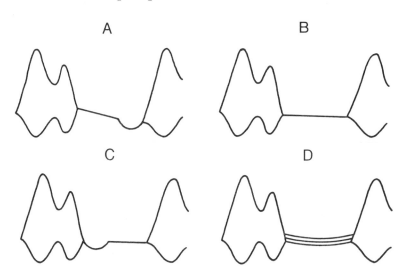

A   B

C   D

104

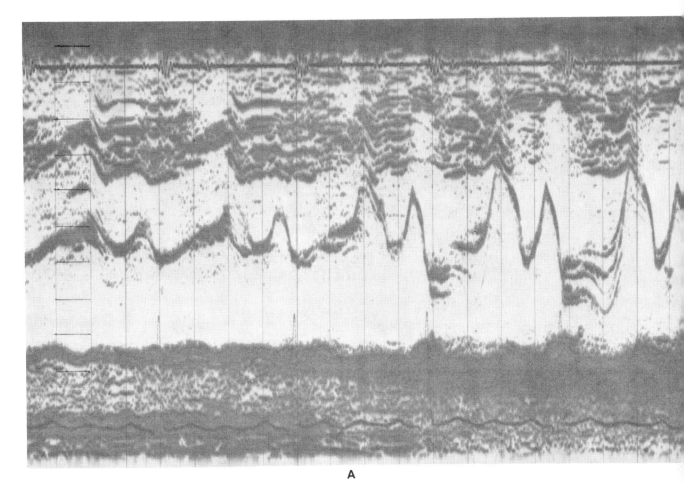

A

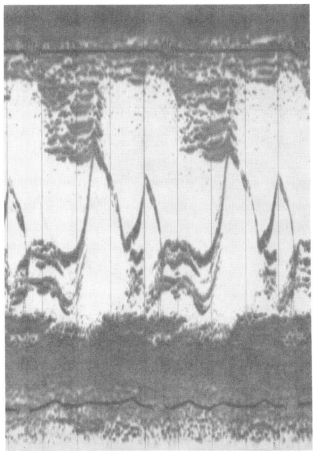

B

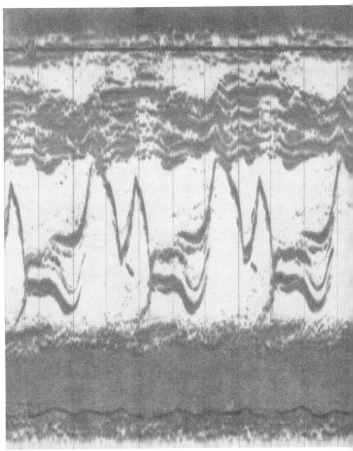

C

105

ANSWERS TO CASE 18
Late Systolic Prolapse of the Mitral Valve

ANSWERS

1. This echocardiogram shows the classic pattern of late systolic prolapse of the mitral valve. The mitral echoes move abruptly posteriorly in midsystole and return anteriorly prior to diastole. They bow greater than 2 mm posterior to the D point, defined here as when the anterior leaflet moves sharply anteriorly in diastole. As will be discussed below, echo evidence of late systolic prolapse may be associated with a pansystolic murmur.

2. Amyl nitrite can be useful in exaggerating mitral valve prolapse by decreasing left ventricular volume and allowing the mitral valve with its chordae of fixed length to prolapse further into the left atrium. With amyl nitrite inhalation, late systolic prolapse often begins earlier in systole and may become pansystolic. Accompanying clicks on simultaneous phonocardiograms usually move earlier in systole.[68, 71, 77]

3. (A) 1,2,3,4   (B) 1,2,3,4   (C) 1,2,3,4
   Although a midsystolic click followed by a late systolic murmur is the classic auscultatory finding associated with a prolapsing mitral valve, this association is by no means invariable. Echocardiographic evidence of late systolic prolapse may be associated with a pansystolic murmur, with no murmur or clicks, with midsystolic clicks only, or with the classic midsystolic click and late systolic murmur. Similarly, echo evidence of pansystolic prolapse may be associated with no abnormal auscultatory findings, with a late systolic murmur, with clicks only, or with a pansystolic murmur. This patient, in fact, is an example of the echo pattern of late systolic prolapse occurring with a holosystolic murmur. Even in the presence of auscultatory findings of mitral prolapse, an abnormal mitral echo is not invariably recorded. In studying presumably healthy young women Markiewicz[74] found that 41 per cent of those with auscultatory evidence of mitral prolapse had normal mitral echoes. The great variability of the echo- and phonocardiographic features of this syndrome has been emphasized by DeMaria, et al.[72]

"NOT MITRAL PROLAPSE"

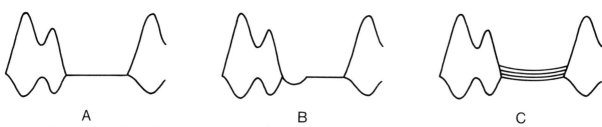

A   B   C

Figure 18–1.   Three echo patterns of the mitral valve that do not correspond to mitral valve prolapse. See text for discussion.

4. Only drawing *A*, which shows an abrupt posterior motion of the mitral valve in mid-systole with bowing greater than 2 mm posterior to the D point, represents an echo pattern of mitral prolapse (see Fig. 17–2). The other patterns do not represent mitral prolapse (Fig. 18–1). A purely horizontal C-D segment, often noticed on parts of the echocardiographic examination in patients with mitral valve prolapse, is not in itself diagnostic of mitral prolapse and should not be read as prolapse.[74] Early bowing of the C-D segment, lasting 20 to 80 msec after the C point, is a normal finding on high quality echocardiograms and does not represent mitral prolapse.[74] It probably represents bulging of the mitral valve toward the left atrium in isovolumetric systole.[71] Multiple systolic lines without bowing posterior to the C-D points likewise do not correspond to phonocardiographic, angiographic, or pathologic evidence of mitral prolapse.[70–72, 74] As discussed in Case 17, these multiple systolic lines can be recorded in normal patients and can result from problems with lateral resolution and the inherent width of the echo beam without prolapse of the mitral leaflets.

Two other echo patterns may resemble late systolic prolapse of the mitral valve without prolapse actually being present. In hypertrophic subaortic stenosis, in which there is prominent systolic anterior motion of the mitral valve in midsystole and abrupt posterior motion in the last third of systole, confusion with late systolic prolapse may occur. However, in hypertrophic subaortic stenosis the mitral valve does not move posterior to the D point in late systole as it does in true late systolic prolapse. In addition, in patients with large pericardial effusions, abnormal mitral echoes showing typical late systolic prolapse, which disappears after removal of the pericardial fluid, may be obtained. This represents a false-positive echo diagnosis for mitral valve prolapse that will be discussed in subsequent cases and which occurs because of excess motion of the entire heart posteriorly in late systole.[204]

CASE 19

This asymptomatic 22-year-old graduate student is referred for an echocardiogram after a systolic click is heard on a routine physical examination. No cardiac murmur is present. An electrocardiogram demonstrates T wave inversion in leads III and AVL.

MEASUREMENTS (Echo tracing A-C)   **Time lines = 200 msec**

cf	=	RV	=
D-E amplitude	=	EDD	=
E-F slope	=	ESD	=

QUESTIONS

1. Which of the following statements is/are correct with regard to the C-D segment of the mitral valve echo obtained from this patient?

   (A) The greater than 2 mm of "hammocking" of the C-D portion of the mitral valve represents the echo pattern of pansystolic prolapse.
   (B) A pansystolic murmur invariably accompanies this abnormality.
   (C) This echocardiographic pattern may accompany other echo findings for ruptured chordae tendineae.
   (D) This echocardiographic pattern may be created artifactually in normal persons by inferior angulation of the transducer.
   (E) The multiple echoes in systole represent separation of the anterior and posterior leaflets and are diagnostic of mitral prolapse.
   (F) This echocardiographic picture may be produced by amyl nitrite inhalation in a patient with late systolic prolapse.
   (G) This echocardiographic pattern and the pattern of late systolic prolapse of the mitral valve may be recorded in the same patient without provocation, even with proper transducer position.

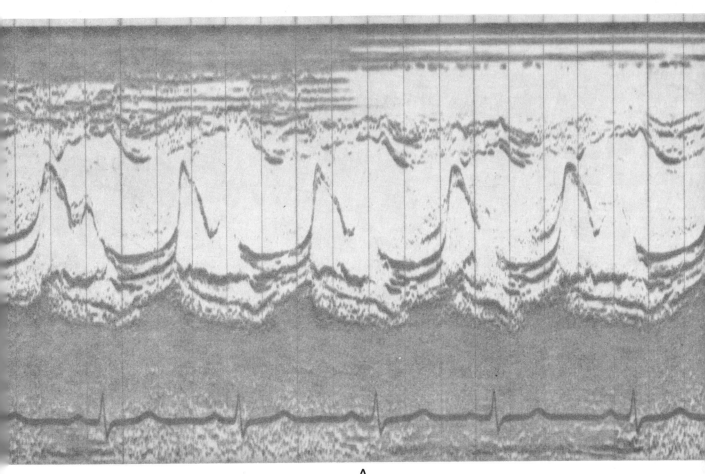

A

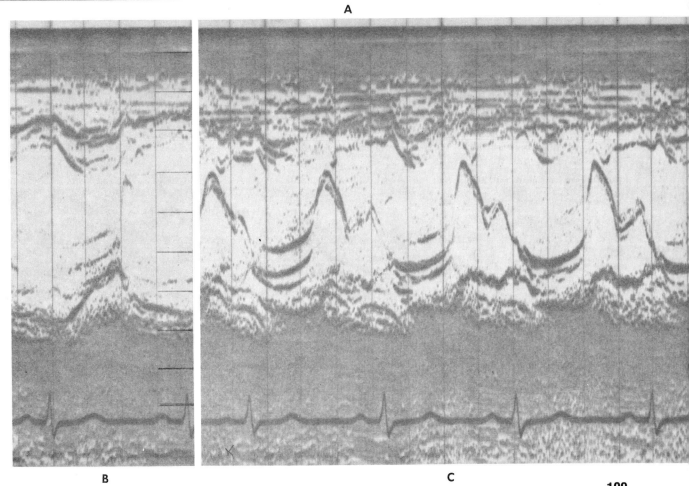

B

C

109

ANSWERS TO CASE 19
Pansystolic Prolapse of the Mitral Valve

MEASUREMENTS

cf	$= 0.95$	RV	$= 0.9$ cm
D-E amplitude	$= 24$ mm	EDD	$= 4.1$ cm
E-F slope	$= 100$ mm/sec	ESD	$= 2.4$ cm

ANSWERS

1. (A), (C), (D), (F), and (G)

(A) The C-D segment of this patient's echocardiogram demonstrates a smooth "hammock-like" sagging of the entire systolic portion of the mitral valve echo (Fig. 19–1). This pattern of pansystolic prolapse is one of the characteristic echo findings in patients with angiographic, anatomic, and phonocardiographic evidence of mitral prolapse (Figure 17–2).[67, 70-74, 78] This type of pansystolic bowing reaches its nadir in midsystole and characteristically is associated with an increased D-E amplitude of the anterior leaflet and with multiple systolic echoes. Markiewicz[74] found that, when the maximum displacement of this pansystolic bowing was greater than 2 mm posterior to an imaginary line drawn between the C and D points, the pattern had a statistically significant correlation with phonocardiographic evidence of mitral prolapse (Fig. 19–1). When the sagging was less than 2 mm, the correlation was not significant. In identifying this pattern of pansystolic prolapse it is important to identify the C and D points positively by recording the leaflets coapting and separating in order to judge whether the C-D segment actually bows posteriorly. Less strict criteria than those advanced by Markiewicz probably will result in high rates of echo false-positives for mitral prolapse.

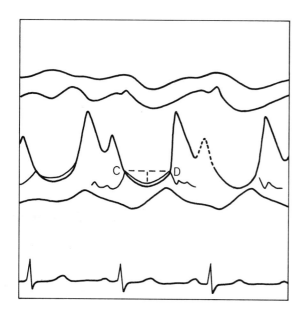

Figure 19–1 (Echo tracing *A*). Pansystolic prolapse of the mitral valve. As per Markiewicz,[74] construction of an imaginary line between the *C* and *D* points that are positively identified by the anterior and posterior mitral leaflets coapting and separating, and demonstration that the systolic portion of the mitral valve bows greater than 2 mm posterior to this line at its nadir are illustrated.

(B) As in late systolic prolapse, a wide range of auscultatory findings may accompany the echocardiographic findings of pansystolic prolapse.[72] Although pansystolic murmurs may be present, the only abnormal auscultatory finding may be midsystolic clicks, as in this patient, or the classic late systolic murmur. In fact, pansystolic prolapse may be recorded echocardiographically in patients with no abnormal auscultatory findings.[72]

(C) Patients with ruptured chordae tendineae to the anterior or posterior mitral leaflets have flail mitral valves, which often demonstrate pansystolic prolapse. Careful scanning of the mitral leaflets should be done in all patients with pansystolic prolapse, looking for additional evidence of ruptured chordae tendineae. Although mitral valve prolapse and ruptured chordae tendineae may be etiologically unrelated problems, they may produce similar motions of the C-D portion of the mitral echocardiogram.[70, 72, 79]

(D) It has recently been recognized that recording from too high an intercostal space with inferior angulation of the transducer is an important potential source of error in the echocardiographic diagnosis of pansystolic mitral prolapse. By so recording the mitral valve from a high intercostal space with inferior angulation of the transducer, very high instances of false-positive pansystolic bowing of the C-D segment of the mitral echocardiogram have been found in normal persons without any abnormal auscultatory findings[80] and in patients with no mitral prolapse on cineangiography.[78] This source of error is consistent with the motion of the normal mitral valve as observed with cross-sectional echocardiography.[75] During ventricular

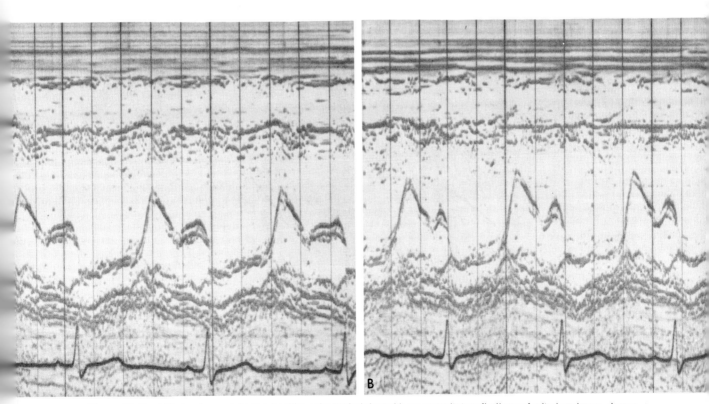

Figure 19-2. Mitral echogram from a healthy echo technician with no auscultatory findings of mitral prolapse, demonstrating how a pattern very similar to pansystolic prolapse can be created artifactually with a high transducer position (*A*). With the transducer perpendicular to the chest wall (*B*) the *C–D* segment is normal, rising slowly throughout systole.

systole the normal mitral ring moves *inferiorly* and the closed mitral valve forward. If the transducer is located too high on the chest wall, the mitral valve may move primarily away from the transducer during systole, and the transducer will record this motion as pansystolic mitral prolapse. In patients with thin chest configurations that often permit recording the mitral valve from high intercostal spaces, it is easy to produce this abnormality artifactually. To avoid this source of error in the diagnosis of mitral prolapse, extreme care must be taken to record the mitral valve with the transducer perpendicular to the chest wall with no inferior angulation of the transducer.

Figure 19–2 illustrates how a false-positive echo for pansystolic prolapse can be created in a perfectly healthy echo technician with no evidence of cardiac clicks or murmurs in several different positions after amyl nitrite inhalation or during hand grip exercise. By recording from the second intercostal space with marked inferior angulation of the transducer, pansystolic bowing of the mitral valve very similar to pansystolic prolapse was consistently demonstrated. However, with the transducer perpendicular to the chest wall in the fourth intercostal space, the C-D segment of the mitral echo was perfectly normal, rising slowly from posterior to anterior throughout systole without any posterior bowing. Thus it is extremely important to ensure that the transducer is perpendicular to the chest wall to avoid this technical source of error in the diagnosis of pansystolic prolapse.

(E) Although multiple echoes in systole are commonly recorded in mitral valve prolapse, they are nonspecific findings and occur in normal patients as well as in those with a variety of cardiac disorders. Their presence is due to the width of the ultrasonic beam, which encounters the mitral valve tangentially. The near edge of the beam comes in contact with the mitral valve before the far edge of the beam, making it appear that parts of the mitral valve are anterior to others. Thus, because the ultrasonic beam has a discrete width, several lines may be produced by each leaflet and leaflets may actually be coapting but appear separated.[71-73, 78]

(F) Amyl nitrite inhalation usually moves late systolic prolapse earlier in systole and may, in fact, change the echo pattern of late systolic prolapse to pansystolic prolapse.[68, 71, 77] This change probably occurs because of a decrease in left ventricular volume, allowing the mitral valve leaflets to prolapse earlier in systole.

(G) Cross-sectional echocardiography has demonstrated that the entire spectrum of M-mode abnormalities from late systolic to pansystolic mitral prolapse can exist in the same patient at the same time.[75] In addition, in patients with late systolic prolapse by single crystal echo, pansystolic prolapse very often can be detected on some portion of the mitral valve as viewed by cross-sectional techniques. Thus, these different echo patterns do not represent different types of prolapse, but rather are a spectrum of patterns dependent in part on that portion of the prolapsing mitral valve traversed by the single crystal echo beam.

CASE 20

A 38-year-old executive secretary is referred because of frequent, sequential, premature ventricular contractions demonstrated on a recent treadmill test. The patient has a history of a "functional" murmur noted in her teens and of occasional palpitations dating from her college years. On physical examination, a grade II/VI late systolic murmur which increases in intensity on standing is noted.

Echo tracings A and B are mitral echoes from this patient recorded with the transducer perpendicular to the chest wall. In echo tracing C, amyl nitrite was administered, and tracing D is recorded with slight superior angulation of the transducer.

QUESTIONS

(Echo tracings A-C)   Time lines = 200 msec

1. Which of the following observations are present on this patient's echocardiogram?

   (A) Abrupt posterior bowing of the terminal portion of the C-D segment
   (B) Mitral valve prolapse moving slightly earlier following amyl nitrite inhalation
   (C) Anterior leaflet collapsing into the left atrial wall at the beginning of systole
   (D) Pansystolic mitral prolapse

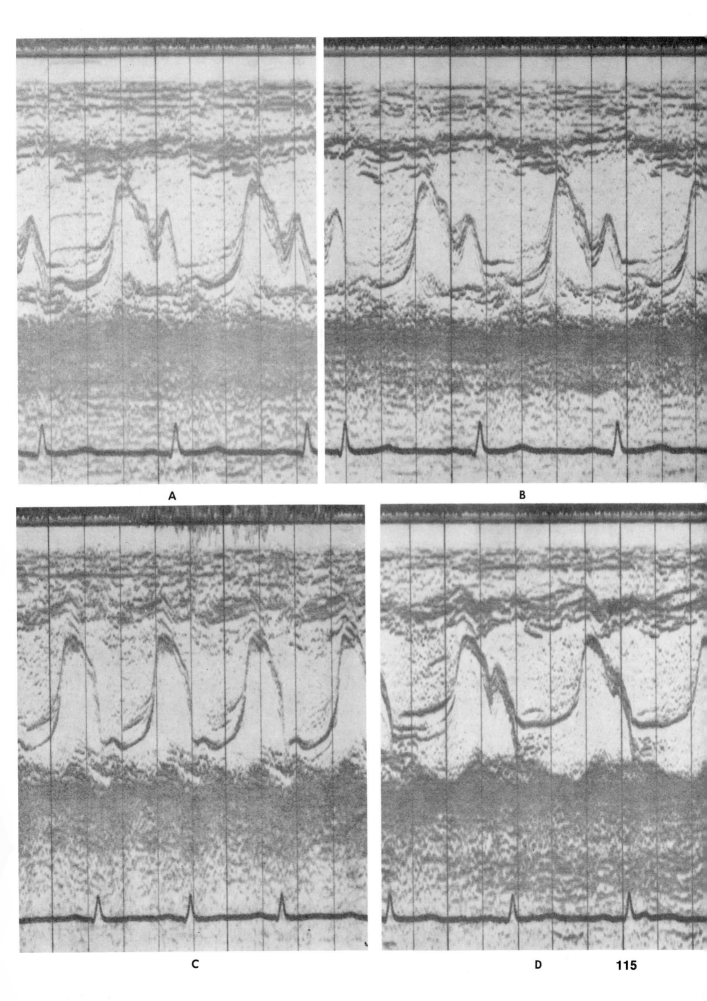

A

B

C

D   115

ANSWERS TO CASE 20
Late Systolic Prolapse of the Mitral Valve
Collapse of the Anterior Leaflet into the Left Atrial Wall

ANSWERS

1. (A), (B), (C) This patient's mitral echogram demonstrates the abrupt posterior motion in mid-systole, with bowing posterior to the D point that is consistent with the echo pattern of late systolic prolapse. After amyl nitrite inhalation in echo tracing *C* this finding becomes slightly more prominent and occurs earlier in systole.[68, 71, 77]

   In addition, on echo tracing *D*, with slight superior angulation of the transducer into the left atrium, the anterior mitral leaflet is observed to collapse precipitously into the left atrial wall after the A point (Fig. 20–1). DeMaria, et al.,[72, 73] have reported this pattern of the anterior leaflet plunging into the left atrial wall as part of the variable spectrum of echo abnormalities that may be observed in mitral prolapse (Fig. 17–2). In their experience this localized abnormality usually was accompanied by echo evidence of generalized pansystolic prolapse. However, they did find it the predominant echo disorder in five patients with angiographic evidence of mitral prolapse in whom the C-D segment was otherwise either flat or bowed only minimally in other parts of the echo tracing. Although collapse of the anterior leaflet into the left atrial wall is observed in the patient from this case, the predominant pattern of the C-D segment is late systolic rather than pansystolic prolapse.

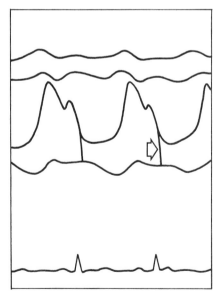

Figure 20–1 (Echo tracing *D*). Collapse of the anterior mitral leaflet into the left mitral wall at the beginning of systole (*open arrow*), one of the echo patterns observed in mitral valve prolapse (see Fig. 17–2).

CASE 21

A tall six-year-old girl is referred for an echocardiogram because of a harsh systolic apical murmur. She is active, keeps up with her peers, but notes that her heart pounds heavily when she runs. She wears glasses and is self-conscious about her large hands and feet. Height = 52 inches, Weight = 45 lbs. BSA = 0.9 m².

MEASUREMENTS (Echo tracings *A-E*)   **Time lines = 200 msec**

cf	=		EDD	=	(2.4–3.8 cm)*
Ao	=	(13–22 mm)*	ESD	=	
Ao valve opening	=	(0.9–1.6 cm)*	Ejection fraction	=	
C-E amplitude	=		Percentage change	=	
D-E amplitude	=		IVS amplitude	=	
RV	=	(0.4–1.5 cm)*	LVPW amplitude	=	

*Normal values for children based on weight (26–50 lbs).[1,3]

QUESTIONS

1. Which of the following observations are present on this patient's echocardiogram?
   (A) Pansystolic mitral prolapse
   (B) Tricuspid prolapse
   (C) Abrupt midsystolic, posterior motion of the C-D segment of the mitral valve
   (D) Paradoxic IVS motion
   (E) RV dilatation
   (F) Dilated aortic root
   (G) Evidence for aortic insufficiency
   (H) LV cavity dilatation

2. These observations are most consistent with which one of the following diagnoses?
   (A) Tetralogy of Fallot
   (B) Atrial septal defect
   (C) Marfan's syndrome
   (D) Common A-V valve

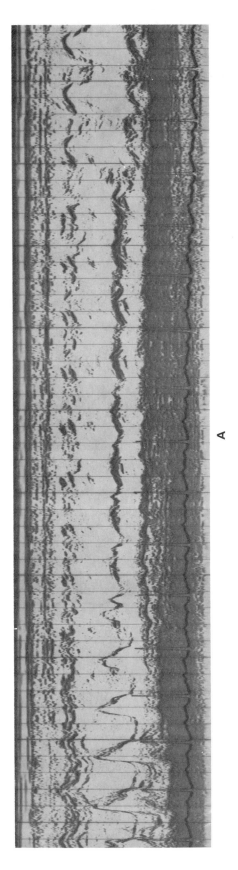

A

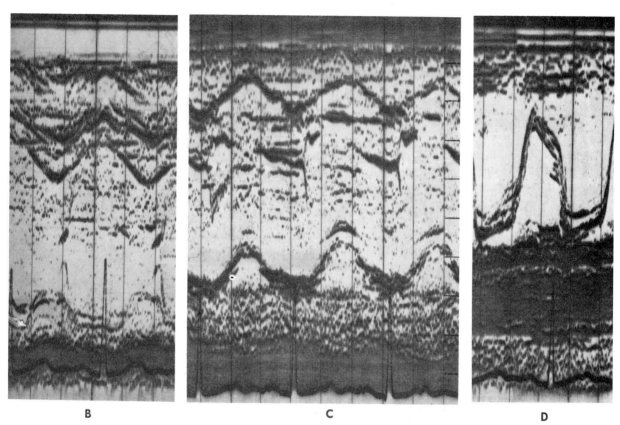

B   C   D

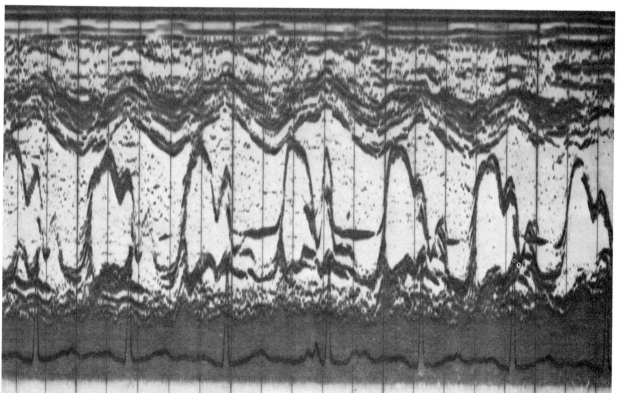

E

ANSWERS TO CASE 21
Marfan's Syndrome with Dilated Aortic Root and Late Systolic Mitral Prolapse

MEASUREMENTS

cf	= 0.96	ESD	= 4.5 cm (2.4–3.8 cm)*
Ao	= 43 mm (13–22 mm)*	ESD	= 2.7 cm
Ao valve opening	= 1.5 cm (0.9–1.6 cm)*	Ejection fraction	= 71%
C-E amplitude	= 32 mm	Percentage change	= 40%
D-E amplitude	= 31 mm	IVS amplitude	= 11 mm
RV	= 0.8 cm (0.4–1.5 cm)*	LVPW amplitude	= 9 mm

*Normal values for children based on weight (25–60 lbs).[1,3]

ANSWERS

1. (C), (F), (H) On echo tracing *E* (Fig. 21-1) the mitral valve is observed to move abruptly posteriorly toward the left atrial wall in mid-systole and to bow prominently posterior to the D point during late systole. This pattern, of course, is consistent with late systolic prolapse of the mitral valve.

   The aortic root, seen on echo tracings *A* and *C*, and identified as two parallel lines moving anteriorly in systole and posteriorly in diastole, is grossly dilated. The aortic cusps open normally without evidence of stenosis. When the aortic root or cusps are markedly dilated, the left atrial dimension often appears compromised as is shown on echo tracings *A* and *C*.

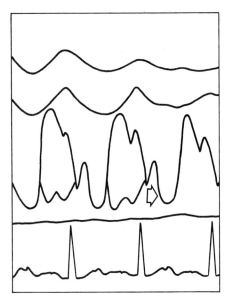

Figure 21-1 (Echo tracing *E*). Late systolic prolapse of the mitral valve (*open arrow*).

As judged by the published normal values for children, the left ventricular cavity is dilated based on this patient's weight.[1, 3]

The C-D segment of the mitral valve does not bow posteriorly throughout systole in a pattern of pansystolic prolapse. The tricuspid valve, on echo tracing D, shows no evidence of systolic prolapse. The right ventricle is of normal size, and the interventricular septal motion is appropriately timed, as seen on echo tracing B. Although the aortic root is grossly dilated, there is no evidence of aortic insufficiency from the anterior mitral leaflet.

2. (C). Aortic root dilatation and mitral valve prolapse are most consistent with Marfan's syndrome, a connective tissue disease commonly associated with both these cardiac abnormalities.[81, 82] Brown, et al.,[81] found echo evidence of both aortic root dilatation and mitral valve prolapse in 97 per cent of a group of 35 patients with Marfan's syndrome. Aortic root dilatation alone was found in 60 per cent of this group and mitral valve prolapse, usually of a pansystolic pattern, in 91 per cent. Only about one-half of these patients had auscultatory evidence of mitral prolapse. Likewise, there was no consistent relationship between a murmur of aortic insufficiency and echo evidence of aortic root dilatation, as is illustrated by the patient in this case without aortic insufficiency but with a grossly dilated root. Given the difficulty in detecting aortic root dilatation in this syndrome by the routine chest x-ray, echocardiography may be more sensitive than other noninvasive methods in detecting cardiac involvement of the aortic root and mitral valve in Marfan's syndrome.

Clinically, the patient shown in this case has the body habitus typical of Marfan's syndrome. At cardiac catheterization, left ventricular dilatation and moderate mitral regurgitation were documented. The mitral valve was very mobile, had pronounced scalloping of its free edge, and prolapsed prominently into the left atrium during systole. Marked aneurysmal dilatation of the three aortic sinuses with dilatation of the ascending aorta unassociated with aortic insufficiency was seen on a thoracic aortogram.

CASE 22

This 25-year-old lineman recently experienced two episodes of "feeling faint" while up on a telephone pole. He did not lose consciousness and has otherwise been asymptomatic. The company physician detects a normal carotid pulse and a normal S1 followed by an early systolic ejection sound. No systolic murmur is heard and the second sound also is normal. He does hear a grade II/VI early diastolic blowing murmur along the left sternal border and refers the young man for evaluation. The electrocardiogram is normal.

MEASUREMENTS (Echo tracings A-C)   **Time lines = 200 msec**

cf	=	C-E amplitude	=
Ao	=	D-E slope	=
LA	=	E-F slope	=
Aortic valve opening =			

QUESTIONS

1. This patient most probably has which of the following diagnoses?

   (A) Marfan's syndrome
   (B) Aortic vegetation secondary to endocarditis
   (C) Bicuspid aortic valve
   (D) Congenital aortic stenosis
   (E) Pansystolic mitral prolapse

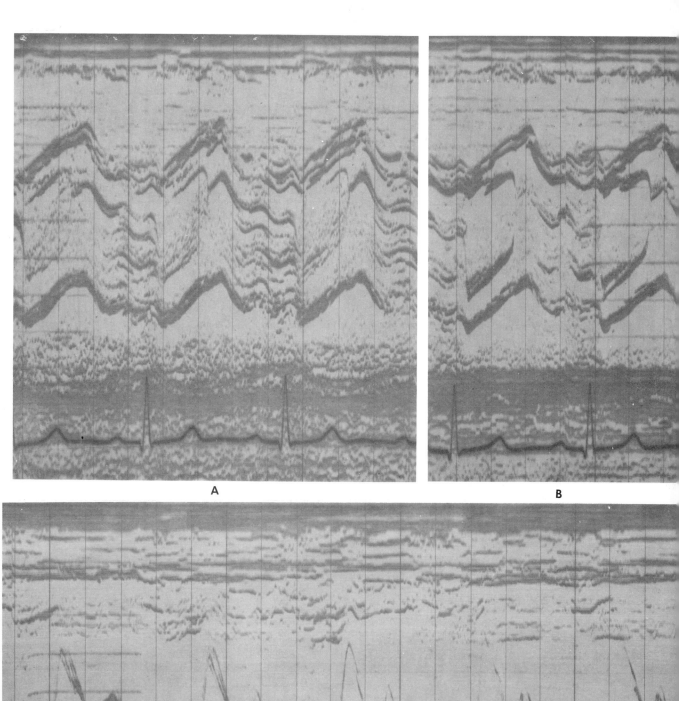

A

B

C

ANSWERS TO CASE 22
Bicuspid Aortic Valve/
Pansystolic Mitral Prolapse

MEASUREMENTS

cf	= 1.0	C-E amplitude	= 32 mm
Ao	= 40 mm	D-E slope	= 460 msec
LA	= 2.4 cm	E-F slope	= 170 msec
Aortic valve opening	= 2.0 cm		

ANSWERS

1. (C), (E) Eccentric closing of the aortic cusps is noted on echo tracings *A* and *B*, and calculation of the Eccentricity Index (1/2 [Ao internal diameter] / minimal distance between closed cusps and Ao wall = 1/2 [35 mm]/8 mm) reveals an

elevated valve of 2.1, strongly suggesting that this young man has a bicuspid aortic valve[15, 16] (see Case 3 for details of this calculation). As is common with bicuspid aortic valves, multiple linear echoes are recorded within the aortic root during diastole. In the absence of the clinical setting of endocarditis, such echo densities should not be read as aortic valvular vegetations. Even though a bicuspid aortic valve may be associated with aortic stenosis, there is no suggestion of that diagnosis in this young man with no systolic murmur, normal carotid pulses and second sound, and no left ventricular hypertrophy on the electrocardiogram.

The mitral valve, recorded on echo tracing C with the transducer perpendicular to the chest wall, demonstrates the continuous sagging or "hammocking" posterior to the C and D points throughout systole typical of the pattern of pansystolic prolapse. This man is another example of the variability that exists between echocardiographic and phonocardiographic findings in mitral prolapse. Despite the echo pattern of pansystolic prolapse, he has no systolic murmur.

The early systolic sound was thought to be an ejection sound secondary to the bicuspid aortic valve. The lack of fine, high frequency shuddering of the anterior mitral leaflet in the presence of auscultatory evidence of aortic insufficiency is interesting. It probably results from a combination of mild aortic regurgitation with eccentricity of the regurgitant jet which misses the anterior leaflet. The degree of fine shuddering of the mitral valve in aortic insufficiency is related more to the direction of the regurgitant jet than to the magnitude of the regurgitation.

CASE 23

This 33-year-old priest complains of increasing fatigue and vague left-sided chest pains that occur only while he is working at his desk. Occasionally with exercise he will note rapid, regular palpitations, and once he had a short bout of atrial fibrillation documented in an emergency room. Otherwise, he is asymptomatic, jogs three times a week, and has no coronary risk factors. His electrocardiogram now shows sinus rhythm with T wave inversion in the inferior and lateral leads. On physical examination, there is an apical "cooing" systolic murmur.

QUESTION

MEASUREMENTS   (Echo tracings A-C)   Time lines = 200 msec

cf	=	E–F slope	=
Ao	=	D–E amplitude	=
Ao valve opening	=		
LA	=		

1. How does this echocardiogram help explain the patient's symptoms, physical findings, and electrocardiographic abnormalities?

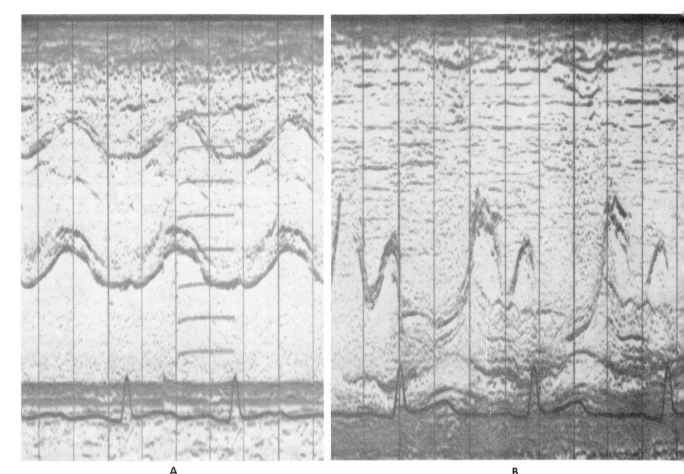

A

B

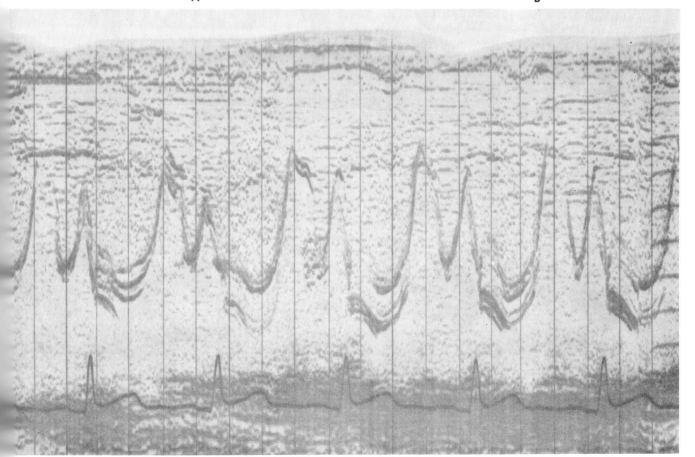

C

127

ANSWER TO CASE 23
Late Systolic Prolapse of the Mitral Valve

MEASUREMENTS:

cf	= 1.09	E–F slope	= 110 mm/sec
Ao	= 37 mm	D–E amplitude	= 35 mm
Ao valve opening	= 2.2 cm		
LA	= 3.9 cm		

ANSWER

1. The echocardiogram demonstrates late systolic prolapse of the mitral valve with a prominent D-E amplitude and a normal-sized left atrium.

Clinical Applications. Because of the variable clinical spectrum with which mitral valve prolapse without ruptured chordae tendineae may be associated, echocardiography often can be very helpful in establishing the etiology of certain, often confusing, signs and symptoms. Although a classic mid-systolic click and late-systolic murmur may be present, this syndrome also is associated with a pansystolic murmur similar to that heard in rheumatic mitral regurgitation, systolic clicking sounds without any murmur, a systolic murmur that is delayed just after the first heart sound and is unassociated with any clicks, and unusual "hooking" or "cooing" musical murmurs.

In addition, vague atypical anterior chest pain which often has a highly neurotic aspect is common in these patients with mitral prolapse. Sometimes this pain may be so disabling as to suggest coronary artery disease. In fact, this syndrome may be associated with T wave changes in the inferior and lateral leads of the electrocardiogram, even in the absence of coronary artery disease, adding to the difficulty of evaluating these patients. Many patients with mitral prolapse previously thought to have ischemic heart disease can be reassured as to the benign nature of their chest pain and ECG abnormalities. Mitral prolapse can also be the explanation for recurrent atrial and ventricular arrhythmias. These arrhythmias usually are considered to have a benign prognosis, although there are reports that the ventricular arrhythmias very rarely may be associated with sudden death.

Because of an increased incidence of endocarditis in this syndrome, patients with auscultatory evidence of mitral prolapse, especially when this is associated with echo evidence of prolapse, should receive antibiotic prophylaxis during dental work and similar types of invasive procedures. The meaning and natural history of echo evidence of mitral prolapse without any auscultatory abnormalities is unknown, but apparently very prevalent in females.[74] Consequently, antibiotic prophylaxis is not currently recommended in this large group without systolic clicks or murmurs.

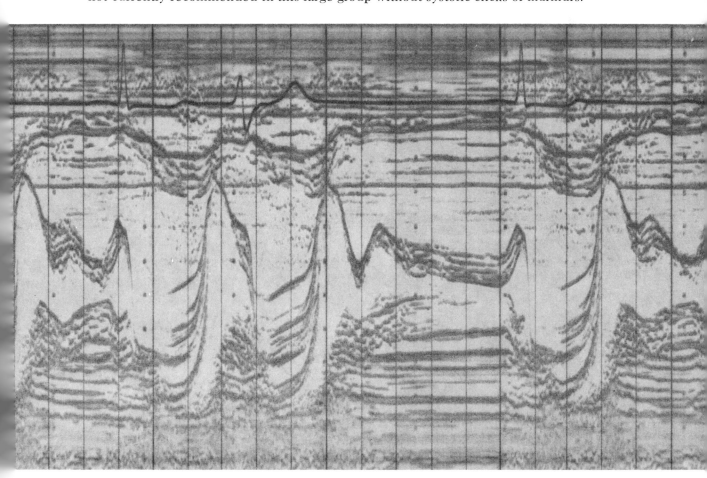

Figure 23–1. Echocardiogram illustrating prominent pattern of systolic mitral prolapse in a patient with a holosystolic murmur. This patient's teenage daughter has late systolic mitral prolapse by echo associated with a midsystolic click with late systolic murmur.

CASE 24

This 50-year-old investment counsellor with the history of "rheumatism" as a child and a "heart attack" six months ago consults a physician because dyspnea, fatigue, and chest pain have recently forced him to discontinue his rehabilitation exercise class. An echocardiogram is ordered to delineate the etiology of a systolic murmur noted on physical examination.

QUESTIONS

(Echo tracing A)   **Time lines = 100 msec**

1. Which of the following observations are present on this echo?
   (A) Echo-dense mitral valve
   (B) Echo-dense mitral annulus
   (C) Increased C-E amplitude
   (D) Posterior bowing of the mitral valve in systole
   (E) Increased D-E slope
   (F) Coarse, jagged E-F portion of the anterior mitral leaflet
   (G) Fine, high frequency diastolic shuddering of the anterior mitral leaflet

2. Using the above observations, which one of the following is the best explanation for this patient's murmur?
   (A) Rheumatic mitral regurgitation
   (B) Aortic insufficiency
   (C) Pansystolic prolapse of the mitral valve
   (D) Late systolic prolapse
   (E) Flail mitral valve with ruptured chordae tendineae to the anterior mitral leaflet

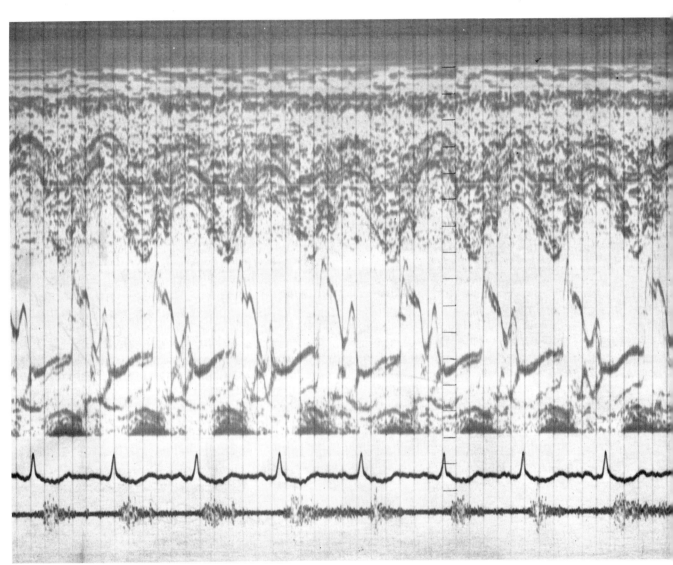

A

ANSWERS TO CASE 24
Ruptured Chordae Tendineae to the Anterior Mitral Leaflet
(RCT-AML)

ANSWERS

1. (C), (E), (F)   2. (E)

From this echo of the mitral valve, we observe that the E point of the anterior leaflet is sharply peaked and that the subsequent E-F portion of the leaflet has a coarse, jagged, and erratic appearance (Fig. 24–1, *open arrow*). This pattern, observed in a thin, nonrheumatic anterior leaflet, is the characteristic echo finding of a flail mitral valve secondary to ruptured chordae tendineae to the anterior leaflet.[1, 70, 83] This grossly irregular contour usually begins with a sharply peaked E point and is usually, but not always, accompanied by an increased mitral amplitude and opening slope. In this case, the D-E amplitude and slope are increased to 35 mm and greater than 500 mm/sec, respectively. Such an irregular and jagged E-F portion of the anterior mitral leaflet differs from the regular, fine, high frequency diastolic vibrations seen in aortic insufficiency (Fig. 24–2).[20, 23]

However, because the diastolic vibrations in aortic insufficiency sometimes are quite irregular, it may be very difficult to make the distinction between these two entities from the echo alone (Fig. 24–3). Consequently, a grossly irregular diastolic portion of the anterior leaflet should be interpreted with knowledge of whether mitral or aortic regurgitation is clinically evident. Usually the mitral vibrations secondary to a flail anterior leaflet occur only in the E-F portion of the anterior leaflet, whereas in aortic insufficiency the high-frequency vibrations usually extend throughout diastole and involve both the E and A points. These types of abnormal diastolic motion of the anterior mitral leaflet are easily distinguished from the slow undulations of the anterior leaflet seen with atrial fibrillation (Fig. 24–2). These slower motions are especially evident with longer cycle lengths, may be observed in both mitral leaflets, and also may occur in the tricuspid valve during diastole in the presence of atrial fibrillation.

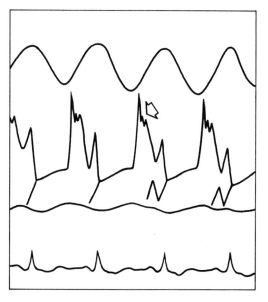

Figure 24–1(Echo tracing *A*). Ruptured chordae tendineae to the anterior mitral leaflet resulting in a flail mitral valve. Note the coarse, jagged, and erratic motion of the diastolic portion of the anterior leaflet (*open arrow*) and its sharply peaked *E* point.

Figure 24-2. Illustration of the characteristic abnormal diastolic motion of the anterior mitral leaflet in aortic insufficiency (*AI*), ruptured chordae tendineae to the anterior leaflet (*RCT—AML*) and atrial fibrillation (*AF*). In aortic insufficiency, the mitral leaflet typically shows a fine, high frequency shuddering in diastole. This motion should be distinguished from the coarse, jagged, and erratic type of motion typically seen with a flail anterior mitral leaflet. In contrast, slower undulations typically are seen in the anterior leaflet in the presence of atrial fibrillation.

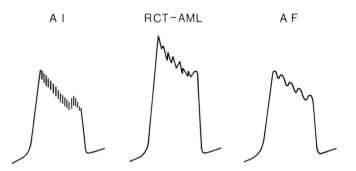

On this echo, neither the mitral valve nor annulus is echo-dense, and the C-D portion of the valve is normal in that it rises slowly from posteriorly to anteriorly throughout systole without posterior bowing. Thus, there is no evidence of rheumatic mitral regurgitation or of pansystolic or late systolic prolapse as previously described.

Technical Hints. In recording a flail anterior leaflet, the typical jagged E-F portion of an anterior leaflet with ruptured chordae tendineae may be very difficult to record and the abnormality may be very subtle.

(1) Scan diligently the distal tip of the anterior leaflet, where this abnormality is

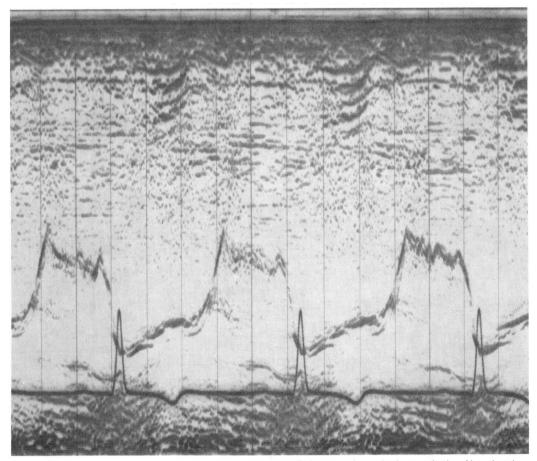

Figure 24-3. Echocardiogram of a patient with aortic insufficiency and no mitral regurgitation. Note that the vibrations of the anterior mitral leaflet (*AML*) may be very coarse and irregular in aortic insufficiency.

most obvious. Recording more proximally often will show normal anterior and posterior mitral leaflets, even in the presence of ruptured chordae to the anterior leaflet.

(2) Use the minimal amount of gain necessary to record the E-F portion of the anterior leaflet. Too much gain often will obscure the characteristic jagged contour of the anterior leaflet, especially when it is subtle.

This gentleman's cardiac catheterization demonstrated severe mitral regurgitation. At cardiac surgery for mitral valve replacement he had several ruptured chordae tendineae to the central portion of the anterior leaflet. The chordae posterior to the leaflet were intact.

CASE 25

A 61-year-old carpenter presents with a three-month history of progressive dyspnea at work, and when seen in the office he is found to have pulmonary edema. He denies chest discomfort and syncope as well as any previous illness. A parasternal heave is present. A Grade III/VI harsh systolic ejection murmur at the aortic area with radiation to both carotids and a Grade III/VI apical holosystolic murmur are heard. The carotid upstroke is within normal limits, but S2 is soft and single. No diastolic sounds are appreciated. The clinical impression is aortic stenosis and mitral regurgitation with pulmonary edema.

MEASUREMENTS (Echo tracings A-E)		Time lines = 200 msec	
cf	=	EDD	=
Ao valve opening	=	ESD	=
LA	=	Ejection fraction	=
E-F slope	=	Percentage change	=
D-E amplitude	=	IVS amplitude	=
D-E slope	=	LVPW amplitude	=
		IVS thickness	=

QUESTIONS

1. Does the echo support the clinical impression of aortic stenosis and mitral regurgitation?

2. What observations from the echo explain the patient's murmurs, and what etiology do they suggest?

3. Surgical correction of this patient's valvular abnormality is being considered. What observations can be made from this echo to help decide whether surgery will lead to significant improvement in this patient's congestive heart failure or whether continuing difficulty with cardiac failure is likely postoperatively?

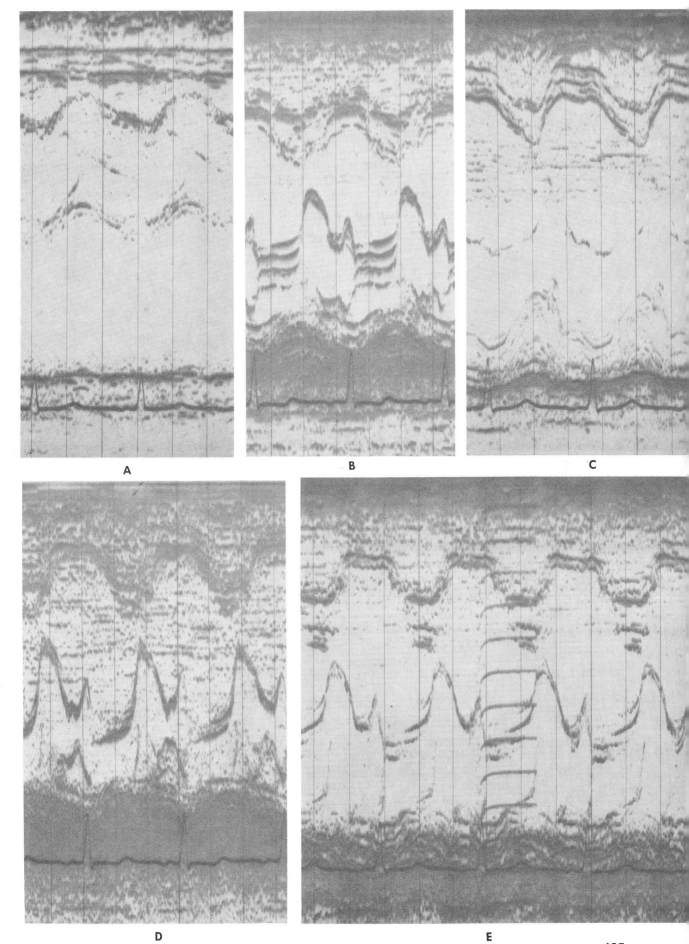

A

B

C

D

E

ANSWERS TO CASE 25
Ruptured Chordae Tendineae to the Posterior Mitral Leaflet (RCT-PML)

MEASUREMENTS

cf	= 1.14	EDD	= 7.0
Ao valve opening	= 1.8 cm	ESD	= 4.4
LA	= 5.0 cm	Ejection fraction	= 65%
E-F slope	= 100 mm/sec	Percentage change	= 37%
D-E amplitude	= 29 mm	IVS amplitude	= 12 mm
D-E slope	= 340 mm/sec	LVPW amplitude	= 16 mm
		IVS thickness	= 10 mm

ANSWERS

1. This echo does not support the clinical impression of aortic stenosis because the aortic cusps are thin and open normally and the aortic root is not echo-dense. However, there is echo evidence of mitral regurgitation secondary to ruptured chordae tendineae to the posterior mitral leaflet, as is discussed below.[1, 70, 79, 83] Clinically, it is common for the murmur of a flail posterior mitral leaflet to radiate to the aortic area, simulating the murmur of aortic stenosis.

2. The mitral echo shows a thin mitral valve with abnormal, paradoxic anterior motion of a portion of the posterior mitral leaflet in early diastole (echo tracings *D* and *E*). This is seen as a thin line that moves sharply anteriorly in early diastole, posterior to, but separate from, the D-E portion of the anterior leaflet (Fig. 25–1, *open arrow;* Fig. 25–2). This "flicking" type of anterior motion of the posterior leaflet in early diastole is highly characteristic of nonrheumatic mitral regurgitation secondary to ruptured chordae tendineae to the posterior mitral leaflet.[1, 70, 79, 83] When the posterior leaflet is recorded throughout the rest of diastole, as in this case, it is seen to remain primarily anterior and in some cases even horizontal in diastole before it moves posteriorly toward the left atrial wall with the beginning of the next systole.

   This type of "flicking" anterior motion of the posterior leaflet in early diastole is to be distinguished from the anterior motion of the posterior leaflet in mitral stenosis. In rheumatic disease, of course, the mitral valve is echo-dense, and the posterior leaflet moves anterior from the D point. In nonrheumatic mitral regurgitation secondary to a flail posterior leaflet, the mitral valve is of normal echo density and the thin posterior leaflet moves rapidly anterior in early diastole from a point posterior to the D point of the anterior leaflet.

   In addition, with ruptured chordae tendineae to the posterior leaflet, the flail leaflet occasionally can be recorded well within the left atrium during ventricular

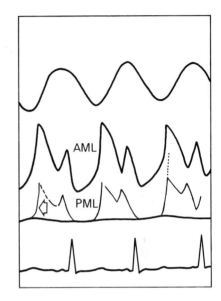

Figure 25–1 (Echo tracing *D*). Ruptured chordae tendineae to the posterior mitral leaflet showing the sharp "flicking" anterior motion of the posterior leaflet in early diastole (*open arrow*). The motion of the posterior leaflet is also shown during the rest of diastole. Note that if the initial plane of motion of the posterior leaflet in early diastole is extended (*dotted line*), it usually remains separate from the *D–E* portion of the anterior leaflet in this entity.

FLAIL MITRAL VALVE

RCT–AML   RCT–PML

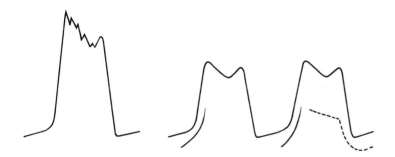

Figure 25–2. Illustration of the characteristic echo patterns in ruptured chordae tendineae to the anterior mitral leaflet (*RCT–AML*) and in ruptured chordae tendineae to the posterior mitral leaflet (*RCT–PML*).

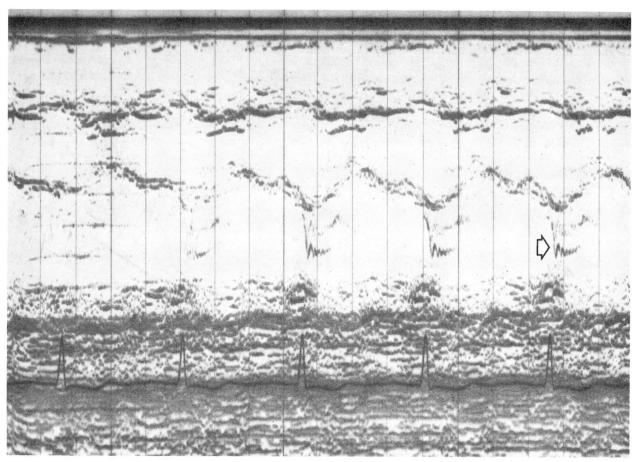

Figure 25–3. Echo showing a flail posterior mitral leaflet seen well within the left atrium as a thin, vibrating structure (*open arrow*) in another case of surgically confirmed ruptured chordae to the posterior leaflet.

systole on M-mode scanning between the aorta and mitral valve.[70, 79] Then the posterior leaflet is appreciated as a thin echo with high frequency vibrations seen within the left atrium only during ventricular systole (Fig. 25–3, *open arrow*). Although more specific than the previous pattern for ruptured chordae tendineae to the posterior leaflet, this sign is recorded much less frequently.

When there is echo evidence of pansystolic or late systolic prolapse, echoes very similar to this "flicking" anterior motion of the posterior leaflet seen behind the anterior leaflet in early diastole may be obtained in the absence of a flail posterior leaflet. We have found the following four points helpful, but not infallible, in making this distinction.

First, with ruptured chordae tendineae to the posterior leaflet, as opposed to prolapse without rupture, the posterior leaflet moves anteriorly in early diastole shortly *after* the anterior leaflet, and therefore appears separate from the anterior leaflet. It is often helpful to draw a line extending the initial plane of motion of the posterior leaflet in early diastole in order to appreciate this difference in timing (Fig. 25–1, *dotted line*). In prolapse without rupture, this dotted line usually merges with the D-E portion of the anterior leaflet.

Second, a flail posterior leaflet often begins its anterior motion in early diastole from a point that is very posterior near the left atrial wall in distinction to a prolapsing leaflet without rupture, which is more anterior.

Third, identifying the posterior leaflet as a thin, high frequency vibrating echo well within the left atrium during systole strongly favors ruptured chordae tendineae to the posterior mitral leaflet.[70, 79]

Fourth, the E point of the anterior leaflet may be rounded or may have a slight high frequency shuddering with a flail posterior leaflet, as opposed to prolapse without rupture, when this point usually is normal.

Cross-sectional echocardiography confirms these signs of ruptured chordae tendineae to the posterior mitral leaflet.[84] As is illustrated in Figure 25–4, at the end of systole the flail portion of the posterior leaflet lies along the posterior left atrial wall. At the beginning of diastole, just after the anterior leaflet moves anteriorly into the left ventricle, the flail portion of the posterior leaflet leaves the posterior left atrial wall and moves slightly anterior toward the transducer before it opens into the left ventricle. This anterior motion of the flail portion of the posterior leaflet toward the transducer produces the anteriorly "flicking" echo seen posterior to and slightly separated from the anterior leaflet.

This diagram also explains why this anterior "flicking" echo often appears to move anteriorly from deep within the left atrium along the posterior atrial wall. With cross-sectional imaging, this motion of the posterior leaflet resembles that of a "bull whip" flipping into the left ventricle. With ventricular systole, the flail portion again moves back into the left atrium.

On echo tracing *B* in this case, the mitral valve echo shows multiple parallel lines during systole. Such patterns occasionally are seen in different types of mitral regurgitation. However, this is a nonspecific finding and because similar echoes may be obtained in normals, it should not be considered indicative of mitral regurgitation. Note that the multiple systolic lines seen in this echo are not characteristic of pansystolic prolapse in that they do not bow posterior to a line connecting the C and D points as described in previous cases.

3. Although the left ventricular cavity is significantly dilated, the calculated ejection fraction and percentage change of the minor diameter are normal. In addition, the

amplitudes of motion of the septum and the left ventricular posterior wall are increased.

These findings suggest that hemodynamically significant mitral regurgitation is present, that the myocardium is compensating relatively well for this left ventricular volume overload, and that the patient is likely to have significant improvement in his cardiac failure after surgical correction of the valvular abnormality. In patients with mitral regurgitation, a grossly dilated left ventricle with low wall amplitudes and decreased ejection indices, significant myocardial dysfunction is suggested. Poor surgical results are likely in such patients, even though the valvular abnormality is corrected.

Clinical Application.   Echocardiographic measurement of left ventricular function can be quite helpful in patients with mitral regurgitation to assess whether any disability may result from myocardial dysfunction and, therefore, be unlikely to be improved by surgery.[169a, 295]

In addition, echo detection of a flail posterior leaflet (Fig. 25–2) as the cause of significant mitral regurgitation may have important surgical implications. It is often possible for a surgeon to successfully plicate the posterior leaflet if ruptured chordae tendineae to this leaflet are producing the mitral regurgitation and thus avoid prosthetic valve replacement. On the other hand, if there are ruptured chordae tendineae to the anterior leaflet, prosthetic valve replacement is always required. Therefore, echo evidence of only a flail posterior leaflet implies that there is a reasonable chance of avoiding prosthetic valve replacement if surgery is performed.

However, when there is echo evidence for a flail posterior leaflet, it is not always possible to exclude a concomitant abnormality of the anterior leaflet by echo. This difficulty occurs because ruptured chordae tendineae to the posterior leaflet may be associated with nonspecific abnormalities of the anterior leaflet and because the sign of ruptured chordae tendineae to the anterior leaflet may be subtle and difficult to demonstrate. Similarly, even though there is a flail posterior leaflet, the regurgitation may result primarily from stretched chordae to the anterior leaflet without rupture, from a cleft anterior leaflet or from a flail anterior leaflet that may not be detected. Despite these limitations, the echo abnormalities seen in ruptured chordae tendineae to the posterior leaflet are useful in recognizing from the echo

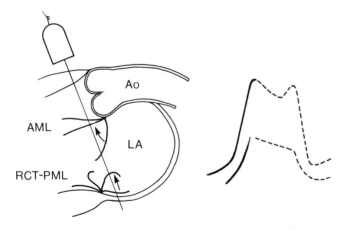

Figure 25–4.   Illustration of the motion of the flail portion of the posterior mitral leaflet with ruptured chordae tendineae (*RCT–PML*) and of the anterior leaflet (*AML*) during the *initial part of diastole only*. Note that at the beginning of diastole the flail portion of the posterior leaflet lies within the left atrium. Just after the anterior leaflet opens the flail portion of the posterior leaflet first moves anteriorly toward the transducer before it moves into the left ventricle. This anterior motion of the posterior leaflet produces the anteriorly "flicking" echo seen posterior to and separate from the *D–E* segment of anterior leaflet when chordae tendineae to the posterior leaflet are ruptured.

different patterns of mitral regurgitation and in suggesting that the liability of a prosthetic valve may be avoided if surgery is performed.

Cardiac catheterization and left ventricular cineangiography in this patient revealed severe mitral regurgitation with a mean pulmonary artery wedge pressure of 28 mm Hg and a "v wave" of 50 mm Hg. On a cineangiogram the left ventricle was dilated and showed good contractility, but no definite mitral prolapse could be identified. The left ventricular end-diastolic pressure was 12 mm Hg. At surgery, several chordae tendineae to the central portion of the posterior leaflet were found to be ruptured. Because the rest of the mitral valve was intact, the posterior leaflet was successfully plicated without prosthetic replacement. Postoperatively, no murmur was present, and the patient has resumed cabinet making without symptoms of cardiac failure.

CASE 26

This 59-year-old florist with the history of paroxysmal atrial tachycardia for over 30 years was active and able to perform her housework and shopping until five months ago. While at her cabin in the mountains, she noted the onset of progressive dyspnea on exertion and fatigue associated with increasing palpitations. On physical examination, an apical III/VI holosystolic murmur is noted. Because of the disabling nature of her symptoms, despite medical therapy, a cardiac catheterization is planned and an echocardiogram is ordered to help delineate the etiology of her presumed mitral regurgitation.

QUESTIONS

(Echo tracings *A-D*)   Time lines = 200 msec

1. Which of the following observations are both present on this echo *and* are also helpful in establishing an etiology of this patient's mitral regurgitation?

   (A) Echo-dense mitral valve
   (B) Thin mitral valve that is not echo-dense
   (C) Multiple mitral echoes in systole
   (D) Abnormal anterior motion of the posterior mitral leaflet in early diastole
   (E) Pansystolic mitral "hammocking"
   (F) Mitral vegetation
   (G) Echo-dense mitral annulus

2. What etiology of the mitral regurgitation does the echo suggest?

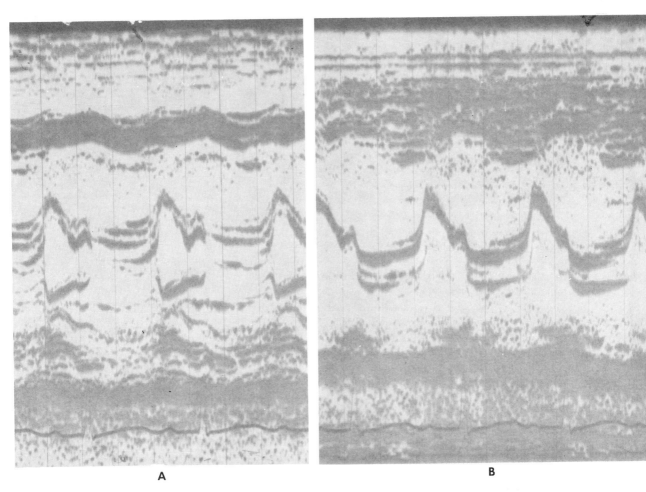

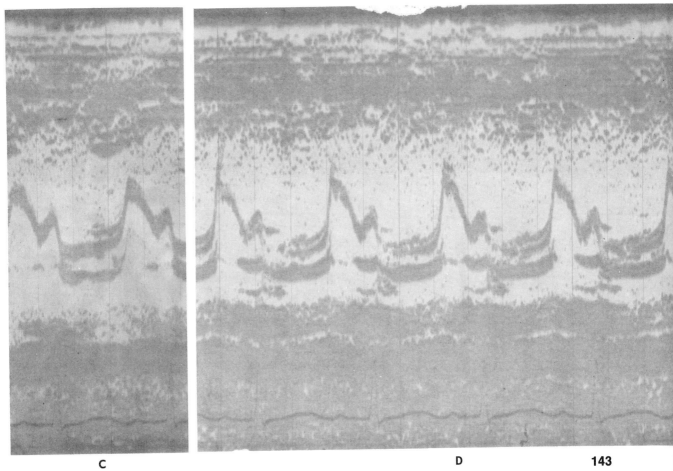

A

B

C

D

143

ANSWERS TO CASE 26

Ruptured Chordae Tendineae to the Posterior Mitral Leaflet (RCT-PML)

ANSWERS

1. (B) and (D).

2. An anterior mitral leaflet that is not echo-dense indicates a nonrheumatic cause of the mitral regurgitation. The abnormal anterior motion of the posterior mitral leaflet in early diastole seen "flicking" anteriorly just behind the D-E portion of the anterior leaflet suggests a ruptured chordae tendineae to the posterior leaflet (Fig. 26–1, *open arrow*).[1, 70, 79, 83] If only a few chordae tendineae to the posterior leaflet are ruptured, it is not unusual to obtain some mitral echoes with the posterior leaflet moving appropriately, as seen in echo tracing A in this patient. Therefore, it is important to scan the entire mitral valve in order to detect the abnormalities characteristic of a flail posterior leaflet.

Multiple mitral echoes in systole are also present on echo tracing A, but these are not helpful in establishing an etiology of the patient's mitral regurgitation. Signs of pansystolic mitral hammocking, mitral vegetations, or an echo-dense mitral annulus are not present.

After moderately severe mitral regurgitation was documented at cardiac catheterization, this patient underwent cardiac surgery. Although ruptured chordae tendineae to the posterior leaflet with intact chordae within several millimeters on either side were discovered, the major cause of the mitral regurgitation was stretched and elongated chordae tendineae to the anterior leaflet, which also had a small cleft. There were no ruptured chordae to the anterior leaflet. Mitral valve replacement was performed with a porcine heterograft. Pathologic examination documented myxomatous degeneration of the mitral valve.

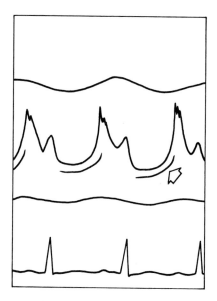

Figure 26–1. (Echo tracing *D*). Ruptured chordae tendineae to the posterior mitral leaflet. Abnormal anterior motion of the posterior mitral leaflet is seen "flicking" anteriorly just behind and separate from the *D-E* portion of the anterior leaflet (*open arrow*).

Although this abnormal pattern of an echo "flicking" anteriorly in early diastole is a reliable sign of ruptured chordae tendineae to the posterior mitral leaflet, there are several limitations to its use. First, as is illustrated by this case, when only a few chordae to the posterior leaflet are ruptured, causing part of the leaflet to be flail, a normal mitral echo of both leaflets may be obtained from those parts of the valve that coapt properly. This occurs more commonly when the ruptured chordae are to the lateral portions of the posterior leaflet, rather than to its central portion. In order to record this type of flail posterior leaflet the entire mitral valve must be diligently scanned.

Second, in patients with late systolic prolapse of the mitral valve, occasionally an abnormal echo may be recorded "flicking" anteriorly in early diastole in the absence of ruptured chordae tendineae to the posterior leaflet. Consequently, this echo pattern is an unreliable sign of a ruptured posterior chordae tendineae in the presence of late systolic mitral prolapse. A third limitation of this abnormal echo pattern is that even though a flail posterior mitral leaflet is detected it is not always possible to exclude a concomitant abnormality of the anterior leaflet. In fact, the undetected abnormality of the anterior leaflet, such as stretched, elongated chordae without rupture or a cleft, may be the primary cause of the mitral regurgitation.

Because the E-F portion of the anterior leaflet may have a slight irregularity with ruptured chordae tendineae to the posterior leaflet, even with intact chordae to the anterior leaflet, it may be difficult to exclude an associated flail anterior leaflet in the presence of ruptured chordae to the posterior leaflet. Even though there are certain limitations to its use, the echo pattern of a flail posterior leaflet as discussed in this case and in the preceding case remains a valuable echo sign of ruptured chordae tendineae to the posterior mitral leaflet.

CASE 27

This 20-year-old college student with a history of a murmur and previous cardiac catheterization presents to the student health service complaining that for one month he has felt very hot and had chills during football practice. He goes to bed for about one hour, his temperature climbs to 102 degrees, he sweats profusely, and then feels perfectly well until the next day's practice. Three months ago he was given penicillin for several days after a tooth was extracted. An echocardiogram is ordered to help delineate the cause of a Grade III/VI harsh systolic murmur heard at the apex and axilla as well as at the base of the heart and in the neck.

MEASUREMENTS (Echo tracings *A-F*)   **Time lines = 40 msec**

cf	=	LVPW amplitude	=
Ao valve opening	=	EDD	=
LA	=	ESD	=
D-E amplitude	=	Ejection fraction	=
D-E slope	=	Percentage change	=
RV	=	Ejection time	=
IVS amplitude	=	Vcf	=

QUESTIONS

1. Which of the following abnormal observations are present on this echo?

   (A) Eccentric aortic valve closing with an abnormal Eccentricity Index
   (B) Fine, high frequency diastolic shuddering of the anterior mitral leaflet
   (C) Early closure of the anterior mitral leaflet
   (D) Increased D-E amplitude
   (E) Increased D-E slope
   (F) Coarse, jagged E-F portion of the anterior mitral leaflet
   (G) Pansystolic mitral bowing
   (H) Anterior motion of the posterior mitral leaflet in early diastole
   (I) Echo-dense posterior mitral leaflet
   (J) Increased septal amplitude

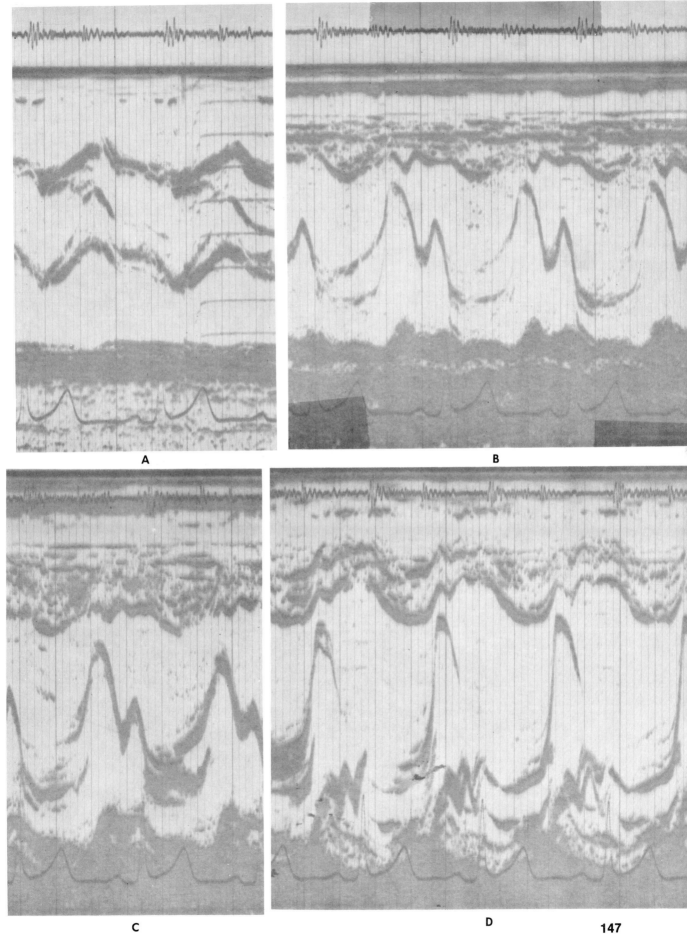

A

B

C

D

2. From the above observations and measurements, with which of the following descriptions is this echo consistent? More than one may apply.

   (A) Bicuspid aortic valve
   (B) Aortic insufficiency
   (C) Aortic vegetation
   (D) Late systolic prolapse
   (E) Pansystolic prolapse
   (F) Ruptured chordae tendineae to the anterior mitral leaflet
   (G) Ruptured chordae tendineae to the posterior mitral leaflet
   (H) Vegetation of the posterior mitral leaflet
   (I) Rheumatic mitral disease
   (J) Left ventricular volume overload
   (K) Left atrial enlargement

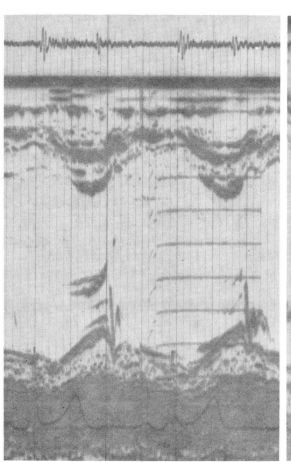

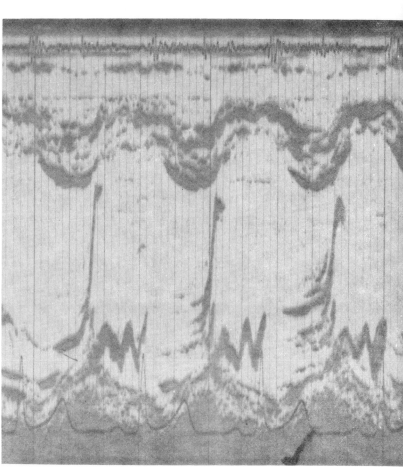

E

F

ANSWERS TO CASE 27

Ruptured Chordae Tendineae to the Posterior Mitral Leaflet (RCT-PML)
Pansystolic Mitral Prolapse (PSP)
Vegetation of the Posterior Mitral Leaflet

MEASUREMENTS

cf	= 1.14	LVPW amplitude	= 10 mm
Ao leaflet opening	= 1.9 cm	EDD	= 6.3 cm
LA	= 3.3 cm	ESD	= 4.1 cm
D-E amplitude	= 45 mm	Ejection fraction	= 63%
D-E slope	= 750 mm/sec	Percentage change	= 35%
RV	= 1.2 cm	Ejection time	= 250 msec
IVS amplitude	= 15 mm	Vcf	= 1.40 circ/sec

ANSWERS

1. (D), (E), (G), (H), (I), (J)
2. (E), (G), (H), (J)

This young man's mitral echo is abnormal and is consistent with a nonrheumatic type of mitral regurgitation as the cause of his systolic murmur. The following three descriptions of this mitral valve are supported by the echo:

(1) Ruptured chordae tendineae to the posterior mitral leaflet, as evidenced by the anterior "flicking" motion of the posterior leaflet early in diastole seen just posterior to the D-E portion of the anterior leaflet (Fig. 27–1, *open arrow*).[1, 70, 79, 83]

(2) Pansystolic prolapse, as evidenced by the prominent posterior bowing of the mitral valve throughout systole in echo tracing D.[70-74] The C-D portion of the valve is seen to bow posteriorly to an imaginary straight line connecting the C and D points. In this echo, the D point cannot be positively identified because the posterior leaflet is ruptured and is not seen to separate from the anterior leaflet at the beginning of diastole. Such pansystolic prolapse commonly accompanies ruptured chordae tendineae to the posterior leaflet.

(3) Vegetation of the posterior mitral leaflet. Observe the very prominent echodense posterior leaflet with unrestricted motion in diastole (Fig. 27–1, *closed arrow*). This pattern is similar to that which has been described for vegetation of the posterior leaflet.[26, 70] In a clinical setting compatible with endocarditis, i.e., a fever and cardiac murmur following a dental extraction, as in this case, such a finding suggests a vegetation of the posterior leaflet (Table 2–1).

Increased D-E amplitude of the anterior mitral leaflet, as seen in this patient, may be seen with a flail anterior or posterior leaflet and with pansystolic prolapse without rupture. We have also observed patients with increased D-E amplitude of the anterior leaflet as the only echo abnormality of the mitral valve who at surgery had an enlarged anterior leaflet with stretched, elongated chordae without actual rupture.[70] Pathologic examination revealed myxomatous degeneration of both leaf-

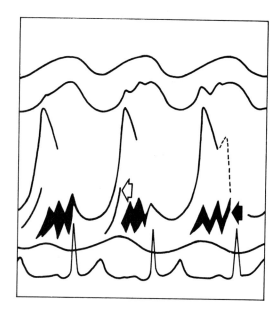

Figure 27–1. Ruptured chordae tendineae to the posterior mitral leaflet (**open arrow**) with echo density of the posterior leaflet consistent with a vegetation (*closed arrow*), and with evidence for pansystolic prolapse of the mitral valve.

lets and chordae. Thus, an increased opening amplitude and slope of the anterior leaflet may be the only echo evidence for mitral regurgitation secondary to this type of degenerative disease.

In the present case, the increased D-E amplitude probably results from the flail posterior leaflet with pansystolic prolapse, although accompanying stretched chordae to the anterior leaflet cannot be excluded. The E-F portion of the anterior leaflet is not jagged and irregular and thus there is insufficient echo evidence to support a diagnosis of ruptured chordae tendineae to the anterior leaflet.

Examination of the left ventricle reveals that there is dilatation of this cavity and increased amplitude of motion of the septum, findings compatible with left ventricular volume overload (Table 2–2). There is no echo evidence of an aortic vegetation, aortic insufficiency, or of rheumatic mitral thickening. The Eccentricity Index of the aortic valve is normal according to the values of both Nanda[15] and Radford,[16] and thus there is no echo evidence for a bicuspid aortic valve.
diagnosis of ruptured chordae tendineae to the anterior leaflet.

Technical Hints. The importance of scanning the entire mitral valve in order to define all the abnormalities that may be present is again illustrated by this case. Note that if only echo tracings *B* and *C* of the mitral valve had been obtained, evidence for pansystolic prolapse and the vegetation of the posterior leaflet would have been missed. It is also important to realize that different patterns of mitral regurgitation may be recorded in the same patient, and that the entire valve should be scanned to delineate all abnormalities that may be present.

Three years prior to this echo, this young man had a late systolic murmur without click that became pansystolic after amyl nitrite inhalation, documented on physical examination and on a phonocardiogram. Prolapse of the posterior mitral leaflet was also demonstrated by left ventricular cineangiography with 1–2+ mitral regurgitation. When he was seen for the present episode, his murmur had increased in intensity and had become pansystolic at rest. When blood cultures were positive for alpha-hemolytic Streptococcus, a diagnosis of bacterial endocarditis was made; he responded well to intravenous penicillin therapy.

CASE 28

This 45-year-old salesperson with the history of a murmur for over 10 years has noted dyspnea, light-headedness, and substernal pain which occasionally radiates down her left arm during exertion for the last year. Despite treatment with digitalis, nitroglycerin and increased doses of diuretics, the patient has recently become increasingly disabled. Physical examination reveals blood pressure of 120/70, elevated venous pressure, bibasalar rales, and a Grade III/VI harsh systolic ejection murmur at the base. A diagnosis of aortic stenosis and congestive heart failure is made, and an echo is ordered to evaluate the mitral valve and left atrial size prior to a planned trans-septal left heart catheterization.

MEASUREMENTS   (Echo tracings A-B)   **Time lines = 200 msec**

cf   =   D-E amplitude   =
Ao leaflet opening=   E-F slope   =
LA   =   IVS thickness   =
                                    LVPW thickness   =

QUESTIONS

1. Match the lettered echo abnormalities below (A-F) and the subsequent numbered statements (I-VII) that correlate best. More than one letter may be appropriate, and letters may be used more than once. The lettered abnormalities may or may not be present.

   (A) Asymmetric septal hypertrophy (ASH)
   (B) Systolic anterior motion (SAM) of the mitral valve
   (C) Partial midsystolic closure of the aortic valve
   (D) "B-bump" on the mitral valve
   (E) Decreased initial opening of the aortic valve
   (F) Low E-F slope of the anterior mitral leaflet

   _____   I.   Illustrated on this echo
   _____   II. The echo abnormality virtually always present at rest in this patient's disease
   _____   III. A sign on this echo of loss of left ventricular compliance
   _____   IV. May be produced by amyl nitrite inhalation
   _____   V.   Seen in valvular aortic stenosis
   _____   VI. The finding most predictive of the degree of left ventricular–aortic gradient in this patient's disease
   _____   VII. The abnormality reported to decrease following operation for this disease

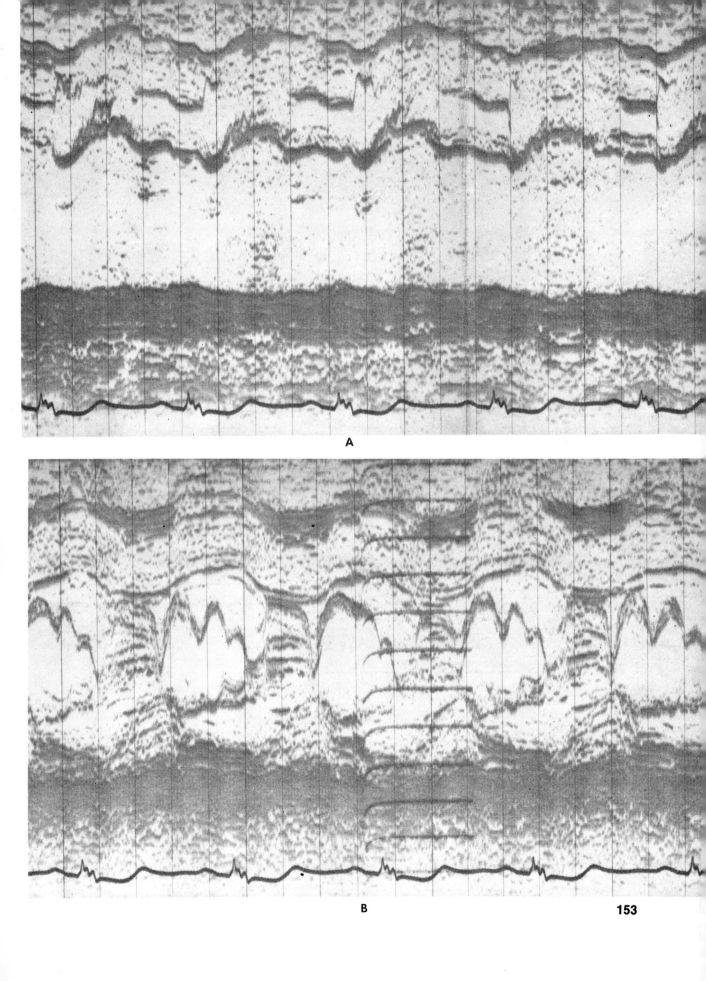

A

B

153

2. Which one of the following explanations for the patient's systolic murmur does this echo establish?

    (A) Valvular aortic stenosis
    (B) Left atrial myxoma
    (C) Discrete membranous subvalvular aortic stenosis
    (D) Hypertrophic subaortic stenosis
    (E) Valvular vegetations

3. Simultaneous cardiac catheterization in this patient would be most likely to show which of the following?

    (A) 90 mm Hg systolic gradient between the left ventricle and the aorta without change following isoproterenol infusion

    (B) 50 mm Hg systolic gradient between the left ventricle and the aorta, which increases to 100 mm Hg following amyl nitrite inhalation

    (C) No resting gradient but a 20 to 30 mm gradient between the left ventricle and aorta following a PVC, Valsalva maneuver, or amyl nitrite inhalation

    (D) No left ventricular to aortic gradient at rest or following the above maneuvers

ANSWERS TO CASE 28
Hypertrophic Subaortic Stenosis

MEASUREMENTS

cf	= 1.01	D-E amplitude	= 22 mm
Ao leaflet opening	= 1.9 cm	E-F slope	= 110 mm/sec
LA	= 4.5 cm	IVS thickness	= 21 mm
		LVPW thickness	= <10 mm

ANSWERS

1. I. (A), (B), (C), and (D). The following abnormalities are illustrated on this echo and establish the diagnosis of hypertrophic subaortic stenosis (Table 28–1):

(A) *Asymmetric septal hypertrophy* (ASH),[117-119] i.e., thickening of the interventricular septum that is disproportionate to the thickening of the left ventricular posterior wall. On this echo, the septal thickness equals 21 mm and the left ventricular posterior wall equals about 10 mm. Although a precise measurement of the left ventricular posterior wall cannot be made on the echo strip shown, the thickness of the free wall of the left ventricle is certainly not in the same range as that of the septum. From these measurements, we obtain an IVS thickness/LVPW thickness ratio equal to about 2.1. Henry, et al.,[114, 115, 123] and others[116] have found that, in all cases of hypertrophic subaortic stenosis proved at catheterization, this ratio of IVS thickness/LVPW thickness as determined by echocardiography always exceeds 1.3, regardless of whether a resting gradient is present. On the contrary, the ratio of septal thickness to left ventricular posterior wall thickness was always less than 1.3 in normal adult patients and in adult patients with congestive cardiomyopathy or

TABLE 28–1.   Hypertrophic Subaortic Stenosis

Criteria for Diagnosis:
   (1) Asymmetric septal hypertrophy (ASH)
      (a) Abnormally thickened septum (greater than 15 mm)
      (b) Disproportionate thickening of septum*

$$\frac{\text{IVS thickness}}{\text{LVPW thickness}} > 1.3$$

   (2) Systolic anterior motion of AML (SAM)

±*Associated Findings:*
   (1) Decreased systolic septal thickening (<30%) and reduced septal amplitude
   (2) Abnormal anterior position of mitral valve
   (3) Small LV cavity
   (4) Partial midsystolic closure of the aortic valve
   (5) Decreased E-F slope of the AML

*Rarely LVPW may secondarily hypertrophy, producing a ratio less than 1.3.

valvular aortic stenosis with left ventricular hypertrophy. However, a ratio of greater than 1.3 has also been described in patients with pulmonary hypertension and no evidence of hypertrophic subaortic stenosis,[120, 220] transiently in normal infants in the neonatal period,[3, 121] and in some forms of congenital heart disease such as pulmonic stenosis, tetralogy of Fallot, and ventricular septal defect.[120, 270] Thus, asymmetric septal hypertrophy is not pathognomonic of hypertrophic subaortic stenosis.[123, 124]

(B) *Systolic anterior motion* (SAM) of the mitral valve (Fig. 28–2, *closed arrow*).[125-129] Shortly after the onset of systole, the anterior mitral leaflet (C-D segment) begins to move anteriorly, bulging into the left ventricular outflow tract toward the hypertrophied septum. After reaching its peak anterior position at the beginning of the second third of systole, it remains anterior until at the beginning of the final third of systole it moves *posteriorly* to coapt with the posterior leaflet at the D point. During this anterior systolic bulging, the mitral valve may or may not contact the septum. These characteristic details of timing and motion of the anterior mitral leaflet are important in avoiding false-positive diagnoses for systolic anterior motion.

Using cross-sectional echocardiography, Henry, et al.,[130] concluded that the obstruction in hypertrophic subaortic stenosis is secondary to two factors: (1) the mitral valve being located more anteriorly within the left ventricular outflow tract at the onset of systole and (2) hydrodynamic forces that are generated in the narrowed left ventricular outflow tract and that pull the anterior leaflet forward in systole by the Venturi effect.

If a carotid pulse is recorded simultaneously with the echo, the early systolic dip seen in the pulse tracing in some patients with hypertrophic subaortic stenosis will correspond with the peak of the systolic anterior motion of the mitral valve, and the subsequent tidal wave of the carotid pulse will occur as the anterior mitral leaflet moves posteriorly in late systole.[125, 126]

(C) *Partial midsystolic closure of the aortic valve.* Shortly after an initial, normal opening, the anterior aortic leaflet is seen to close partially in midsystole[129, 131] (Fig. 28–1, *open arrow*). Usually it then reopens prior to closing completely at the end of

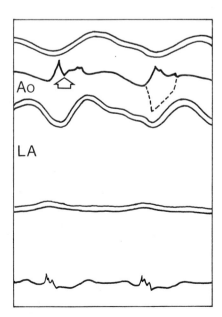

Figure 28–1 (Echo tracing *A*). Partial midsystolic closure of the aortic valve in hypertrophic subaortic stenosis (*open arrow*).

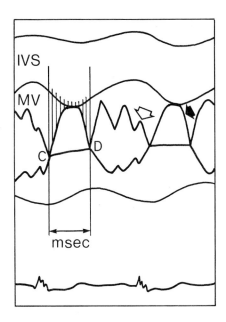

Figure 28–2 (Echo tracing *B*). Hypertrophic subaortic stenosis with systolic anterior motion of the anterior mitral leaflet (*solid arrow*) and a thickened interventricular septum. Calculation of the Obstructive Index[114] is illustrated; see text for details. A "B bump" is also present on the mitral valve (*open arrow*).

systole. This partial midsystolic aortic closing may result from an alteration in the flow dynamics of ejection in this disease rather than an actual reduction in flow secondary to obstruction.[132] A similar abnormality of partial early closure has been described in discrete subvalvular aortic stenosis, where there is apparently no sudden reduction in flow across the aortic valve.[3, 281]

(D) *"B bump" on the mitral valve.* During diastole after the atrium contracts producing the A point on the mitral valve echo, the closing motion of the anterior mitral leaflet is interrupted by a small horizontal plateau or bump before the leaflet reaches its closed position at the C point (Fig. 28–2, *open arrow*). This abnormality is called the "B bump" and is thought to be caused by a stiff or noncompliant left ventricle producing a delay in the flow of blood from the left atrium to the left ventricle late in diastole, thus interrupting the closing of the anterior mitral leaflet.[162] This sign will be discussed in subsequent cases.

II. (A) The echo abnormality virtually always present in hypertrophic subaortic stenosis is *asymmetric septal hypertrophy* (ASH), an abnormality present in both the obstructive and nonobstructive forms of the disease.[114, 116, 123] It is true that some cases of obstructive hypertrophic subaortic stenosis have been reported in which the left ventricular posterior wall is thickened to such an extent that there is loss of asymmetric septal hypertrophy—i.e., an IVS thickness/LVPW thickness ratio of less than 1.3.[120, 124] This hypertrophy of the left ventricular free wall is thought to be secondary to long-standing subaortic obstruction. In all these cases, the diagnosis of hypertrophic subaortic stenosis was still evident from the excessively thickened septum which had a reduced percentage of systolic thickening and from the prominent systolic anterior motion of the mitral valve.

Systolic anterior motion of the anterior mitral leaflet may or may not be present, depending on whether there is obstruction to flow. If systolic anterior motion is thought to be present in the absence of a thickened septum, the causes of "false-positive SAM" (discussed later) should be considered. Partial midsystolic closure of the aortic valve is an uncommon and nonspecific finding. It also may be seen in discrete subvalvular aortic stenosis, and we have observed a similar abnormality in several patients with severe mitral stenosis and low cardiac outputs.

III. (D) The "B bump" is the only sign of loss of left ventricular compliance present on this echo. Although a low E-F slope of the anterior mitral leaflet may be a sign of reduced left ventricular compliance and is commonly seen in this disease,[116, 125-127] this measurement is normal on this echo.

IV. (B) In hypertrophic subaortic stenosis, systolic anterior motion (SAM) of the mitral valve may be produced by amyl nitrite inhalation if this sign is absent, or increased if it is only minimally apparent.[125, 126, 131] Creation of this echo abnormality results from amyl nitrite's ability to decrease the volume of the left ventricle, both by lowering systemic resistance and pressure and by decreasing venous return. In this way, amyl nitrite increases the subaortic gradient and the degree of SAM. Although it has not been reported, amyl nitrite might also induce partial midsystolic closure of the aortic valve if systolic anterior motion of the mitral valve became pronounced enough to alter flow dynamics across the outflow tract.

V. (D), (E), (F) In contrast to hypertrophic subaortic stenosis, valvular aortic stenosis is associated with decreased initial opening of the aortic valve. A low E-F slope and a "B bump" of the anterior mitral leaflet also may be seen as reflections of decreased left ventricular compliance secondary to symmetric left ventricular hypertrophy.[114]

VI. (B) In hypertrophic subaortic stenosis, the systolic anterior motion of the mitral valve correlates best with the amount of left ventricular–aortic gradient measured simultaneously at cardiac catheterization.[123, 125, 126, 128] The thickness of the septum has a very poor correlation with this gradient. For example, there may be very pronounced septal thickening but, in the absence of systolic anterior motion of the mitral valve, no resting gradient will be recorded. Although partial closure of the aortic valve is more likely to be seen with severe gradients, it likewise is a poor predictor of severity.[132]

VII. (B) Ventriculoseptalmyectomy usually abolishes the resting gradient in hypertrophic subaortic stenosis and is associated with complete absence or marked improvement in the abnormal systolic motion of the mitral valve.[117, 129, 133, 134] Henry, et al., found that within minutes after myectomy, the anterior mitral leaflet assumed a more posterior position in reference to the septum and that there was disappearance of systolic anterior motion.[117, 130] They likewise reported absence of systolic anterior motion in patients with hypertrophic subaortic stenosis studied two to 11 years after myectomy. However, the degree of asymmetric septal hypertrophy or reduction in the E-F slope of the anterior mitral leaflet has been found to be unaltered within one year of this operation.[133] There are data to suggest that the thickness of the left ventricular posterior wall may decrease with time after the operation.[134]

2. (D) Hypertrophic subaortic stenosis is established by asymmetric septal hypertrophy with an IVS thickness/LVPW thickness ratio of 2.2[114-116, 123] and by the prominent systolic anterior motion (SAM) of the anterior mitral leaflet (Table 28–1).[116, 125, 126] Septal thickening, usually in excess of 15 mm, is an integral part of this diagnosis. Asymmetric septal hypertrophy or hypertrophic subaortic stenosis should *not* be diagnosed solely on the basis of an IVS thickness/LVPW thickness ratio of greater than 1.3 in the absence of septal thickening. It is possible to obtain an abnormally elevated ratio in normal individuals if a low value is obtained for the thickness of the left ventricular free wall.

3. (B) By recording the echo of the anterior mitral leaflet simultaneously with measurement of the left ventricular-aortic gradient at cardiac catheterization in patients

with hypertrophic subaortic stenosis, Henry, et al.,[114] devised a regression formula whereby this gradient could be predicted noninvasively from the echo. This prediction is based on the assumption that the magnitude of the gradient is inversely proportional to the distance between the septum and the anterior mitral leaflet during systole and directly proportional to the time during which these structures are in close proximity. These authors published the following two formulae:

(A) Obstructive Index = $\dfrac{\text{Duration of Narrowing}}{\text{Average Septal–Mitral Distance}}$

(B) Estimated Gradient = (1.8 Obstructive Index) − 35

where the duration of narrowing is measured in milliseconds, the average septal–mitral distance in millimeters, the obstructive index in milliseconds/millimeters, and the gradient in millimeters of mercury. Standard error of the estimated gradient is reported as ± 14 mm Hg.

To calculate the obstructive index, the average septal–anterior mitral leaflet distance is obtained (Fig. 28–2). The distance between the septum and anterior mitral leaflet is measured in millimeters every 30 milliseconds, beginning where the anterior mitral leaflet starts to move forward in early systole and continuing until the leaflet returns to its most posterior point in late systole. All these distances are summed and divided by the number of data points to obtain the average septal–anterior mitral leaflet distance. The duration of the narrowing is the time in milliseconds between the first and the last lines. Thus, the ratio of duration of narrowing to average septal–mitral distance is the obstructive index. The estimated left ventricular–aortic gradient in mm Hg is then obtained by using formula B. These authors[114] found a high correlation (r = 0.95) between the obstructive index and the gradient measured simultaneously at cardiac catheterization and concluded that the echo can be used to quantitate the gradient in hypertrophic subaortic stenosis. They stressed that these measurements must be made from a tracing that includes a recording of both the anterior and posterior mitral leaflets and that the tip of the mitral valve should be recorded before concluding that there is no systolic anterior motion of the mitral valve. They have stated that mild degrees of systolic anterior motion may or may not be associated with a resting gradient and that the obstructive index and estimated gradient must be calculated before an accurate gradient can be predicted.

Applying these formulae to the patient in this case (Fig. 28–2):

(A) Obstructive Index = $\dfrac{350 \text{ msec}}{87 \text{ mm/12 data points}} = 47;$

(B) Estimated Gradient = (1.8) (47) − 35 = 51 mm Hg.

Because the gradient in IHSS is not fixed and would be expected to increase with provocative measures like amyl nitrite inhalation, answer (B) becomes the most appropriate answer to this question.

Calculation of this Obstructive Index affords a useful approximation of the degree of subaortic stenosis in most patients with this disease.[114, 124-126, 135] However, two groups[124, 135] have reported a total of six patients in whom the obstructive index predicted gradients ranging from 20 to 87 mm Hg when no resting gradient was detected at cardiac catheterization done simultaneously with the echo. This discrepancy has been attributed to a variable degree of proximity between different parts of the mitral valve and the septum during systole.[124, 135] The echo with its single-plane, ice-pick view may detect a severely narrowed portion of the left ventricular outflow tract, when, in fact, most of the outflow tract is not narrowed and there is, therefore, no resting gradient.

At cardiac catheterization, this patient, who has an older brother with hypertrophic subaortic stenosis, had a peak systolic gradient between the left ventricular cavity and the subaortic valvular area of 64 mm Hg at rest. This gradient increased following amyl nitrite inhalation and premature ventricular contractions. The left ventricular cineangiogram was characteristic of hypertrophic subaortic stenosis, and the left ventricular end-diastolic pressure equaled 16 mm Hg.

CASE 29

A 23-year-old social worker is concerned because her 17-year-old brother died suddenly following a workout involving weight lifting and jogging. She has been told of a heart murmur and wants to be evaluated.

MEASUREMENTS (Echo tracings *A* and *B*)   **Time lines = 200 msec**

cf	=	Ejection fraction	=
E-F slope	=	Percentage change	=
RV	=	IVS thickness	=
EDD	=	LVPW thickness	=
ESD	=	IVS/LVPW thickness	=

QUESTIONS

1. What abnormality is shown on this echo, and which of the following disease states may be associated with this abnormality?

   (A) Aortic stenosis
   (B) Hypertrophic subaortic stenosis
   (C) Systemic hypertension
   (D) Pulmonary hypertension

2. What additional maneuver(s) should be done during the echo examination to characterize this patient's disease?

3. Which of the following resting gradients between the left ventricle and aorta would this patient most likely have at cardiac catheterization?

   (A) 100 mm Hg
   (B) 50 mm Hg
   (C) 25 mm Hg
   (D) No gradient

4. This patient recently was married and is planning a family. What would be the likelihood of her children's inheriting her abnormality?

   (A) None; not hereditary
   (B) 50%; with male:female ratio = 4:1
   (C) 50%; equal sexual distribution
   (D) 25%

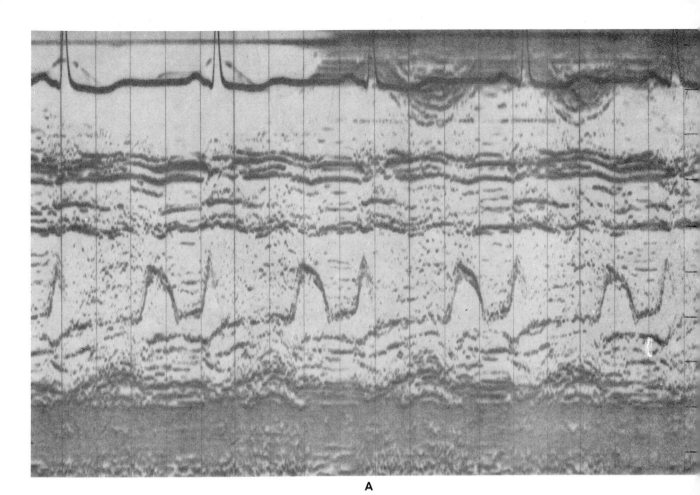

A

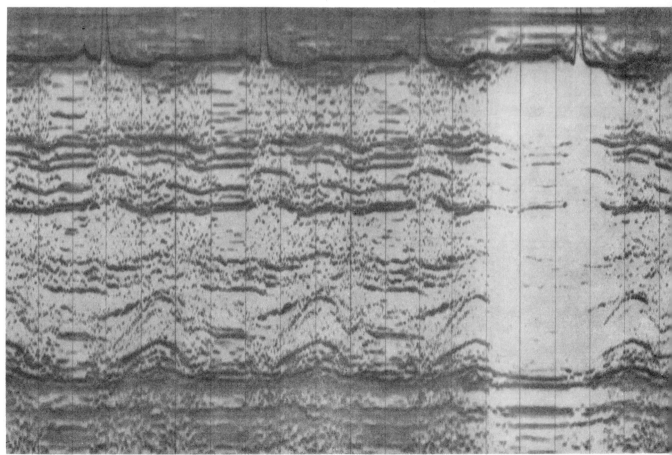

B

ANSWERS TO CASE 29
Asymmetric Septal Hypertrophy without Systolic Anterior Motion of the Mitral Valve

MEASUREMENTS

cf	= 0.83	Ejection fraction	= 71%
E-F slope	= 25 mm/sec	Percentage change	= 39%
RV	= 1.7 cm	IVS thickness	= 15 mm
EDD	= 3.1 cm	LVPW thickness	= 8 mm
ESD	= 1.9 cm	IVS/LVPW	
		thickness	= 1.9

ANSWERS

1. (B) and (D). This echocardiogram shows asymmetric septal hypertrophy (ASH)—i.e., thickening of the septum that is disproportionate to the thickening of the left ventricular posterior wall (Fig. 29–1). Both hypertrophic subaortic stenosis [114-117, 119] and pulmonary hypertension [220] could cause this abnormality, whereas aortic stenosis and systemic hypertension would be expected to cause symmetric left ventricular hypertrophy. If pulmonary hypertension is associated with this abnormality, right ventricular dilatation is also usually present.

2. When asymmetric septal hypertrophy is seen without systolic anterior motion of the mitral valve, as in this echo, or when slight systolic anterior motion of the mitral valve is seen and hypertrophic subaortic stenosis is suspected, a Valsalva maneuver and amyl nitrite inhalation should routinely be done while recording the mitral valve, concentrating especially on the C-D portion. These provocative maneuvers have been found to bring out or exaggerate systolic anterior motion of

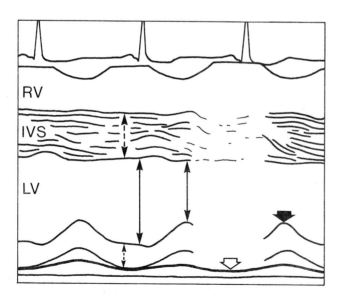

Figure 29–1 (Echo tracing *B*). Asymmetric septal hypertrophy. The maneuver of quickly decreasing the total gain to identify the left ventricular epicardium (*open arrow*) is shown. Using this maneuver, the epicardium and endocardium (*closed arrow*) of the left ventricular posterior wall can be positively identified so that an accurate measurement of the left ventricular free wall thickness can be obtained. Increasing the dampening control is an alternative method of positively identifying these structures. The proper places for measuring septal and left ventricular posterior wall thickness and the diastolic and systolic left ventricular cavity dimensions also are illustrated. Note that the left ventricular free wall is measured in mid-diastole prior to the QRS and prior to any presystolic thinning of the left ventricular posterior wall.

the mitral valve in hypertrophic subaortic stenosis, but not in other forms of symmetric left ventricular hypertrophy.[125, 126, 131] Thus, these maneuvers can be extremely useful in making a diagnosis of hypertrophic subaortic stenosis and in determining the degree of provocative gradient that may be present. In the patient shown in this case, amyl nitrite inhalation transiently produced a small amount of systolic anterior motion of the mitral valve.

3. (D) In patients with hypertrophic subaortic stenosis without systolic anterior motion (SAM) of the mitral valve at rest or after provocation, no resting or provokable gradient has been found at simultaneously performed cardiac catheterization.[116, 117, 125, 130] Those patients with asymmetric septal hypertrophy and a small amount of SAM, but with a calculated Obstructive Index indicating no significant resting gradient, have been found to have a significant gradient (greater than 30 mm Hg) only following provocation with amyl nitrite inhalation or isoproterenol infusion.[130]

4. (C) Studying first-degree relatives of 30 consecutive patients with echocardiographic and catheterization-proved hypertrophic subaortic stenosis, Henry, et al.,[120, 136] showed that 50 per cent of these relatives had an abnormally increased ratio of septal to left ventricular posterior wall thickness as determined by echo. There was equal prevalence among males and females. These findings suggest the abnormality of asymmetric septal hypertrophy (ASH) is inherited as an autosomal dominant trait. These authors noted that, on the basis of the history, physical examination, and electrocardiogram, over 20 per cent of these relatives would probably have been judged completely normal, approximately 60 per cent would have been recognized as abnormal but only in nonspecific diagnostic terms, and only 16 per cent could have been confidently diagnosed as having hypertrophic subaortic stenosis. However, because the fate of asymptomatic people with asymmetric septal hypertrophy and no provokable systolic anterior motion of the mitral valve is unknown, they should not be classified as having a disease at the present time.

CASE 30

This 44-year-old high school coach has been followed by his physician for the last 10 years, after a cardiac murmur was discovered on a multiphasic screening exam. At present, he is asymptomatic except for occasional excess dyspnea with jogging. An echocardiogram is ordered to evaluate the course of his disease.

MEASUREMENTS (Echo tracings A-C)   **Time lines = 200 msec**

cf	=	Ejection fraction	=
Ao leaflet opening	=	Percentage change	=
LA	=	IVS thickness	=
E-F slope	=	LVPW thickness	=
RV	=	IVS/LVPW ratio	=
EDD	=	Percentage systolic	
ESD	=	septal thickening	=

QUESTIONS

1. Which of the following abnormalities are present on this echocardiogram? More than one may apply.

   (A) Partial midsystolic closure of the aortic valve
   (B) Late systolic mitral prolapse
   (C) Decreased E-F slope of AML
   (D) Echo-dense mitral valve
   (E) Abnormal motion of the PML in diastole
   (F) Large RV cavity
   (G) Hypertrophy of the LVPW
   (H) Hypertrophy of the IVS
   (I) Abnormal ratio of IVS thickness/LVPW thickness
   (J) Decreased systolic septal thickening

2. Which of the following diagnoses should be made from the above observations? More than one may apply.

   (A) Rheumatic mitral disease
   (B) Late systolic prolapse
   (C) Pulmonary hypertension
   (D) Hypertrophic subaortic stenosis

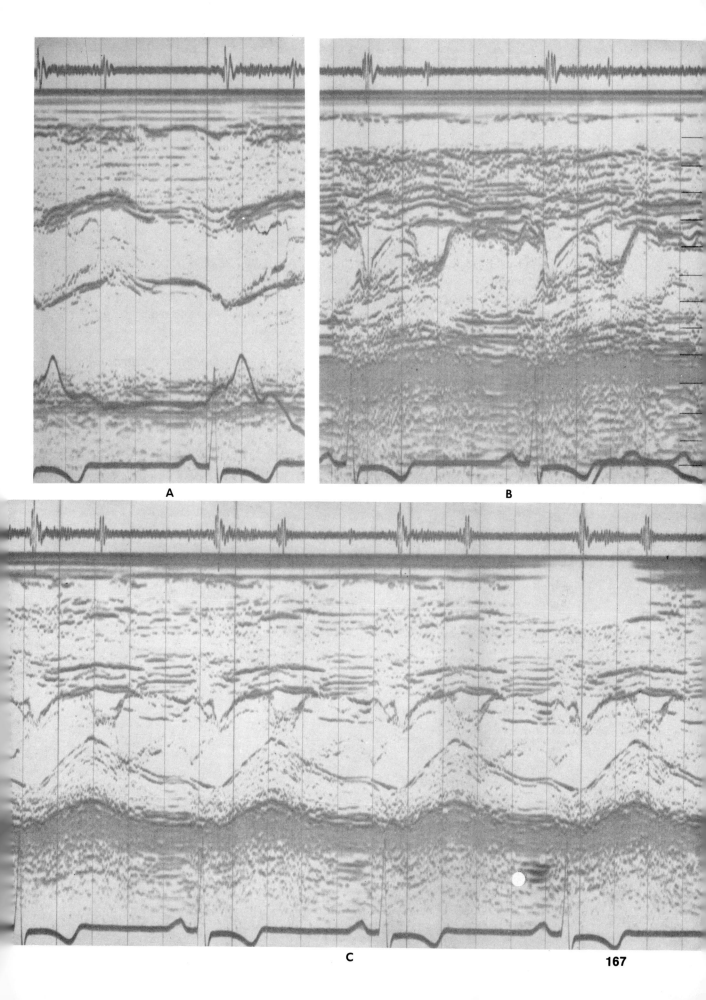

A

B

C

3. Opposite each of the following echo abnormalities found in hypertrophic subaortic stenosis, list one *other* diagnosis that may also be associated with each abnormality other than hypertrophic subaortic stenosis.

   (A) Asymmetric septal hypertrophy (ASH):
   (B) Partial closure of the aortic valve during systole:
   (C) Small LV cavity:
   (D) Systolic anterior motion of the mitral valve (SAM):

4. For each lettered statement below, indicate whether the statement is true or false. If it is true, also list one illustrative condition for which the statement is correct.

	Check One		If Statement is True, List One Illustrative Condition:
	True	*False*	
Example: A decreased E-F slope of the AML occurs without HSS	X		Mitral Stenosis
(A) HSS occurs without SAM			
(B) SAM occurs without HSS			
(C) HSS occurs without ASH			
(D) ASH occurs without HSS			

ANSWERS TO CASE 30
Hypertrophic Subaortic Stenosis

MEASUREMENTS

cf   = 1.39
Ao leaflet opening = 2.0 cm
LA   = 4.1 cm
E-F slope   = 10 mm/sec
RV   = 1.2 cm
EDD   = 3.5 cm
ESD   = 1.8 cm

Ejection fraction   = 80%
Percentage change   = 49%
IVS thickness   = 27 mm
LVPW thickness   = 14 mm
IVS/LVPW ratio   = 1.9
Percentage systolic
    septal thickening = 0–10%

ANSWERS

1. (A), (C), (G), (H), (I), (J). 2. (D).

The interventricular septum is greatly hypertrophied and has a markedly decreased amplitude of motion and percentage of systolic thickening. It thus represents the classic type of septum seen in hypertrophic subaortic stenosis.[114, 116, 120, 123, 124, 137-140] Even though asymmetric septal hypertrophy (ASH) is present with a ratio of IVS/LVPW thickness of 2.7, the left ventricular posterior free wall itself is also hypertrophied. This latter hypertrophy is thought to be secondary to long standing subaortic obstruction, in distinction to the primary myopathic process producing septal hypertrophy in this disease.[124] Continued hypertrophy of the left ventricular posterior wall could account for those cases of obstructive hypertrophic subaortic stenosis in which the septum is greatly hypertrophied, but because of hypertrophy of the left ventricular posterior wall the ratio of IVS/LVPW thickness is less than 1.3.[124] In such cases, hypertrophic subaortic stenosis occurs with symmetric left ventricular hypertrophy, although the proper diagnosis is still evident from the prominent degree of systolic anterior motion of the mitral valve.

In addition, prominent systolic anterior motion (SAM) of the mitral valve touching the septum is shown on echo tracing B.[124-129] This indicates an obstructive type of hypertrophic subaortic stenosis with a resting gradient, as calculation of the Obstructive Index and estimated gradient also suggest (Obstructive Index = 60; estimated gradient = 75 mm Hg).[114] Partial midsystolic closure of the anterior leaflet of the aortic valve, an abnormality occurring in some cases of obstructive hypertrophic subaortic stenosis, is also present (echo tracing A).[131] The E-F slope of the mitral valve is decreased, with the anterior leaflet lying against the septum throughout most of diastole. Because this diastolic slope may be reduced only because its motion is restricted by the septum, it probably is not a reliable indicator of decreased mitral flow in such cases.

Late systolic prolapse of the mitral valve is not present, as the C-D portion of the mitral valve does not move posterior to the D point in late systole (Fig. 17–2). Likewise, mitral stenosis is not present, as the mitral valve is thin and the posterior leaflet moves appropriately in diastole, as seen on echo tracing C. With a normal size right ventricle, there is no evidence for pulmonary hypertension.[220]

Cardiac catheterization in this patient substantiated the diagnosis of hypertrophic subaortic stenosis by both pressure measurements and left ventricular cineangiography ten years prior to this echo. At that time, the resting left ventricular–aortic gradient equaled 40 mm Hg with increases to 100 mm Hg with a Valsalva and 130 mm Hg post-PVC. Five years later, a repeat catheterization showed little change in this gradient that equaled 60 mm Hg at rest, 82 mm Hg with isoproterenol infusion, and 126 mm Hg post-PVC. More recently, the patient has been followed with serial echocardiograms.

3. (A) Asymmetric septal hypertrophy (ASH) may also occur in pulmonary hypertension,[120, 220] transiently in the neonatal period[3, 121] and in some forms of congenital heart disease such as pulmonic stenosis, tetralogy of Fallot, and ventricular septal defect.[3, 121]

(B) Partial systolic closure of the aortic valve is also seen in discrete membranous subaortic stenosis.[281] Usually in this type of fixed subaortic stenosis, the aortic valve partially closes abruptly in early systole almost immediately after opening and remains partially closed throughout the rest of systole. In hypertrophic subaortic stenosis, on the other hand, partial closure usually occurs in midsystole, has a more gradual posterior motion, and reopens in late systole prior to closing completely at the end of systole,[129, 131] as is illustrated on echo tracing A of this case.

(C) A small left ventricular cavity may also be seen in pulmonary hypertension with marked right ventricular dilatation,[220] in Ebstein's anomaly, and in causes of hypoplastic left heart, i.e., aortic and/or mitral atresia.[3, 289, 290]

(D) The echo pattern of systolic anterior motion of the mitral valve (SAM) may occur in the absence of hypertrophic subaortic stenosis (HSS) and has been termed "false-positive SAM" or "pseudo-SAM." This type of echo pattern can be recorded in each of the following circumstances in the absence of HSS (Table 30–1).

First, in *late systolic prolapse* the mitral valve may appear to move prominently anteriorly in early to mid-systole, because in late systole it prolapses so posteriorly (Fig. 30–1, A). This pattern is particularly evident in the presence of tachycardia. In the SAM that occurs with hypertrophic subaortic stenosis, the mitral valve does not move posterior to the D point in late systole, and consequently true systolic anterior motion of the mitral valve should not be read if there is evidence for late systolic mitral prolapse.

Second, in significant *pericardial effusion,* systolic anterior motion of the mitral valve can be observed. This disappears with relief of the effusion. Presumably, this is related to excessive motion of the heart within the effusion and merely means that in mid-systole the algebraic sum of the motion of the heart as a whole and the mitral valve is more toward the transducer than in the absence of effusion.

Third, if the *annular portion of the mitral valve* is recorded, slight degrees of exaggerated systolic anterior mitral motion often will be seen in normal individuals

TABLE 30–1. Causes of "False-Positive SAM"

1. Late systolic prolapse of mitral valve.
2. Pericardial effusion.
3. Recording the annular portion of mitral valve.
4. "Verticalization" of posterior aortic wall and the mitral valve.
5. "Verticalization" of the LVPW and the mitral valve.
6. Possible excess catecholamine stimulation.

"FALSE-POSITIVE SAM"

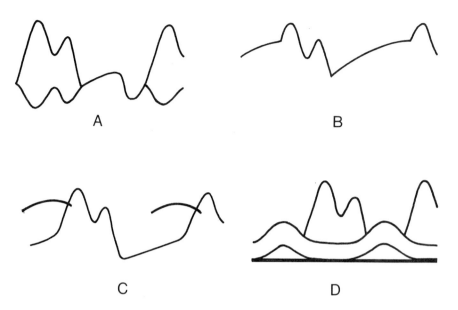

Figure 30–1. The patterns of four causes of "false-positive SAM."

   A, Late systolic prolapse.

   B, Recording the annular portion of the mitral valve.

   C, "Verticalization" of the posterior aortic wall and mitral valve.

   D, "Verticalization" of the LVPW and the mitral valve.

(Fig. 30–1, *B*). This results because the normal motion of the mitral annulus and the posterior aortic wall is anterior in systole. Prominent anterior motion can thus be recorded through this annular part of the mitral valve. In addition, the mitral valve and the posterior aortic wall may be detected with different parts of the echo beam and recorded superimposed on each other so that the mitral valve again appears to have prominent anterior systolic motion, which in reality is the superimposed posterior aortic wall (Fig. 30–1, *C* and Fig. 30–2). This occurs because of problems with lateral resolution of the echo beam and because the echo machine electronically "verticalizes" all images—i.e., it displays all echoes seen within the beam as if they were in a straight line (see Case 17). A highly reflective surface like the aortic wall is more likely to be recorded from the lateral edge of an echo beam than a less echo-dense structure. Again, this type of "false-positive SAM" is more likely to occur if the mitral valve is recorded near its base.

Also, there is no doubt that systolic anterior motion of the mitral valve may rarely be seen in *normal individuals,* even with proper transducer position, under certain circumstances. It has been theorized that this may result from strong catecholamine stimulation even in the normal heart.[141] In these cases the prominent anterior motion of the lateral ventricular posterior wall during systole may be "verticalized" with the mitral valve to produce the false impression of systolic anterior motion of the mitral valve (Fig. 30–1, *D*).

"False-positive SAM" secondary to recording the annular portion of the mitral valve can be distinguished from SAM occurring with hypertrophic subaortic stenosis in two ways. First, in "false-positive SAM," the mitral valve does not move posterior to the D point in the latter one-third of systole as it does in systolic anterior motion seen with hypertrophic subaortic stenosis, but rather remains anterior throughout systole until the anterior leaflet opens in diastole (Fig. 30–1). In cases where the mitral valve and aortic wall are recorded superimposed, the aortic wall echo often will move just past the opening of the anterior leaflet into diastole (Fig. 30–1, *C*). These differences in timing and motion are important in distinguishing "false-positive

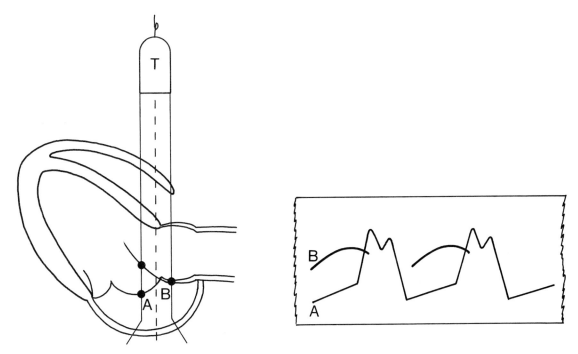

Figure 30–2.   Ilustration of how the mitral valve (A) and the posterior aortic wall (B) can be detected by different parts of the echo beam, verticalized, and displayed on the echo tracing superimposed to create a pattern of "false-positive SAM."

SAM" from the true systolic anterior motion seen with hypertrophic subaortic stenosis. Second, scanning distally on the mitral valve away from its annular portion causes this type of "false-positive SAM" to disappear, whereas the systolic anterior motion seen with hypertrophic subaortic stenosis increases in magnitude with this maneuver. To insure that the annular portion of the mitral valve is not being recorded, the maximally obtainable mitral amplitude and simultaneous recording of the anterior and posterior mitral leaflets should be sought with this scan.

4. All the lettered statements are true.

(A) HSS may occur without SAM in nonobstructive hypertrophic subaortic stenosis.[116]

(B) SAM may occur without HSS in all the conditions producing "false-positive SAM" discussed in the answer above, i.e., late systolic mitral prolapse, pericardial effusion, aiming across the annular portion of the mitral valve, and in normal individuals under certain circumstances, even with proper transducer position (Table 30–1).

(C) HSS may occur without ASH in those advanced cases of obstructive hypertrophic subaortic stenosis in which the left ventricular free wall hypertrophies to such an extent that asymmetric septal hypertrophy is abolished as concentric left ventricular hypertrophy develops.[124]

(D) ASH may occur without HSS in pulmonary hypertension,[120, 220] transiently in the neonatal period,[3, 121] in pulmonic stenosis, tetralogy of Fallot, and ventricular septal defect.[122, 270]

CASE 31

This 65-year-old housewife with severe deforming rheumatoid arthritis is admitted for an operation on her hands. After the history of exertional chest discomfort and palpitations is elicited and a harsh systolic ejection murmur heard, a cardiologist is consulted. He orders an echocardiogram to confirm his impression of aortic stenosis.

MEASUREMENTS   (Echo tracings A-C)   **Time lines = 200 msec**

cf	=	Percentage change	=
LA	=	IVS thickness	=
E-F slope	=	LVPW thickness	=
RV	=	IVS/LVPW thickness	=
EDD	=	Percentage of systolic septal thickening	=
ESD	=	Obstructive Index	=
Ejection fraction	=	Estimated systolic gradient	=

QUESTIONS

1. What maneuver is illustrated in echo tracing C, and what does it reveal?

2. Does the echo of this patient's interventricular septum support the statement that left ventricular function in hypertrophic subaortic stenosis is hyperdynamic?

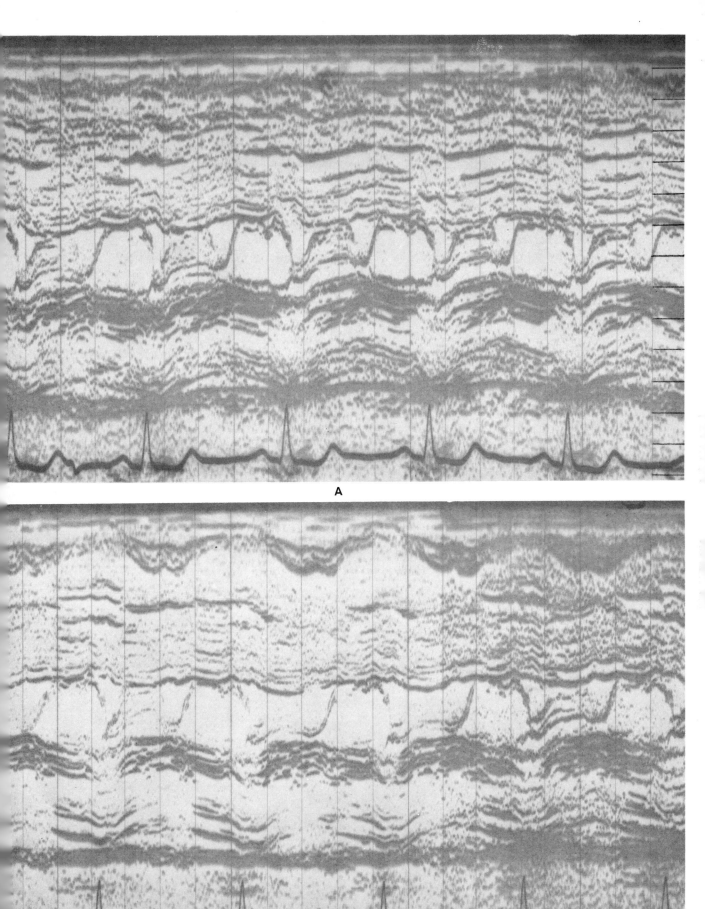

A

B

175

Figure 31 C appears on the opposite page.

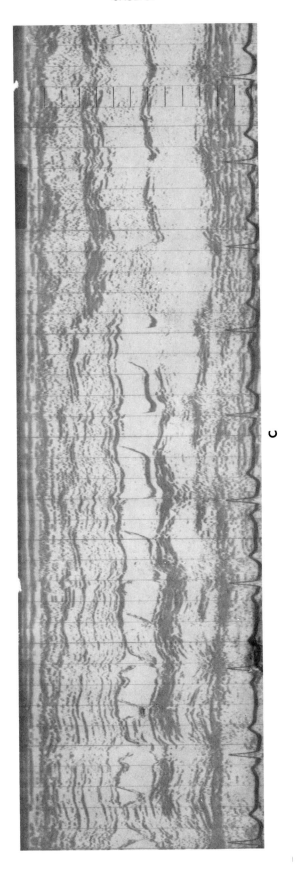

C

ANSWERS TO CASE 31
Hypertrophic Subaortic Stenosis

MEASUREMENTS

cf (echo *A* and *B*)	= 1.20	Percentage change	= 19%
cf (echo *C*)	= 2.15	IVS thickness	= 24 mm
LA	= 3.9 cm	LVPW thickness	= 12 mm
E-F slope	= 3 mm/sec	IVS/LVPW	
RV	= 1.9 cm	thickness	= 2.0
		Percentage of sys-	
EDD	= 4.7 cm	tolic septal thick-	
		ening	= 0–5%
		Obstructive Index	= 78–93
ESD	= 3.8 cm	Estimated systolic	
Ejection fraction	= 36%	gradient	= 100–130 mm Hg

ANSWERS

1. The result of suddenly changing the damping control while recording the mitral valve is shown in echo tracing *B* and Figure 31–1. Notice that, although the mitral valve echo fades while the damping control is at a higher setting, the previously obscured right ventricular side of the septum and, indeed, the epicardium and endocardium of the left ventricular free wall become more obvious. Such a maneuver is often helpful in hypertrophic subaortic stenosis, especially

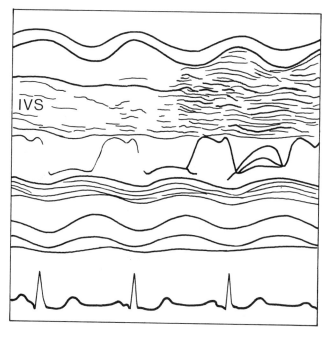

Figure 31–1 (Echo tracing *B*). Hypertrophic subaortic stenosis. Note that at the higher damping control, the right ventricular side of the septum is clear, whereas with a lower damping setting this surface is obscured.

when the anterior septal wall is difficult to define. Decreasing the gain is an alternative maneuver to aid in positively identifying these surfaces.

2. No, the echo of this interventricular septum does not support hyperdynamic left ventricular function. As several groups have shown,[137, 138, 140] the percentage of systolic thickening of the septum in hypertrophic subaortic stenosis, as well as mean velocity of septal motion, is significantly diminished in comparison with normals (Table 29–1). Rossen, et al.,[137] found that in patients with hypertrophic subaortic stenosis, the percentage of systolic septal thickening was always less than 30 per cent, whereas in normals and patients with concentric left ventricular hypertrophy this calculation always exceeded 30 per cent. Cohen[140] made similar observations, but also reported that the left ventricular free wall in hypertrophic subaortic stenosis exhibited increased mean velocity of motion in comparison with normals. All these observations remained statistically significant when normalized for left ventricular cavity size.

Technical Hints. For recording patients with hypertrophic subaortic stenosis:
(1) Positively identify the right ventricular side of the septum by using multiple settings of the damping control and multiple adjustments of the near and total gain. This identification, as well as positive identification of the epicardium and endocardium of the left ventricular free wall, is crucial to the proper detection of asymmetric septal hypertrophy (ASH).
(2) Avoid identifying a right ventricular trabecula or part of the tricuspid valve as the right ventricular side of the septum. This differentiation usually can be made, because right ventricular trabecula and tricuspid chordae tendineae usually have a motion slightly different from that of the septum, whereas the true septal endocardium parallels the motion of the rest of the septum. However, it is sometimes impossible to be absolutely sure of the right ventricular side of the septum, even though the septum is obviously thickened greatly out of proportion to the left ventricular free wall.

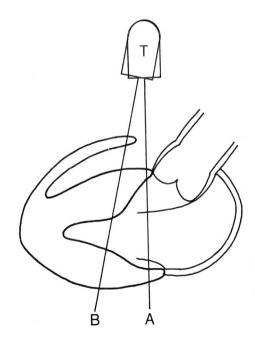

Figure 31–2. Hypertrophic subaortic stenosis. Proper transducer positions for recording the left ventricular posterior wall (Position *A*) and the interventricular septum (Position *B*) for the detection of asymmetric septal hypertrophy (*ASH*). In Position *A*, the posterior mitral leaflet should be visible; in Position *B*, the mitral valve should not be visible.

(3) Record the septal and left ventricular posterior wall thickness in the proper places (Fig. 31–2). Henry[120] has pointed out that because the septum in hypertrophic subaortic stenosis is thicker in its mid-portion than more superiorly, the entire septum should be scanned and the thickest portion recorded for calculation of the ratio of septal to left ventricular posterior wall thickness. Citing studies in normals, he has stated that different angles of the transducer will not spuriously change septal thickness by more than 2 mm. This thickest portion of the septum will be found just inferior to the anterior mitral leaflet. Therefore, to detect asymmetric septal hypertrophy (ASH), the septum should be recorded at B in Figure 31–2 without anterior leaflet in view. On the other hand, Henry's group states that the proper place to record the left ventricular free wall for calculation of septal/LVPW thickness ratio is behind the posterior mitral leaflet at A in Figure 31–2, where the left ventricular free wall is thinnest. Such careful attention to the angle of the transducer is more important in patients with equivocal or borderline findings for hypertrophic subaortic stenosis than in cases where the diagnosis is obvious. As was previously stated, septal and left ventricular posterior wall thicknesses are measured in mid-diastole before presystolic thinning occurs.

(4) Record the mitral valve distally with both the anterior and posterior leaflets in view, away from the annular portion of the mitral valve, in order to detect the presence and the maximal degree of systolic anterior motion (SAM). This is well illustrated on echo tracing C in this case, where on M-mode scan from the mitral valve to the aortic valve SAM is not seen proximally on the mitral valve but is very obvious more distally, where it indeed touches the septum. This type of scan is also useful in avoiding those causes of "false-positive SAM" that result from recording

the mitral valve near its annular portion, as was discussed in Case 30. This type of "false-positive SAM" diminishes as the scan moves distally on the mitral valve, whereas SAM seen with hypertrophic subaortic stenosis increases and becomes more obvious.

(5) Use the provocative maneuvers of amyl nitrite inhalation and Valsalva while recording the C-D portion of the mitral valve in order to exaggerate equivocal degrees of SAM and to detect those patients who only have gradients with provocation.

Clinical Applications. Echocardiography's primary use in hypertrophic subaortic stenosis is in diagnosis, especially in patients in whom the diagnosis of valvular aortic stenosis or mitral regurgitation is clinically suspected. It is not uncommon for hypertrophic subaortic stenosis to masquerade clinically as valvular aortic stenosis or as mitral regurgitation only to be detected in the echo laboratory. However, it should be remembered that valvular aortic stenosis and hypertrophic subaortic stenosis may coexist in the same patient, and, indeed, their combined detection by echo has been described.[139, 142, 143]

In patients whose symptoms are not severe enough to require surgery, an echocardiogram that unequivocally shows hypertrophic subaortic stenosis may make immediate cardiac catheterization unnecessary.

Echocardiography also can be used in hypertrophic subaortic stenosis to separate patients into an obstructive group at rest or after provocation or into a nonobstructive category.[116, 118] It is the author's opinion that the Obstructive Index and calculated estimated gradient usually provide a reasonable, although rough, estimate of the gradient across the left ventricular outflow tract but should not be taken as an exact mm Hg prediction.

CASE 32

This 63-year-old college professor with slowly progressive congestive heart failure has had to retire prematurely because of dyspnea, weakness, and fatigue. Orthopnea and nocturnal dyspnea recently have been relieved by furosemide, 40 mg daily. The patient is normotensive, has no history of chest pain, rheumatic fever, or alcoholism. Marked cardiomegaly is present on x-ray. An echocardiogram is ordered to help delineate the etiology of an apical systolic murmur, present at least for five years.

MEASUREMENTS (Echo tracings A-C)   Time lines = 200 msec

cf	=	RV	=	
Ao	=	IVS amplitude	=	
Ao valve opening	=	LVPW amplitude	=	
LA	=	EDD	=	
Ao amplitude	=	ESD	=	
C-E amplitude	=	Ejection fraction	=	
D-E amplitude	=	Percentage change	=	
E-F slope	=	Ejection time	=	
		VCF	=	

QUESTIONS

1. What etiology of this patient's systolic murmur does the echo suggest?

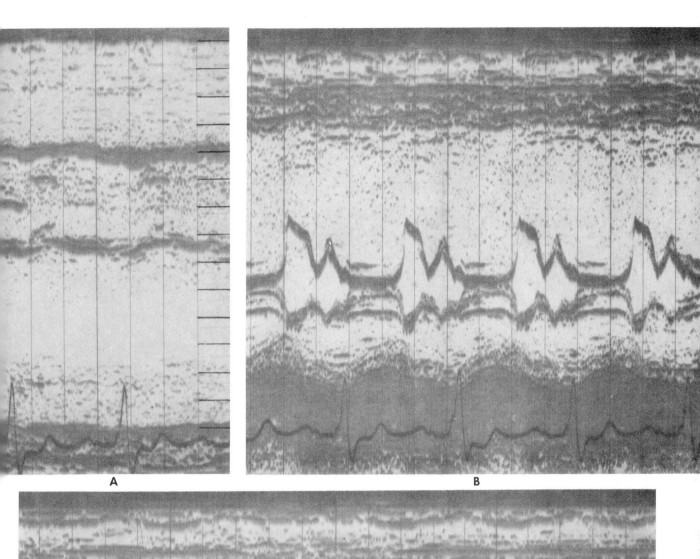

A

B

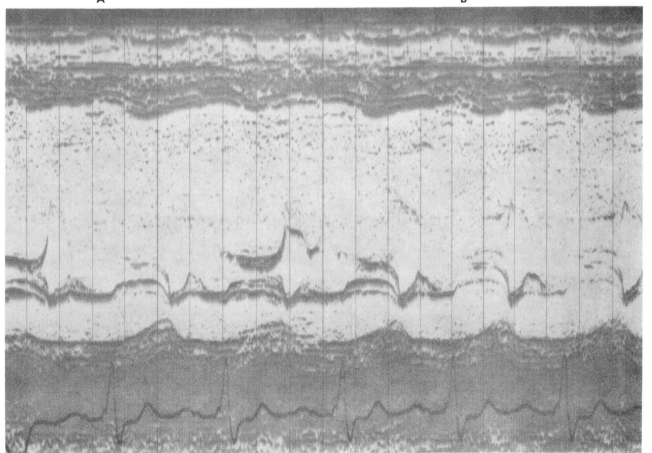

C

183

2. Complete the following measurements from the echo tracings. Then match each echo observation (A-G) with the hemodynamic condition (1-3) with which it is typically associated. More than one echo observation may be appropriate for each hemodynamic condition, and the observations may be used more than once.

Echo Observations:

(A) Ao amplitude   =
(B) E-F slope   =
(C) "B-bump"
(D) "Double-diamond" mitral
     valve

(E) Ejection fraction   =
(F) Percentage change =
(G) VCF   =

Hemodynamic Conditions:

	Typical echo observations in the hemodynamic conditions to the left.
(1) Decreased LV compliance; increased left ventricular end diastolic pressure	
(2) Low cardiac output	
(3) Mitral regurgitation	

3. From the standpoint of the echo, which statement best describes the role of mitral replacement in this patient's management?

    (A) Low risk operation with excellent chance of symptomatic relief
    (B) High risk operation with excellent chance of symptomatic relief
    (C) Moderate risk operation with moderate hope of benefit
    (D) High risk operation with little hope of symptomatic improvement

ANSWERS TO CASE 32
Left Ventricular Dilatation and Dysfunction
"Double-diamond" Mitral Valve
"B-bump"

MEASUREMENTS

cf	= 1.37	RV	= 1.0 cm
Ao	= 34 mm	IVS amplitude	= 4 mm
Ao valve opening	= 1.7 cm	LVPW amplitude	= 7 mm
LA	= 6.7 cm	EDD	= 8.6 cm
Ao amplitude	= 1–3 mm	ESD	= 7.5 cm
C-E amplitude	= 26 mm	Ejection fraction	= 26%
D-E amplitude	= 25 mm	Percentage change	= 13%
E-F slope	= 50 mm/sec	Ejection time	= 290 msec
		VCF	= 0.45 circ/sec

ANSWERS

1. On echo tracing *B*, the mitral valve echo is abnormal and consists of a "double-diamond" configuration seen within a significantly dilated and poorly functioning left ventricle (Fig. 32–1). This type of "double-diamond" pattern of the mitral valve[70] may be seen in patients with diffuse coronary or noncoronary cardiac disease who have significant left ventricular dilatation and dysfunction. It is commonly associated with mitral regurgitation thought to be secondary to left ventricular dilatation and dysfunction, i.e., so-called "papillary muscle dysfunction." However, it may be seen in patients with dilated left ventricles who have no evidence of mitral regurgitation, and, thus, this "double-diamond" pattern primarily reflects impaired left ventricular function rather than mitral regurgitation per se.

TABLE 32–1. Echocardiographic Measurements in Patients with Left Ventricular Dilatation and Dysfunction, and a "Double-Diamond" Pattern of the Mitral Valve

	Normals		"Double-Diamond" Mitral Valve n = 18	
	Range	Mean	Range	Mean
C-E amplitude (mm)	23–32	28	18–30	23
C-D amplitude (mm)	5–11	7	0–2	0.6
E-IVS distance (mm)	0–5	3	10–28	21
IVS amplitude (mm)	4–8	6.6	0–5	2
EDD (cm)	3.8–5.5	4.8	6.3–8.8	7.1
Ejection fraction (%)	53–77	66	19–44	25
Percentage change (%)	24–46	36	11–20	15
D-E slope (mm/sec)	240–380	300	275–800	512
E-F slope (mm/sec)	80–150	100	55–285	134

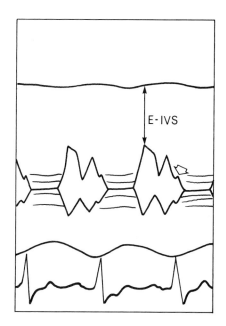

Figure 32–1 (Echo tracing *B*). "Double-diamond" pattern of the mitral valve seen in left ventricular dilatation and dysfunction. The increased distance between the *E* point of the anterior leaflet and the septum (*E − IVS*), a typical finding in this pattern, is indicated. In this patient the *E − IVS* distance = 32 mm. A "B-bump" during mitral closing is also shown (*open arrow*).

When Burgess, et al.,[70] first described this "double-diamond" pattern in patients with papillary muscle and left ventricular dysfunction, they found that it consists of the following characteristics of both the mitral valve and the left ventricle (Table 32–1).

(1) A reduced overall mobility of the mitral valve with a reduced and usually horizontal C-D portion and with a D-E amplitude of the anterior leaflet that is usually reduced or at the lower limits of normal.

(2) A distinct "double-diamond" configuration of the mitral valve in which, because of reduced mitral mobility, the anterior and posterior mitral leaflets have amplitudes of motion that are almost equal (Fig. 32–1). This pattern is in sharp distinction to the normal mitral valve, in which the amplitude of the posterior leaflet is much less than that of the anterior leaflet and the mitral valve thus does not resemble a true diamond.

(3) An increased distance between the E points of the anterior leaflet and the interventricular septum (E-IVS distance) (Fig. 32–1).

(4) A dilated left ventricular cavity with both an increased end-diastolic diameter and increased end-systolic diameter.

(5) Reduced left ventricular ejection fraction and percentage change of the minor diameter.

(6) Reduced amplitude of motion of the septum, which occasionally has a passive, paradoxically timed motion.

In addition, the mean E-F and D-E slopes and the mean left atrial dimension were higher in patients with this "double-diamond" mitral valve than in normals. It should be emphasized that increased distance between the E point of the anterior leaflet and septum and a dilated, poorly functioning left ventricle are *essential* parts of this pattern of a "double-diamond" mitral valve. This mitral valve configuration should not be read unless it occurs within such a left ventricle and represents only one of the abnormal mitral valve patterns seen in patients with left ventricular dilatation and dysfunction.

Two primary theories exist to explain the mitral regurgitation seen with severe left ventricular dilatation—i.e., so-called "papillary muscle dysfunction." According to one theory, when the papillary muscles are diseased by fibrosis, ischemia, or infarction, they no longer contract properly to prevent prolapse of the mitral valve during systole. However, no echo evidence of mitral valve prolapse is evident in this type of mitral regurgitation.[70] The multiple systolic lines often seen in this echo pattern do not meet the criteria for mitral prolapse and probably represent the echo beam traversing the malpositioned chordae tendineae or the mitral leaflets at different places. On the other hand, the dominant echo findings in these patients are an enlarged left ventricular cavity and reduced over-all mobility of the mitral valve (low C-E amplitude and horizontal C-D portion), with both leaflets having a "double-diamond" configuration. Such findings are in concert with an alternative mechanism of abnormal position and anchoring of the papillary muscle, producing mitral regurgitation in these patients. Normally, the papillary muscles arise near the apex of the left ventricle and exert a vertical pull on the chordae tendineae during systole. When the papillary muscles are displaced basely, as in a dilated left ventricle, the pull of the chordal–papillary apparatus on the mitral leaflet is in a more oblique and lateral direction. Such an abnormal tethering of the mitral leaflet by the malpositioned papillary muscles could account for the subnormal mitral valve mobility and flat C-D portion and could potentially cause imperfect mitral coaptation, with resultant mitral regurgitation. Undoubtedly, the low cardiac output in these patients with significant left ventricular dysfunction also contributes to the decreased over-all mitral motion and the flat C-D portion of the mitral valve.

2. (1) (B) and (C). Both a reduced initial diastolic slope (E-F) and "B-bump" on the A-C portion of the anterior leaflet[162, 163] may be seen in patients with an elevated left ventricular end-diastolic pressure and loss of left ventricular compliance. As previously discussed in Case 28 these hemodynamic conditions can prolong the flow of blood from the left atrium to the left ventricle that occurs both with the initial rapid filling wave and after atrial systole. Consequently, there may be a reduction in the mitral E-F slope and a delay or small plateau of the anterior leaflet as it closes at the end of diastole. Both of these abnormalities are seen on echo tracing *B* of this case (Fig. 32–1). In fact, the "B-bump" is seen on both the anterior and posterior mitral leaflets. The presence of first degree heart block in this patient prevents proper interpretation of the interval between the A point of the anterior leaflet and when the mitral valve closes (C point). Although these two abnormalities do not always occur in patients with compromised left ventricular function, the "B-bump" has been reported to occur more often in those patients with left ventricular dysfunction and loss of left ventricular compliance who had an elevated left atrial pressure and a large A wave of the left ventricular diastolic pressure trace.[162, 164]

(2) (A), (B), (D), (E), (F), and (G). Calculation of the ejection fraction, percentage change of the minor diameter, and VCF reveals significant reduction in all these parameters of left ventricular function and are the typical observations seen in patients with low cardiac output. The "double-diamond" pattern of the mitral valve would be expected if there was also significant left ventricular dilatation, as in this patient. Because of low cardiac output and reduced flow, the E-F slope of the mitral valve and the amplitude of aortic root motion also may be reduced.

(3) (D). The only echo observation above that is typical of mitral regurgitation is the "double-diamond" configuration of the mitral valve.[70] As discussed, this is the pattern of the nonrheumatic type of mitral regurgitation occurring in some patients with left ventricular dilatation and dysfunction. However, it should be emphasized

that this pattern may also occur in patients with left ventricular dilatation and no evidence of mitral regurgitation; it therefore does not necessarily imply mitral regurgitation.

3. (D). In this patient with no clinical evidence of coronary artery disease, marked left ventricular cavity dilatation and significantly compromised ejection fraction, percentage change of the minor diameter, and VCF indicate that he has very poor myocardial function.[151-154, 156-158, 165] Even if the mitral regurgitation were corrected surgically, this myocardial dysfunction would remain and would significantly limit the chances of improving the patient's congestive heart failure.

CASE 33

This 43-year-old, hard-working advertising executive with a history of several myocardial infarctions underwent a quadruple aorto-coronary bypass operation one year ago. Although he recovered well from the surgery, within the last six months progressive symptoms of dyspnea on exertion and at rest have occurred despite increasing doses of diuretics. Mild exertional angina has also returned. On physical examination, the venous pressure is elevated, bibasalar rales are present in the lungs and a grade III/VI systolic murmur with an S3 gallop is noted along the left sternal border and at the apex. An echocardiogram is ordered to evaluate this patient's left ventricular function.

MEASUREMENTS (Echo tracings *A-E*)   **Time lines = 200 msec**

cf	=	EDD	=
Ao	=	ESD	=
Ao valve opening	=	Ejection fraction	=
Ao amplitude	=	Percentage change	=
LA	=	IVS amplitude	=
C-E amplitude	=	IVS thickness	=
D-E amplitude	=	LVPW amplitude	=
E-F slope	=	LVPW thickness	=
RV	=		

QUESTIONS

1. Which of the following observations are present on this echo?

   (A) Echo-dense aortic root
   (B) Decreased opening of the aortic valve
   (C) Left atrial enlargement
   (D) Anatomic aortic-mitral discontinuity
   (E) Multiple mitral valve echoes in systole
   (F) "Double-diamond" mitral valve
   (G) RV enlargement and abnormally timed IVS motion
   (H) LV cavity dilatation and dysfunction

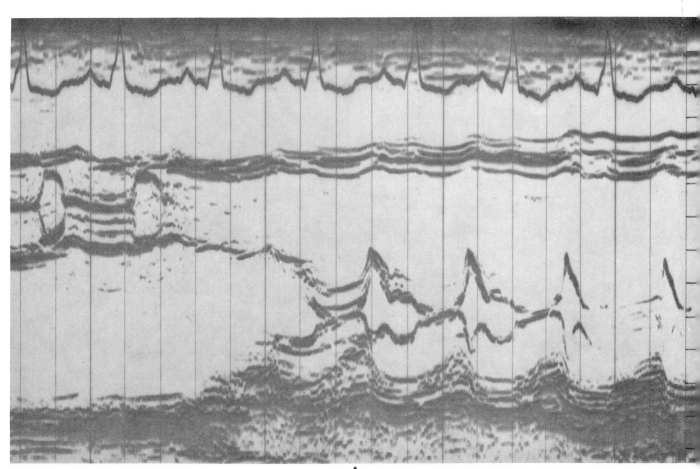

A

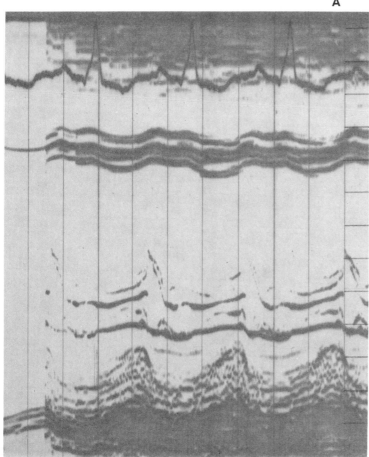

B

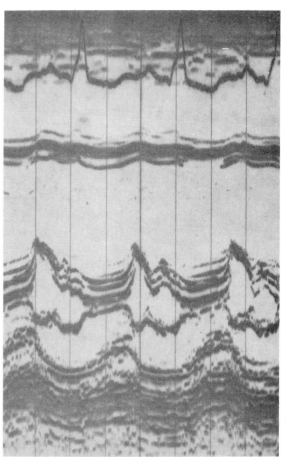

C

2. What etiology of this patient's murmur do these observations suggest?

   (A) Aortic stenosis
   (B) Mitral prolapse
   (C) Tricuspid regurgitation
   (D) Mitral regurgitation
   (E) Pulmonic insufficiency
   (F) Congenital heart disease

3. What observations and measurements of this mitral valve echo are consistent with left ventricular dysfunction?

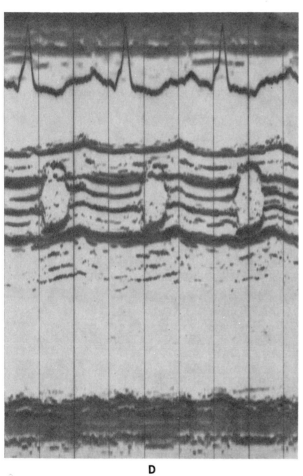

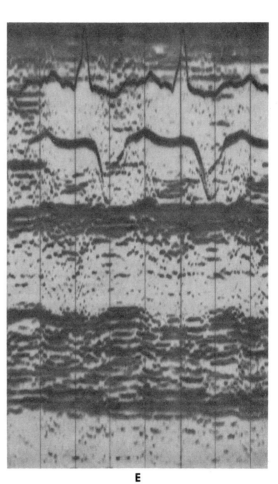

D   E

ANSWERS TO CASE 33
Left Ventricular Dilatation and Dysfunction
"Double-Diamond" Mitral Valve
Abnormal PR-AC Interval

MEASUREMENTS

cf	= 1.14	EDD	= 6.6 cm
Ao	= 26 mm	ESD	= 5.4 cm
Ao valve opening	= 1.6 cm	Ejection fraction	− 37%
Ao amplitude	= 2	Percentage change	= 18%
LA	= 5.2 cm	IVS amplitude	= 3 mm
C-E amplitude	= 20 mm	IVS thickness	= 10 mm
D-E amplitude	= 18 mm	LVPW amplitude	= 11 mm
E-F slope	= 80–90 mm/sec	LVPW thickness	= 10 mm
RV	= 1.7 cm	PR-AC interval	= 0.02–0.04 sec

ANSWERS

1. (A), (C), (E), (F), and (H)
2. (E)

The mitral valve echo fulfills the characteristics of a "double-diamond" mitral valve as discussed in Case 32 (Table 32–1).[70] There is reduced over-all mitral mobility, with a decreased C-D amplitude. The D-E amplitudes of the posterior and anterior leaflets are closer in magnitude than normal. The resulting "double-diamond" configuration of the mitral valve is present within a dilated left ventricular cavity in which the distance between the E-point of the anterior leaflet and the interventricular septum is increased (24 mm) and in which the ejection fraction and percentage change of the minor diameter are decreased. This pattern of the mitral valve may be associated with the type of mitral regurgitation that occurs as a result of left ventricular dilatation and dysfunction. In this patient, its presence suggests mitral regurgitation as the etiology of his systolic murmur.

Although multiple mitral echoes are seen during systole and are common in this type of mitral pattern, they do not fulfill the criteria for mitral valve prolapse. The aortic root is echo dense, but, because the aortic cusps open normally, aortic stenosis is not suggested. This aortic root echo is an excellent example of why aortic stenosis is not read solely on the basis of increased echo densities in the absence of aortic cusps that clearly show decreased opening. No gradient was present across this patient's aortic valve at cardiac catheterization. Right ventricular volume overload, i.e., tricuspid regurgitation and pulmonic insufficiency, is not suggested because the right ventricle is not dilated and the septal motion is not abnormally timed. Likewise, congenital heart disease is not suggested by this echo. The anterior mitral leaflet is displaced considerably, more posteriorly away from the transducer than is the posterior aortic wall, although the echoes of these two structures apparently merge with each other. Such posterior displacement does not necessarily imply true anatomic discontinuity, and in this case merely means that with left ventricular dilatation the mitral valve is displaced posteriorly so that it is a greater distance from the transducer than is the posterior aortic wall. The different causes of displacement of

TABLE 33–1. Patterns of the Mitral Valve in Left Ventricular Dysfunction

1. "Double-diamond" pattern (Cases 32,33).
2. Reduced E-F slope.
3. "B-bump" (Cases 28,32 and 33).
4. Abnormal PR-AC interval (Case 33).
5. Large A (Fig. 33–2).
6. Early mitral closure (Case 2).

the aortic walls, septum, and mitral valve as recorded by the echo and the relation of these patterns to true anatomic discontinuity and to the transducer position will be discussed in a subsequent case.

3. Several patterns of the mitral valve have been observed in patients with left ventricular dysfunction (Table 33–1). In this patient, the "double-diamond" configuration of the mitral valve with increased distance between the E point of the anterior leaflet and the septum (24 mm) implies left ventricular dysfunction.[70]

In addition, the calculated PR-AC interval, a measurement of mitral closure reported to reflect left ventricular dysfunction, is abnormally low (Fig. 33–1).[164] Konecke, et al.,[162] reported the essentially empirical observation that patients with both elevated left ventricular end-diastolic pressures of 20 mm Hg or greater and an amplitude of the atrial component of the left ventricular diastolic pressure of greater than 8 mm Hg had a prolonged A to C interval of the mitral valve echo. However, because increased atrioventricular conduction time will produce a similar effect, this A-C interval must be related to the PR interval (Table 33–2). In all 14 of their patients with the above two hemodynamic conditions, the PR-AC interval was less than 0.06 sec. In 19 other patients with a normal end-diastolic pressure or with an atrial component of the left ventricular diastolic pressure of less than 8 mm Hg, the PR-AC interval was greater than 0.06 sec. In patients with PR intervals of less than 0.14 sec, the normal PR-AC interval is reported to be greater than 0.05 sec.[166] Currently, the normal value of the PR-AC interval in patients with first degree heart block is unknown. To explain this observation of a prolonged PR-AC interval, Konecke, et al.,[162] postulated that in patients with reduced left ventricular compliance the left ventricular end-diastolic pressure exceeds the left atrial pressure earlier than normal. As a result, the mitral valve begins to close earlier and the A-C interval is prolonged. If there is sufficiently impaired left ventricular function, it may also take longer to generate enough left ventricular pressure to overcome the elevated left atrial pressure. Consequently, mitral valve closure may be delayed. Both an earlier A point and a delayed C point apparently contribute to the increased A-C interval. Mitral valve closure may be interrupted by a plateau or "B-bump" on the mitral echogram.

TABLE 33–2. Normal Values of PR-AC Intervals[162,166]

	PR-AC
PR = 0.14 − 0.20	> 0.06 sec
PR < 0.14	> 0.05 sec
PR > 0.20	???

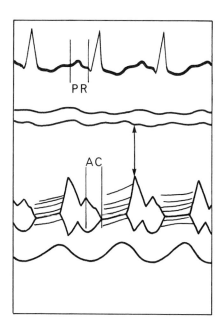

Figure 33–1 (Echo tracing C). Abnormal PR-AC interval, a pattern of the mitral valve in left ventricular dysfunction. The proper place of measuring these intervals is illustrated. The mitral valve also has a "double-diamond" pattern, with an increased distance between its *E* point and the septum (*double-headed arrow*).

Feigenbaum has stressed that an abnormal PR-AC interval must be measured to be reliably detected and that one should take care not to mistake a "B-bump" or closing plateau for the A point of the anterior mitral leaflet.[166] His group has found that an abnormal PR-AC interval, i.e., a prolonged A-C interval, is more sensitive than the "B-bump" in detecting left ventricular dysfunction.

Although not present in this patient, another pattern of the mitral valve that may be seen in patients with left ventricular dysfunction is a large A point greatly exceeding the E point, as is shown in three other patients in Fig. 33–2.[162] This pattern of a large A usually is associated with a reduced D-E slope of less than 240 mm/sec. Although the cause of this pattern is not completely understood, it may be related to a high initial left ventricular diastolic pressure in which the rate of filling of the left ventricle is reduced (low D-E slope) and a larger percentage of mitral flow occurs as a result of left atrial systole. In our experience it is often seen in patients with com-

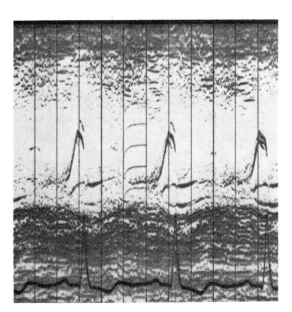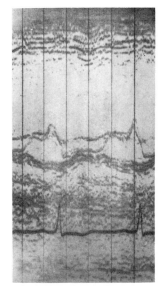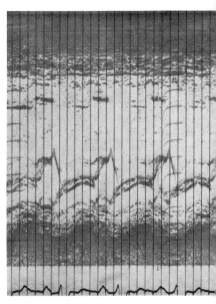

Figure 33–2. Echocardiograms from three different patients showing a large *A* point of the anterior mitral leaflet, a pattern of the mitral valve that may occur in left ventricular dysfunction. All three patients had significant left ventricular dysfunction and combined aortic stenosis and insufficiency proved at cardiac catheterization.

bined aortic stenosis and insufficiency who have poor myocardial function. One could speculate that patients with this mitral valve pattern would have significant hemodynamic embarrassment with the development of atrial fibrillation.

At cardiac catheterization the patient in this case had evidence of biventricular failure, significant pulmonary hypertension, and a low cardiac output. The left ventricular end diastolic pressure was 35 mm Hg and cardiac index 1.2 L/m². The left ventricle was large, with severe and diffuse impairment of contractility, and there was 3+ mitral regurgitation. Consequently, angiography of the coronary arteries or venous bypass grafts were not performed.

CASE 34

This 64-year-old Chinese man on chronic hemodialysis is admitted for recurrent staphylococcal sepsis associated with fever, malaise, and weight loss. Recently, he has developed severe pain and tenderness in the right sacroiliac joint. A Grade III/VI apical systolic murmur is thought to be unchanged. A chest x-ray shows that the heart has increased in size, although the lung fields remain clear. With the differential diagnosis of osteomyelitis, endocarditis, and/or pericarditis, an echocardiogram is ordered to define the etiology of the increased cardiomegaly.

MEASUREMENTS (Echo tracings *A* and *B*)   Time lines = 200 msec

cf	=		Ejection fraction	=
Ao leaflet opening	=		Percentage change	=
LA	=		Ejection time	=
E-F slope	=		Vcf	=
C-E amplitude	=		IVS thickness	=
D-E amplitude	=		IVS amplitude	=
RV	=		LVPW thickness	=
EDD	=		LVPW amplitude	=
ESD	=			

QUESTIONS

1. Which of the following abnormalities explains this patient's cardiomegaly? More than one may apply.

   (A) Left atrial enlargement
   (B) Left ventricular cavity enlargement
   (C) Left ventricular hypertrophy
   (D) Pericardial effusion
   (E) Right ventricular enlargement

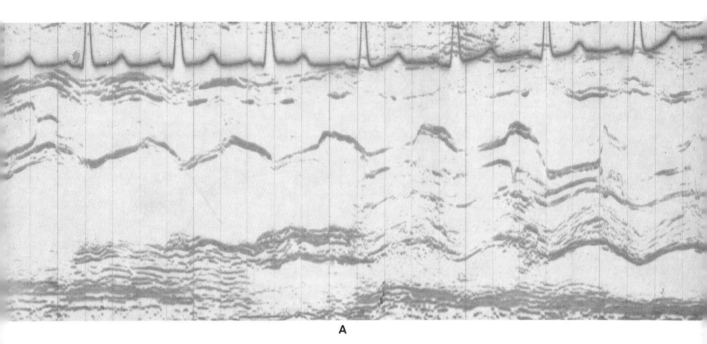

A

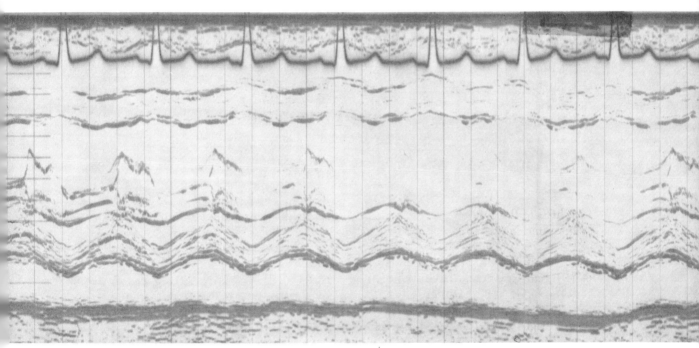

B

ANSWERS TO CASE 34
Pericardial Effusion

MEASUREMENTS

cf	= 1.80	Ejection fraction	= 49%
Ao leaflet opening	= 1.8 cm	Percentage change	= 25%
LA	= 6.5 cm	Ejection time	= 320 msec
E-F slope	= 135 mm/sec	Vcf	= 0.78 circ/sec
C-E amplitude	= 20 mm	IVS thickness	= 15 mm
D-E amplitude	= 14 mm	IVS amplitude	= 6 mm
RV	= 2.1 cm	LVPW thickness	= 14 mm
EDD	= 6.3	LVPW amplitude	= 13 mm
ESD	= 4.7		

ANSWERS

1. (A), (B), (C), (D). The above measurements document that this patient has dilatation of the left atrial and left ventricular cavities, associated with symmetric left ventricular hypertrophy. In addition, an echo-free space is noted in both echo tracings just behind the left ventricular posterior wall during both systole and diastole. The left ventricular wall moves appropriately, but the echo posterior to the echo-free space, which represents the pericardial-lung interspace, remains horizontal. These echo findings indicate that a pericardial effusion is present posteriorly.

The basis for the echo detection of pericardial effusion is that pericardial fluid is acoustically homogeneous and, when present, creates a relatively echo-free space.[1, 185-195] In the absence of pericardial effusion, the echoes from the anterior wall of the right ventricle are in contact with the nonmoving echoes of the chest wall, and the echoes from the left ventricular epicardium are also in contact with the pericardial–lung interface behind the heart. As pericardial effusion begins to accumulate in the sac around the heart, i.e., the pericardium, the left ventricular free wall becomes separated from the pericardial–lung interface by a relatively echo-free space. The left ventricular posterior wall retains its normal motion anteriorly during systole. However, apparently because the pericardial fluid acts as a buffer between the heart and the pericardium, the pericardial–lung interface becomes a flat or almost flat echo as the amount of fluid increases. As even more pericardial fluid accumulates, the anterior wall of the right ventricle also becomes separated from the stationary chest wall by a similar, relatively echo-free space anteriorly.[192]

Two echo patterns have been found to correlate with pericardial fluid present in greater than the normal amount of 15 to 20 cc.[1, 185-195] First, separation of the left ventricular posterior wall and pericardial–lung interface by a relatively echo-free space in both systole and diastole is the basic echo pattern seen in significant pericardial effusions. In this pattern, the left ventricular wall retains its normal anterior motion during systole and the pericardium becomes flat or has only a slight anterior motion in systole. Echo tracing B from this case, as well as tracings from Cases 2 and 6, are illustrations of this pattern. If the motion of the left ventricular wall is excessive, the pericardium might have considerable anterior motion, but it will always be less than

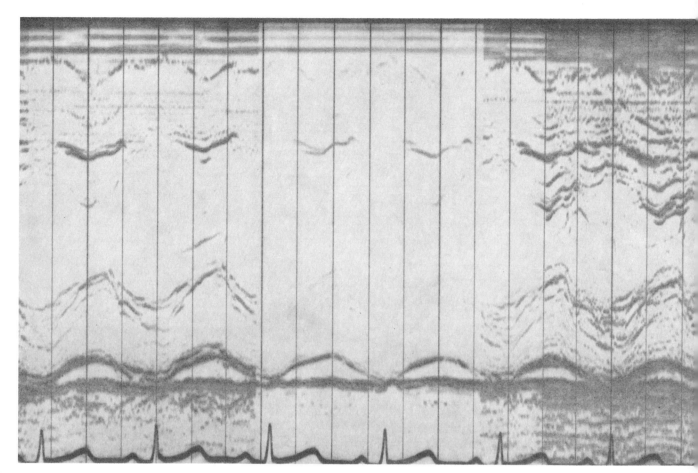

Figure 34–1. Echocardiogram showing the pattern a small pericardial effusion (15 to 100 cc) may present.[194] Note that the pericardial-lung interface is flat and that the posterior echo-free space during systole greatly encroaches on diastole so that the LVPW and pericardium touch only very briefly in diastole.

that of the left ventricular wall. Depending on the size of the heart and pericardial space and on the distribution of the fluid, this pattern may be associated with small to large pericardial effusions (20 cc to greater than 500 cc). Second, a stationary or almost stationary pericardial–lung interface associated with an echo-free space in systole with encroachment of this space on diastole so that the left ventricular wall and pericardium touch only very briefly during diastole.[194] This pattern is illustrated in Figure 34–1 and is associated with small pericardial effusions (15 cc to 100 cc) that dampen the motion of the pericardium and almost create an echo-free space throughout the cardiac cycle. When this pattern is present just below the level of the mitral valve, it often is possible to obtain a small separation during both systole and diastole on M-mode scan toward the apex, where free pericardial fluid tends to accumulate.

Similarly, the following echo patterns have been found unreliable indicators of greater than the normal amount of pericardial effusion: (1) an echo-free space between the left ventricular posterior wall and pericardium only during systole with no encroachment of this systolic echo-free space in diastole and with the pericardium moving slightly anteriorly with the left ventricle;[194] (2) an anterior echo-free space in the absence of a posterior echo-free space;[190, 191, 194, 195] and (3) separation of the left ventricular posterior wall and pericardium by a small echo-free space in

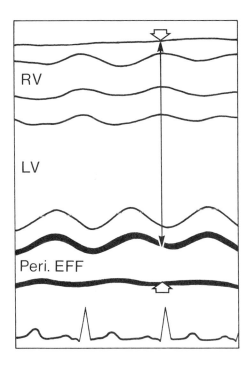

RV

LV

Peri. EFF

Figure 34–2 (*Echo tracing B*). Pericardial effusion posteriorly. Proper places for measuring the total pericardial diameter (*open arrows*) and the total epicardial diameter (*double-headed arrow*) at end-diastole in order to calculate the amount of pericardial effusion by the method of Horowitz, et al.,[194] are shown. See text for formula.

both systole and diastole but with these two surfaces showing equal, parallel motion throughout the cardiac cycle.[194] This pattern was found by Horowitz, et al.,[194] in patients with fibrotic, thickened visceral and parietal pericardia without fluid.

Accurate quantitation of the amount of pericardial effusion present from the echo remains a problem. The size of the echo-free space and whether it is present both posteriorly and anteriorly depend on the relative size of the heart and pericardial space, on the distribution of the fluid within the pericardial space, and on how much fluid is present. For example, in two pericardial spaces of equal size 50 to 75 cc of pericardial effusion might create a prominent posterior echo-free space if the heart is small, whereas if the heart is enlarged, only a small echo-free space probably would be detected. In fact, if this fluid is distributed in the lateral pericardial recesses, no effusion might be detected on echo.

Horowitz, et al.,[194] have proposed a method of roughly quantitating the amount of pericardial effusion from the echo if there is a posterior echo-free space extending throughout the cardiac cycle. Assuming that the pericardial fluid is evenly distributed about the heart, they found that the difference between the cubed diameters of the pericardium and epicardium at end-diastole roughly estimated the volume of pericardial effusion aspirated at surgery or with quantitative pericardiocentesis.

$$\text{Estimated volume of pericardial effusion} = \left(\frac{\text{Pericardial}}{\text{diameter}}\right)^3 - \left(\frac{\text{Epicardial}}{\text{diameter}}\right)^3$$

For this measurement, the diameter of the entire pericardial space is measured in centimeters at end-diastole from the anterior edge of an anterior echo-free space, or from a point 0.5 cm from the chest wall echo if no anterior echo-free space is present, to the posterior pericardium (Fig. 34–2). The epicardial diameter of the whole heart is measured in centimeters at end-diastole from the anterior edge of the right ventricle if an anterior echo-free space is present, or from a point 0.5 cm from

TABLE 34–1. Qualitative Estimate of Pericardial Effusion

Small	20 to 100 cc
Moderate	100 to 500 cc
Large	500 cc or greater

the chest wall echo if no anterior echo-free space is present, to the anterior edge of the posterior left ventricular wall (Fig. 34–2). Both the pericardial and epicardial diameters are cubed as rough estimates of the volume of these spaces. Subtracting the volume of the heart from the total pericardial volume gives an estimate of the volume of pericardial effusion. These authors stress that this method provides only a rough estimate of the amount of pericardial effusion, and at best is only accurate within 100 cc. By applying this formula to this patient, the following rough estimate of pericardial effusion is obtained: $(7.3 \text{ cm} \times 1.80)^3 - (5.9 \text{ cm} \times 1.80)^3 = 250$ cc. This method of calculating the amount of pericardial effusion may be most useful in following a patient with a moderate to large pericardial effusion and determining whether the effusion is increasing or decreasing in amount.

Considering the difficulties in accurate quantitation of pericardial effusion by echo, it probably is preferable at this time only to judge the amount of effusion in a qualitative manner as small, moderate, or large. The values shown in Table 34–1 seem to have a reasonable correlation with this type of estimate. Such a qualitative estimate usually can be made by knowing the pattern a small effusion may present, as described above, by knowing that as more and more effusion accumulates it usually is seen anteriorly as well as posteriorly, and by using the cube method of Horowitz, et al.,[194] as a rough estimate of the amount of effusion.

CASE 35

This 48-year-old bank vault officer consults a physician because dyspnea, excess fatigue, and chest pains recently have limited his golf game. A blood pressure of 190/100, bibasalar inspiratory rales, and a ventricular gallop are noted. Moderate cardiomegaly and pulmonary vascular congestion are present on x-ray. The physician orders an echocardiogram.

MEASUREMENTS (Echo tracing A-C)   **Time lines = 200 msec**

cf	=	Ejection fraction	=
Aorta	=	Percentage change	=
LA	=	IVS thickness	=
C-E amplitude	=	IVS amplitude	=
E-F slope	=	LVPW thickness	=
RV	=	LVPW amplitude	=
EDD	=		
ESD	=		

QUESTIONS

1. What is the cause of this patient's cardiomegaly? More than one may apply.
   (A) Left atrial enlargement
   (B) Left ventricular cavity enlargement
   (C) Left ventricular hypertrophy
   (D) Pericardial effusion, large
   (E) Pericardial effusion, small
   (F) Right ventricular enlargement

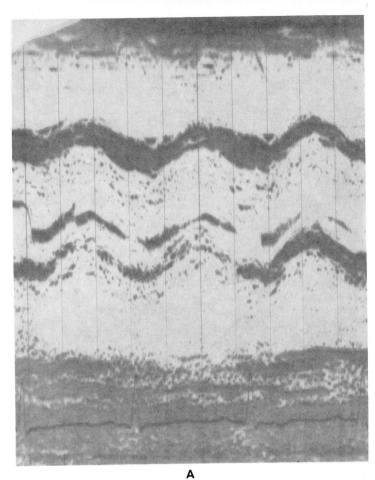

A

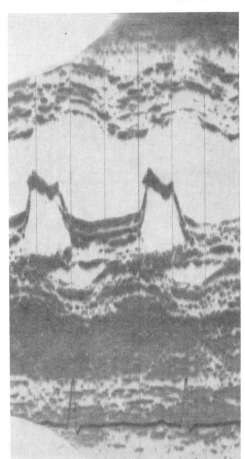

B

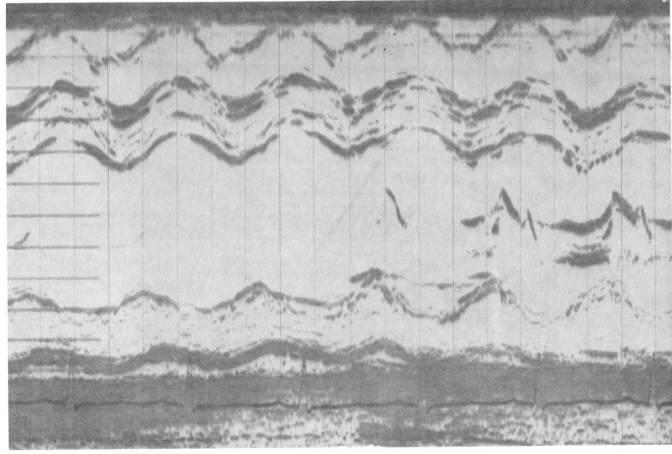

C

ANSWERS TO CASE 35
Pericardial Effusion, Small
Left Ventricular Hypertrophy
Left Ventricular Cavity Dilatation

MEASUREMENTS

cf	= 1.20	Ejection fraction	= 52%
Aorta	= 3.8 mm	Percentage change	= 27%
LA	= 3.8 cm	IVS thickness	= 17 mm
C-E amplitude	= 24 mm	IVS amplitude	= 8 mm
E-F slope	= 60 mm/sec	LVPW thickness	= 16 mm
RV	= 1.6 cm	LVPW amplitude	= 11 mm
EDD	= 5.9 cm		
ESD	= 4.3 cm		

ANSWERS

1. (B), (C), (E). Dilatation of the left ventricular cavity, symmetric left ventricular hypertrophy, and a pericardial effusion are the causes of this patient's cardiomegaly documented by echo. Posteriorly, the pericardium is flat and separated from the left ventricular free wall by an echo-free space throughout the cardiac cycle. Considering the small size of this posterior echo-free space and that the heart is not separated from the chest wall by a similar echo-free space during both systole and diastole, the effusion is best judged to be small (20 to 100 cc).

Several causes of a false-positive echo diagnosis for pericardial effusion have been identified (Table 35–1), some of which will be more fully discussed in subsequent cases. Because the left pleural cavity is contiguous with the posterior pericardium, a left pleural effusion that is large enough to rise behind the heart may very closely simulate pericardial effusion.[187, 193, 197] Even a small pleural effusion that is loculated posterior to the left ventricle may have a similar appearance.[197] Medial angulation of the transducer into the mediastinum can easily produce a false-positive pattern for pericardial effusion.[190, 192, 193, 197] In this case, the left ventricular free wall is recorded moving appropriately with echo-dense, nonmoving mediastinal structures posterior to and separated from it. This pattern can appear as a significant pericardial effusion. In addition, improperly identifying the endocardium, epicardium, chordae tendineae, papillary muscle, or an echo-dense mitral annulus can lead to the mistaken diagnosis of pericardial effusion.[192, 193] An enlarged left atrium bulging posterior to the superior part of the left ventricular free wall has been reported to be another potential source of a false-positive diagnosis for pericardial effusion.[196]

As stated previously, an anterior echo-free space in the absence of a similar space posteriorly should *not* be read as a pericardial effusion.[190, 191, 194, 195] Not only may this pattern be seen in normals without a pericardial effusion, but anterior mediastinal tumors[112] and pericardial cysts[113] have been reported to produce anterior echo-free spaces in the absence of pericardial effusion. It is true, however, that a pericardial effusion may be loculated anteriorly, for example after cardiac surgery, and be recorded only as an anterior echo-free space.

TABLE 35–1. Causes of False-Positive Diagnosis of Pericardial Effusion

1. Left pleural effusion.
2. Medial angulation of transducer.
3. Calcified or echo-dense mitral annulus.
4. Improper identification of endocardium, epicardium, chordae tendineae, or papillary muscle.
5. Enlarged left atrium.
6. Thickened pericardium.
7. Reading an anterior echo-free space only.
8. Acoustically homogeneous tumor posterior to left ventricular posterior wall.

Although echocardiography may detect as little as 16 cc of pericardial effusion, it may fail to detect a significant pericardial effusion if the fluid is loculated to a part of the heart not seen by echo, or if the pericardial fluid is distributed in the lateral recesses of the pericardium.[187, 190, 192-194, 197] Such difficulties may be more common in patients with chronic renal disease or after cardiac surgery. In addition, too high gain settings may obscure a small pericardial effusion. Obesity, emphysema, and edema of the chest wall after cardiac surgery may make the posterior left ventricular wall difficult to visualize adequately.

Technical Hints.   Such difficulties have led to the following technical hints for the proper detection of pericardial effusion by echocardiography:[190, 192, 193, 197, 198]

(1) Aim the transducer inferolaterally through the left ventricular posterior wall just inferior to the tip of the anterior mitral leaflet to detect a possible echo-free space in one of the two basic patterns of a posterior pericardial effusion described in the previous case.

(2) Avoid medial angulation of the transducer, as recording stationary mediastinal structures can produce false-positive patterns for pericardial effusion.

(3) Make several careful M-mode sweeps between the left atrium and the left ventricle, as illustrated on echo tracing A from Case 34. Because a pericardial effusion usually is not seen posterior to the left atrium but begins at the atrioventricular junction just when the mitral valve begins to be recorded, this type of M-mode sweep is helpful in differentiating pericardial from pleural effusions. If the effusion is small, as shown on echo tracing C of Case 35, it may only be detected as this sweep moves distal to the mitral valve toward the left ventricular apex, because pericardial effusion tends to accumulate around the apex.

(4) With the gain set to properly record the left ventricular endocardium, suddenly increase the dampening control to the point that only the pericardial–lung interface is recorded. This will aid in proper identification of structures.

(5) Avoid too high gain settings, as small effusions will be obscured by the excess reverberations. A short recording of the left ventricle should always be made with settings that seem too low at the time of the recording, because these tracings often will reveal small effusions. Of course, if all the recording is made with low settings, the endocardium may not be properly identified.

(6) Positively identify the endocardium, the epicardium, and pericardial–lung interface, the chordae tendineae, and the mitral annulus if it is echo dense, by the above maneuvers of changing the dampening and gain settings, by careful M-mode sweeps and by slight changes of the angle of the transducer.

(7) Review a recent chest x-ray, when appropriate, to detect the presence and extent of any pleural effusion, and to detect any disparity between the size of the heart as seen by x-ray and by echocardiography.

CASE 36

A 34-year-old attorney with multiple episodes of thrombophlebitis—some associated with pulmonary emboli—over the last two years is admitted with pain and swelling in his left popliteal area and vague chest discomfort. A lung scan is compatible with a diagnosis of left lower lobe pulmonary infarction and heparin therapy is initiated. On the fifth hospital day, he suddenly becomes diaphoretic, mildly dyspneic, hypotensive, and obtunded. He is transferred at this time to your hospital for consideration of emergency pulmonary angiography. A portable chest x-ray shows an enlarged heart with clear lung fields. The patient is now clinically in shock with a blood pressure palpable at 60 mm Hg and is peripherally vasoconstricted with an elevated venous pressure. An emergency echo is obtained.

MEASUREMENTS   (Echo tracings *A* and *B*)   **Time lines = 200 msec**

cf	=	EDD	=
Aorta	=	ESD	=
LA	=	Ejection fraction	=
C-E amplitude	=	Percentage change	=
D-E amplitude	=	IVS thickness	=
E-F slope	=	IVS amplitude	=
RV	=	LVPW amplitude	=

QUESTIONS

1. What is the cause of this patient's cardiomegaly?
   (A) Left ventricular cavity dilatation
   (B) Right ventricular dilatation
   (C) Pericardial effusion
   (D) Biventricular enlargement
   (E) Left atrial enlargement

2. What is the most likely diagnosis?
   (A) Massive pulmonary embolus with circulatory collapse
   (B) Acute myocardial infarction and cardiogenic shock
   (C) Gastrointestinal hemorrhage secondary to anticoagulant therapy
   (D) Cardiac tamponade secondary to anticoagulant therapy
   (E) Fulminating myocarditis

3. What is the most appropriate course of management at this time?
   (A) Emergency pulmonary angiography
   (B) Emergency ventilation-perfusion scan
   (C) Dopamine administration
   (D) Pericardiocentesis
   (E) Type and cross-match

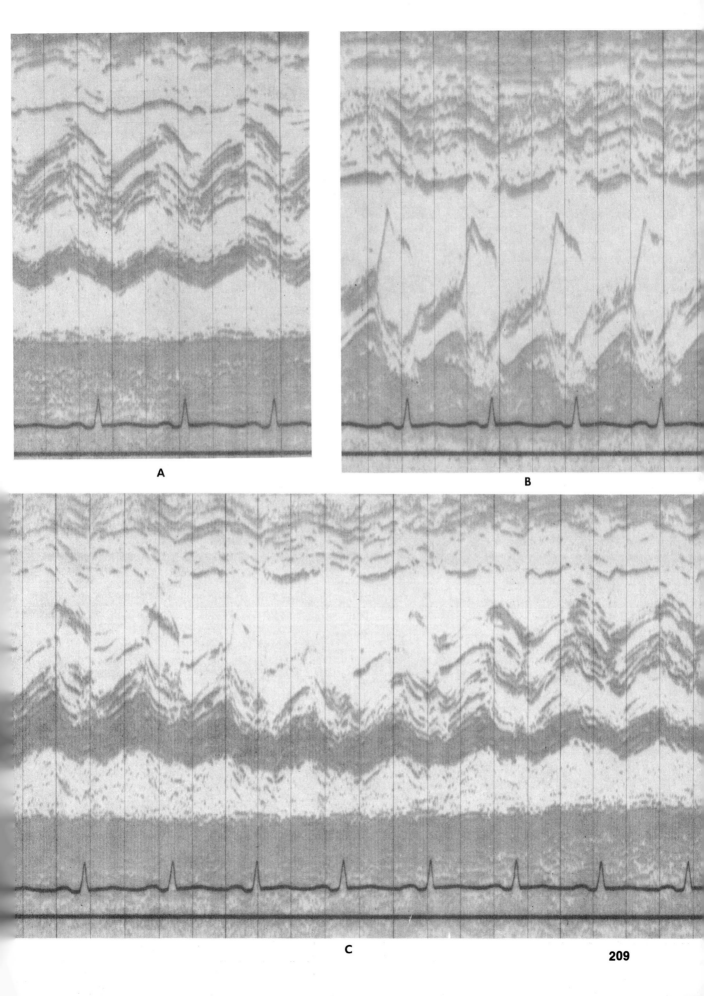

A

B

C

ANSWERS TO CASE 36
Pericardial Effusion with Cardiac Tamponade
Right Ventricular Compression

MEASUREMENTS

cf	= 1.0	EDD	= 3.7 cm
Aorta	= 31 mm	ESD	= 3.0 cm
LA	= 2.5 cm	Ejection fraction	= 41%
C-E amplitude	= 25 mm	Percentage change	= 19%
D-E amplitude	= 22 mm	IVS thickness	= 11 mm
E-F slope	= 115 mm/sec	IVS amplitude	= 4 mm
RV	= 0.3 cm	LVPW amplitude	= 10 mm

ANSWERS

1. (C); 2. (D); and 3. (D).

Echo tracing *C* shows a large, relatively echo-free space posteriorly throughout the cardiac cycle, with the left ventricular free wall retaining its normal motion and the pericardial–lung interface remaining flat (Fig. 36–1). An anterior echo-free space is also present. These findings are most compatible with a large pericardial effusion and suggest that the patient has cardiac tamponade secondary to his anticoagulant therapy as a cause of shock. Estimating the amount of pericardial fluid by the cubing method of Horowitz, et al.,[194] (see Case 34) shows that about 300 cc are present, al-

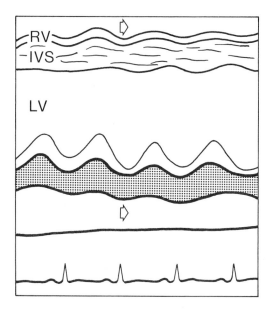

Figure 36–1 (Echo tracing *C*). Pericardial effusion anteriorly and posteriorly (*open arrows*) with right ventricular compression occurring in cardiac tamponade.

though this value may be underestimated because the anterior boundary of the anterior effusion probably is not recorded.

This echo also shows compression of the right ventricular cavity to less than the normal range (Fig. 36–1). In the presence of a significant pericardial effusion, a right ventricle measuring less than 0.7 cm has been suggested as a reliable sign of cardiac tamponade.[199] This sign, of course, depends on there being no inherent cause of right ventricular enlargement, such as chronic lung disease, mitral stenosis, pulmonary hypertension, atrial septal defect, cardiomyopathy, etc. In such cases, cardiac tamponade can occur even with large right ventricular measurements. Others have reported a decreased E-F slope and opening amplitude of the mitral valve during inspiration as a reliable echo sign of cardiac tamponade.[200, 200a] The present echo does not show this sign, despite the patient's being in tamponade. The reason this does not occur in this case is that the heart as a whole does not manifest exaggerated anterior motion with respiration, a condition that probably is necessary to produce the decreased mitral slope and amplitude reported as an echo sign of cardiac tamponade. Others have reported that an exaggerated swing of the heart within the pericardial effusion occurs only in tamponade, although obviously tamponade can occur without such swinging. Thus, there is no completely reliable echo sign of tamponade, and this diagnosis must still be made by clinical assessment of the patient.

An emergency pericardiocentesis was performed in this patient, and more than 500 cc of grossly sanguineous pericardial effusion was withdrawn. During this procedure, the patient's blood pressure rose to normal levels, and his cardiovascular status stabilized.

CASE 37

This 52-year-old former district judge with an old anterior myocardial infarction, congestive heart failure, chronic obstructive airway disease, and metastatic prostatic carcinoma is admitted with extreme weakness and dyspnea. His blood pressure is 85/60. He is peripherally vasoconstricted; the venous pressure is elevated and the heart sounds distant. Slight cardiomegaly with prominent pulmonary vascular congestion and bilateral pleural effusions are noted on x-ray. An echo is ordered to evaluate his left ventricular function.

QUESTIONS

(Echo tracings A and B)   Time lines = 200 msec

1. What technical maneuver is illustrated on echo tracing B? What is its purpose? What conclusion can be drawn from it?

2. Which of the following readings should be made from this echo? More than one may apply.
   (A) Aortic root dilatation
   (B) Left atrial enlargement
   (C) Left ventricular cavity dilatation
   (D) Left ventricular dysfunction
   (E) Right ventricular enlargement
   (F) Pericardial effusion, large
   (G) Pericardial effusion, small
   (H) Pleural effusion

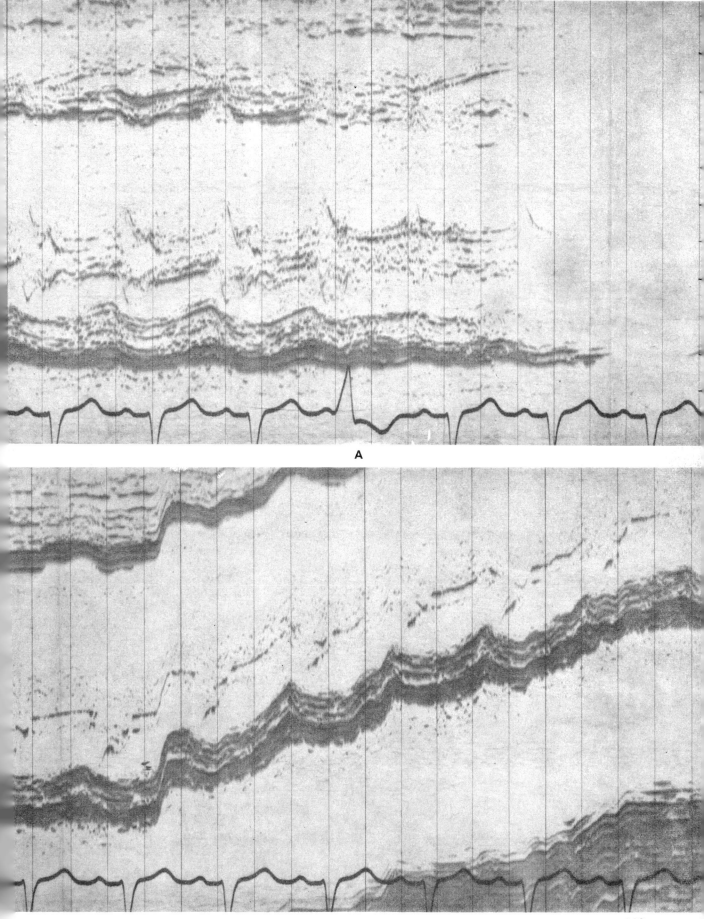

A

B

ANSWERS TO CASE 37
Left Pleural Effusion

ANSWERS

1. Adjustment of the delay control is illustrated on echo tracing *B*. By thus adjusting the starting point of the display of the returning echoes, the depth of an echo-free space behind the left ventricle that is too large to be recorded on the echo tracing can be determined. Because the calibration is not affected by this maneuver, this space can be measured to be 4.6 cm in this patient. If the echo-free space represented a pericardial effusion, the heart size as seen on x-ray should be massive. However, only slight cardiomegaly is present on the chest film, and we can be confident that the posterior echo-free space represents this patient's left pleural effusion present directly behind the heart.

As previously stated, a left pleural effusion large enough to rise behind the heart or one that is loculated directly retrocardiac can simulate the echo picture of a pericardial effusion.[1, 187, 193, 197] When a left pleural effusion creates a smaller echo-free space than in this patient, this differentiation can be very difficult. However, several factors can aid in making this distinction. First, if the echo-free space begins at the atrioventricular junction or at the level of the mitral valve on M-mode sweep from the left atrium to the left ventricle, this favors a pericardial effusion. Such a sweep illustrating a pericardial effusion is shown on echo tracing *A* in Case 34 and on echo tracing *C* in Case 35.

Usually, it is stated that a significant pericardial effusion does not occur posterior to the left atrium, because the pericardium is adherent to the left atrial wall. A left pleural effusion, of course, does not have this restriction. However, recently it has become apparent that a large pericardial effusion may rarely be associated with an echo-free space posterior to the left atrium.[202] The distinctive pattern this produces and how it may help distinguish between pericardial and pleural fluid will be discussed in a subsequent case. Second, with pleural effusions, the posterior border of the echo-free space may vary with respiration, whereas with pericardial effusions it usually remains flat. Third, a large posterior effusion in the absence of an anterior effusion should make one think of the diagnosis of a left pleural effusion. However, large pericardial effusions do occur without any evident anterior echo-free space. Fourth, placing the patient in the left lateral decubitus position to drain pleural effusion from the retrocardiac space may also aid in this differentiation.[190] A pericardial effusion will not vary significantly with this repositioning. Fifth, placing the transducer on the chest in the left posterior axillary line to detect a possible echo-free space separating the chest wall from the echo-dense lung has been proposed as a method of detecting a pleural effusion.[186] Sixth, PA and lateral chest films should be reviewed to detect the presence and the extent of a possible left pleural effusion. A small pleural effusion confined to the costophrenic angle would not cause an echo-free space posterior to the left ventricle. If the x-ray shows a normal sized heart and a large left pleural effusion, a significant echo-free space posterior to the left ventricle is most likely a pleural effusion. If cardiomegaly is present on x-ray and all cardiac chambers have normal dimensions on echo, an echo-free space is most likely a pericardial effusion. Occasionally, both a pericardial and pleural effusion can be detected on echo by identifying two echo-free spaces posteriorly with a flat pericardial echo separating them. However, despite all these points of differentiation, if a left pleural effusion is present, it is not always possible to be sure whether a posterior echo-free space represents a pericardial or pleural effusion.

2. (D) and (H). Although the left ventricular cavity is not dilated (EDD = 5.5 cm and ESD = 5.0 cm) and the amplitude of the left ventricular posterior wall is within normal limits (5 mm), the interventricular septum has poor, and even the suggestion of passive, paradoxic motion. This indicates left ventricular dysfunction and results in a severely depressed calculated ejection fraction (20 per cent) and percentage change of the minor diameter (9 per cent).

CASE 38

This 57-year-old housewife who had bilateral radical mastectomies and postoperative irradiation six years ago for carcinoma presents with a three-week history of increasing dyspnea associated with a hacking, nonproductive cough and rapid, irregular palpitations. Although she has emphysema, she had otherwise been well. On physical examination, the jugular venous pressure is elevated, the blood pressure is 100/70, the heart rate is irregular at 100 per minute, the chest is clear, and the heart sounds are distant. No murmur or rub is heard. A chest film shows an increased heart size since her operation, clear lung fields, and a small right pleural effusion. With the diagnosis of cardiomegaly and congestive heart failure of unknown etiology, an echo is ordered to evaluate left ventricular function and heart size.

MEASUREMENTS   (Echo tracings *A-F*. Tracings *A* and *B* are continuous.)
                  Time lines = 200 msec

cf	=	EDD	=	
Aorta	=	ESD	=	
Ao leaflet opening	=	IVS thickness	=	
LA	=	IVS amplitude	=	
RV	=	LVPW thickness	=	
		LVPW amplitude	=	

QUESTIONS

1. What is the cause of this patient's cardiomegaly noted on x-ray?
   (A) Right ventricular enlargement
   (B) Left ventricular enlargement
   (C) Left atrial enlargement
   (D) Pericardial effusion
   (E) Left pleural effusion

2. Which of the following echo observations are present on these tracings?
   (A) Mitral prolapse
   (B) Tricuspid prolapse
   (C) Right ventricular volume overload
   (D) Left ventricular volume overload
   (E) Left ventricular dysfunction
   (F) Ruptured chordae tendineae

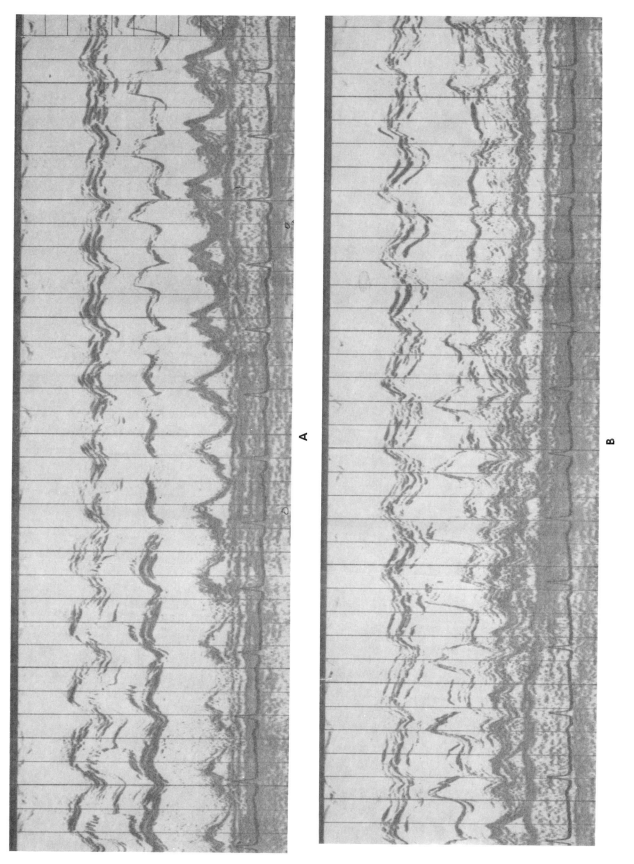

A

B

Illustration continued on following page.

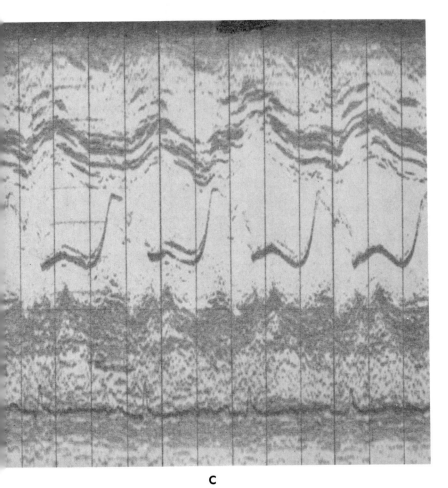

C

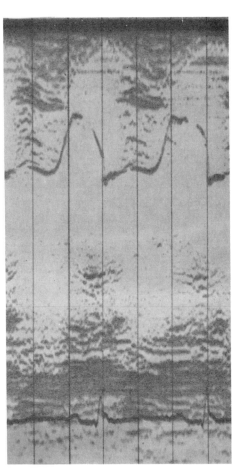

D

Illustration continued on opposite page.

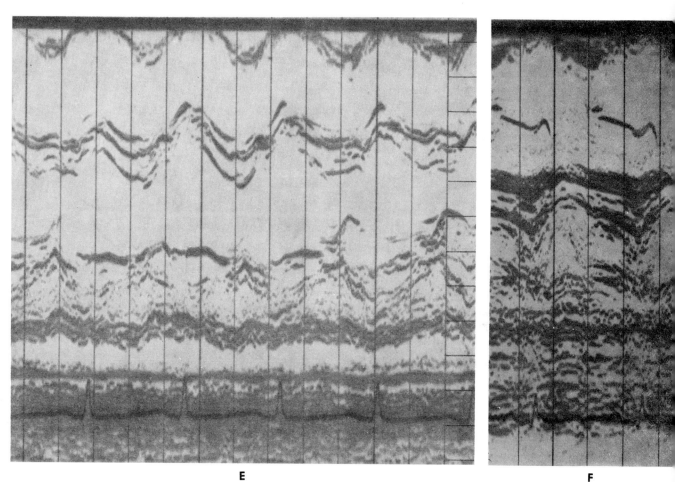

E   F

ANSWERS TO CASE 38

Pericardial Effusion Posterior to the Left Atrium
False Mitral and Tricuspid Prolapse

MEASUREMENTS

cf (echo A and B)	= 1.67	EDD	= 4.2–5.2 cm
cf	= 1.09	ESD	= 2.1–2.7
Aorta	= 33 mm	IVS thickness	= 9 mm
Ao leaflet opening	= 1.7 cm	IVS amplitude	= 8–16 mm
LA	= 2.9–3.7	LVPW thickness	= 12 mm
RV	= 2.2 cm	LVPS amplitude	= 6–12 mm

ANSWERS

1. (A) and (D). On echo tracings *B* and *E*, an echo-free space is observed separating the mobile left ventricular posterior wall from a nonmoving echo throughout the cardiac cycle. A small echo-free space is also seen anteriorly but only during ventricular systole. These show that a pericardial effusion contributes to this patient's cardiomegaly. Although there is variation in its measurement, the right ventricle was slightly enlarged, whereas the left ventricle and left atrium appear normal in size.

   In this patient, who had no radiologic evidence of a left pleural effusion, the continuous M-mode scan on echo tracings *A* and *B* shows that the echo-free space posterior to the left ventricle is continuous with a similar echo-free space posterior to the left atrial wall. This space is even present at the level of aortic valves. As was discussed in Case 37, it usually is thought that a pericardial effusion cannot occur behind the left atrium, because the pericardium is tightly bound to the left atrial wall by its reflections on the pulmonary veins.[1, 2, 198] This limitation of where a pericardial effusion can occur has been helpful in distinguishing pericardial from retrocardiac pleural effusions. However, it is now apparent that occasionally with large pericardial effusions an echo-free space can occur posterior to the left atrial wall in the absence of pleural effusion. Lemire and colleagues[202] reported five patients with large pericardial effusions seen anteriorly and posteriorly in whom on M-mode scan the posterior effusion was continuous with an echo-free space posterior to the left atrial wall. None of these patients had radiologic evidence of left pleural effusion at the time of the echo. These authors presented evidence that the effusion was filling the oblique pericardial sinus behind the left atrium, which is a potential space limited laterally by the pericardial reflection on the pulmonary veins and superiorly by the transverse pericardial sinus. They also observed that in these patients the left atrial wall had prominent anterior motion during systole in unison with the anterior swing of the entire heart. This same type of prominent anterior motion of the left atrial wall, measuring up to 16 mm, is well seen during early systole on echo tracing *A* of this case (Fig. 38–1). Note that it occurs in unison with the exaggerated systolic anterior motion seen in the early part of the C-D portion of the mitral valve echo. This

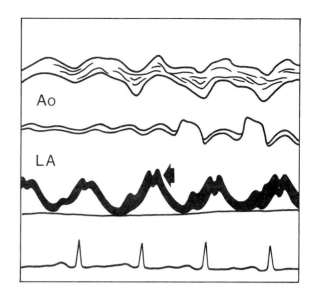

Figure 38–1 (Echo tracing *A***).** Exaggerated anterior systolic motion of the left atrial wall (*arrow*) occurring in a large pericardial effusion that extends behind the left atrial wall. Normal amplitude of left atrial wall excursion is 0 to 5 mm; in this patient this amplitude is 16 mm.

similarity in timing supports the speculation that the excess motion of the entire heart that can occur in early systole with significant pericardial effusion contributes to this prominent anterior motion of the left atrial wall. Kisslo,[203] using a cross-sectional, phased array, multi-element sector scanner, has also observed an echo-free space posterior to the left atrium in patients with large pericardial effusions, but has postulated that this space represents a dilated pulmonary vein. In any case, because pericardial fluid can and does accumulate behind the left atrium in large pericardial effusion, this feature alone can not reliably be used to differentiate pleural from large pericardial effusion.

Lemire, et. al.,[202] suggested that the exaggerated motion of the left atrial wall during ventricular systole may be helpful in distinguishing pericardial from pleural effusions occurring behind the left atrial wall. In pleural effusions, the amplitude of left atrial excursion is normal. We have found this to be 0 to 5 mm.[70] In contrast, when pericardial effusion occurs behind the left atrium, the amplitude of the left atrial wall is greatly increased (Fig. 38–1). Our experience supports the usefulness of this observation in making this distinction between pleural and large pericardial effusions behind the left atrium, although further experience is needed.

2. (A) and (B) On the continuous M-mode scan and on echo tracing *C*, the mitral valve echo shows a posterior bowing in late systole similar to that described in late systolic prolapse (Cases 17 and 18). On echo tracing *D*, late systolic bowing of the tricuspid valve echo also occurs. These patterns undoubtedly do not represent true anatomic mitral and tricuspid prolapse, but occur on the echo tracing because of excess motion of the entire heart within the pericardial fluid.[202, 204-206] Just as there is sometimes exaggerated motion of the entire heart anteriorly in early to mid-systole in significant pericardial effusion, excess posterior motion can occur in late systole. This posterior motion can create the echo pattern of late systolic prolapse of the mitral and tricuspid valves. Such false-prolapse disappears after resolution of the pericardial effusion, as it did in this patient. This pattern merely means that in late systole these valves move away from the transducer. In this case, the pattern occurs because the entire heart moves posteriorly, not because the valves themselves prolapse. Such considerations again illustrate the basic echo principle that the motion of any structure detected by echocardiog-

TABLE 38–1.   Potential Results of Motion of the Entire Heart
in Pericardial Effusion*

1. False late systolic prolapse of mitral and tricuspid valves ("false-LSP").
2. Systolic anterior motion of the mitral valve ("false-SAM").
3. Normalization of abnormal IVS motion in RV volume overload.
4. Creation of abnormally timed IVS motion on echo.
5. Alteration of all slopes and amplitudes of motion of the mitral, tricuspid, and pulmonic valves and of the IVS, LVPW, and LA walls.

*Usually occur in moderately large or large pericardial effusions.

raphy is the algebraic sum of the motion of that structure plus the motion of the heart as a whole in reference to the transducer.

Exaggerated motion of the entire heart within a significant pericardial fluid can affect the echo of intracardiac structures in many ways (Table 38–1). Not only may false mitral and tricuspid prolapse occur, but excess anterior motion of the heart in early systole may create the echo pattern of systolic anterior motion of the mitral valve—i.e., "false-SAM." This is shown on the second C-D portion of the mitral valve on echo tracing *B*. For a similar reason, the abnormal septal motion recorded in right ventricular volume overload states like atrial septal defect and tricuspid insufficiency may be normalized by excess posterior motion of the entire heart during systole in significant pericardial effusion. Abnormal septal motion may even be created because of exaggerated swinging of the heart within significant pericardial fluid. In fact, the increased motion of the heart as a whole can increase or decrease all slopes and amplitudes of the mitral, tricuspid, and pulmonary valves and the septal, left ventricular, and left atrial walls. For example, the mitral E-F slope may appear decreased, and the mitral amplitude increased by excess anterior motion of the heart; the "a wave" of the pulmonic valve may appear falsely increased by excess posterior motion of the heart. The great variation that occurs in the septal and left ventricular posterior wall amplitudes of motion on this echo illustrates this effect. On echo tracing *F* note that, when the septal amplitude is increased, simultaneously there is a slight posterior motion of the left ventricular epicardium and that, when the septal amplitude is at its lowest value, this epicardial surface moves slightly anteriorly.

Although an anterior effusion usually accompanies a significant pericardial effusion, a large pericardial effusion may occur without any anterior space. In this patient, a large enough pericardial effusion occurs to allow the heart exaggerated motion, yet an echo-free space occurs anteriorly only during ventricular systole.

CASE 39

This 26-year-old art student is seen in the emergency room complaining of cramping abdominal pains, nausea, and dyspnea of two days' duration. She gives a history of cardiac catheterization and surgery two and one-half months ago following discovery of a cardiac murmur on routine examination. At present, she is mildly cyanotic and peripherally constricted with a blood pressure of 80/60, heart rate of 100/min and respirations of 40/min. Heart sounds are decreased, and a soft Grade II/VI systolic ejection murmur is heard at the base without radiation to the carotids. The abdomen is diffusely tender without guarding. After cardiomegaly is detected on x-ray, an echocardiogram is ordered.

QUESTIONS

(Echo tracings A-C. Tracings B and C are continuous).   Time lines=200 msec

1. Which of the following is the most appropriate course of management in this patient?
   (A) Aortogram
   (B) Examination of eyes for subluxation of lenses
   (C) Cardiac catheterization for possible congenital heart disease
   (D) Blood cultures with consideration of antibiotic therapy
   (E) Pericardiocentesis
   (F) Thoracentesis

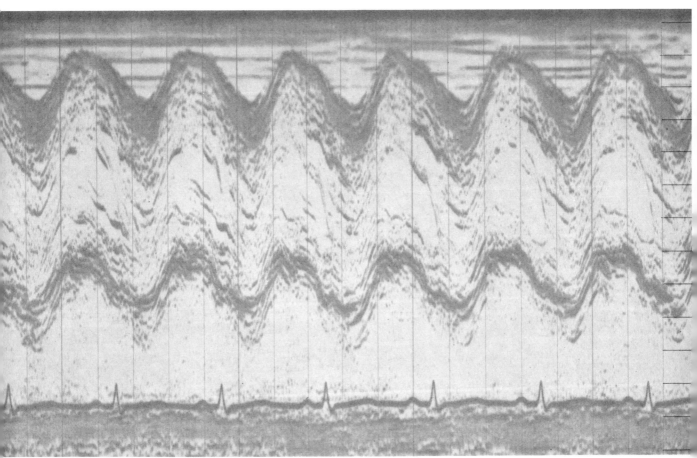

A   *Illustration continued on opposite page*

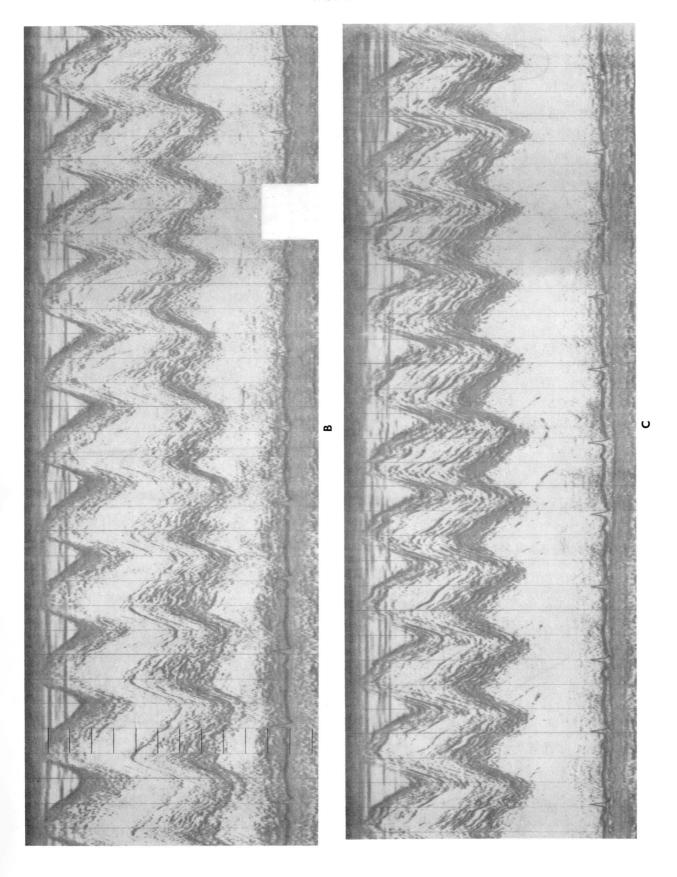

B

C

ANSWERS TO CASE 39
Pericardial Effusion with Cardiac Tamponade

ANSWERS

1. (E) Echo tracing A shows the body of the left ventricle; tracings B and C are a continuous M-mode scan from the base of the heart toward the apex. The entire heart is surrounded by an enormous echo-free space anteriorly and posteriorly. The heart is moving freely within this space, with both the anterior right ventricular wall and the left ventricular posterior wall moving anteriorly with systole in a congruous manner.[195] The pericardium is seen to be stationary posterior to this large echo-free space. All the intracardiac cavities are significantly compressed and, because of the prominent motion of the heart as a whole, it is difficult to distinguish any specific intracardiac structure. This echo demonstrates a massive pericardial effusion with cardiac tamponade. As an emergency pericardiocentesis was being prepared, this patient became markedly hypotensive, had a seizure, and went into ventricular fibrillation. While cardiopulmonary resuscitation was initiated, a subxiphoid incision was made, the tense pericardium opened and a massive amount of straw-colored fluid released. It was grossly estimated as greater than 1 liter. The patient, who recovered, had a postcardiotomy syndrome following removal of a cyst from her pulmonary valve two months previously. The cyst appeared as a filling defect on a right ventricular angiogram done for presumed pulmonic stenosis.

TABLE 39-1.   Motion of the Heart in Pericardial Effusion

Types of Motion	*Potential Results*
1. Swinging of the heart anteriorly with each systole and posteriorly with each diastole.	1. Congruous motion of heart walls. 2. Abnormally timed IVS motion.
2. Excess motion of heart anteriorly in early systole and posteriorly in late systole.	1. "False-LSP." 2. "False-SAM."
3. Swinging of heart anteriorly in a 2:1 or 3:1 ratio with the cardiac cycle.	1. Electrical alternans.
4. Stationary heart.	

TABLE 39–2.   Etiologies of Cardiomegaly Detected by Echocardiography

1. Pericardial effusion.
2. Valvular disease.
3. Congenital heart disease.
4. Systemic hypertension.
5. Pulmonary hypertension.
6. Cardiomyopathy.
7. Coronary artery disease.

From the continuous M-mode scan on echo tracings *B* and *C*, it appears that the diameter of the total pericardial space is about the same at the level of the body of the left ventricle as near the apex. However, the heart itself narrows considerably toward the apex. This variation and where the measurements are taken would, of course, influence the calculation of the amount of pericardial fluid, as suggested by Horowitz, et al.,[194] and as discussed in Case 34. Despite this limitation, estimate of the amount of pericardial effusion by this cubing method shows a very large pericardial effusion between 1100 and 1400 cc.

Four types of motion of the heart as a whole within significant pericardial effusion have been described (Table 39–1). First, the heart may swing anteriorly during each systole and posteriorly in diastole, with the anterior right ventricular wall and left ventricular posterior wall moving parallel or congruously as illustrated in this patient.[195] If such swinging is as prominent as in this case, the motion of the heart as a whole will overshadow the smaller amplitude of motion of the intracardiac structures, and they will become obscured. Although identification of intracardiac structures may be difficult, this pattern should be clearly recognized as a sign of significant pericardial effusion. Second, the heart may move less prominently anteriorly in early systole and posteriorly in late systole, creating the false pattern of late systolic mitral and tricuspid prolapse and systolic anterior motion of the mitral valve, as discussed in Case 38.[202, 204-206] Third, the heart may remain essentially stationary with very little motion even with cardiac tamponade as in Case 36.[195] Fourth, the heart may swing prominently anteriorly after every other cardiac cycle or after every third heartbeat. This type of motion with a two-to-one ratio of cardiac cycle to anterior motion of the heart has been shown to produce the electrical alternans seen in some cases of cardiac tamponade.[192, 193, 195, 208] The volume and viscosity of the pericardial fluid, the configuration and size of the pericardial space, the distance through which the heart can swing with each cardiac cycle and the heart rate have been proposed as the factors that interrelate to produce electrical alternans in pericardial effusion.[208]

Echocardiography also has been helpful in pericardial effusion in suggesting one mechanism for the exaggerated paradoxic pulse seen in this condition.[200, 201] In large pericardial effusions, a transient increase in right ventricular dimension with a corresponding decrease in left ventricular dimension often can be recorded during inspiration. With expiration, the right ventricle decreases in size and the left ventricle returns to its former size. This observation suggests that one cause of the exag-

gerated decrease in arterial pulse during inspiration in significant pericardial effusion is compromise of the left ventricular cavity by a bulging interventricular
septum. Because expansion of the right ventricle is limited by the large pericardial
effusion, the increased venous return during inspiration causes the septum to bulge
into the left ventricle. This decreases left ventricular size and filling and results in a
decrease in stroke volume and exaggeration of the paradoxic pulse.

Clinical Applications. In patients with cardiomegaly, echocardiography is
useful in detecting the etiology of the increased heart size (Table 39–2).[178a] Does a
pericardial effusion contribute to the cardiomegaly? Is left ventricular hypertrophy
or dilatation of the left or right ventricle present? Is there evidence to support congenital heart disease, valvular disease, a diffuse cardiomyopathy, pulmonary hypertension, or coronary artery disease? Or are there several causes of the cardiomegaly? The dilemma that can arise from the plain chest x-ray of deciding whether
the right ventricle, the left ventricle, or indeed both ventricles are enlarged usually
can be settled quickly by echocardiography.

In the area of pericardial effusion, echocardiography is primarily useful in detecting whether more than the normal amount of pericardial fluid is present. In this respect, it has made an outstanding and significant contribution to clinical medicine. In addition, it allows a rough estimate of whether a small (15 to 100 cc), moderate (100 to 500 cc), or large amount (500 cc or greater) of effusion exists. In patients in shock or shocklike states, an emergency echo can establish if a large pericardial effusion is present and perhaps contributing to compromise of the circulation. As discussed in Case 36, certain echo signs, such as right ventricular compression, have been suggested as indicators of cardiac tamponade.[199, 200] The sensitivity of these signs has not been established and, at present, cardiac tamponade properly remains a clinical diagnosis. However, echocardiography can establish if a significant effusion is present and if tamponade is a reasonable diagnosis.

In patients with the diagnosis of pericarditis, the finding of a pericardial effusion, even if it is small, can add credibility to this diagnosis. In our experience, small amounts of pericardial effusion often can be found in these patients, although the sensitivity of this echo finding in pericarditis is not established. It is also very common to find small pericardial effusions in patients with congestive heart failure with no clinical evidence of pericardial effusion or pericarditis.

CASE 40

This active 84-year-old widow consults her physician regarding several recent attacks of irregular palpitations that cause her to feel nervous, dyspneic, and light-headed. He finds her to be in mild congestive heart failure and orders an echocardiogram to delineate the etiology of an apical pansystolic murmur and of the cardiomegaly noted on x-ray.

MEASUREMENTS (Echo tracings A-C)   **Time lines = 200 msec**

cf	=	EDD	=
Aorta	=	ESD	=
LA	=	Ejection fraction	=
D-E amplitude	=	Percentage change	=
D-E slope	=	IVS thickness	=
E-F slope	=	IVS amplitude	=
RV	=	LVPW thickness	=
		LVPW amplitude	=

QUESTIONS

1. What etiology of this patient's murmur does this echo suggest?

2. What cause of this patient's cardiomegaly is demonstrated on the echo? More than one may apply.
   (A) Right ventricular enlargement
   (B) Left atrial enlargement
   (C) Left ventricular cavity enlargement
   (D) Left ventricular hypertrophy
   (E) Pericardial effusion

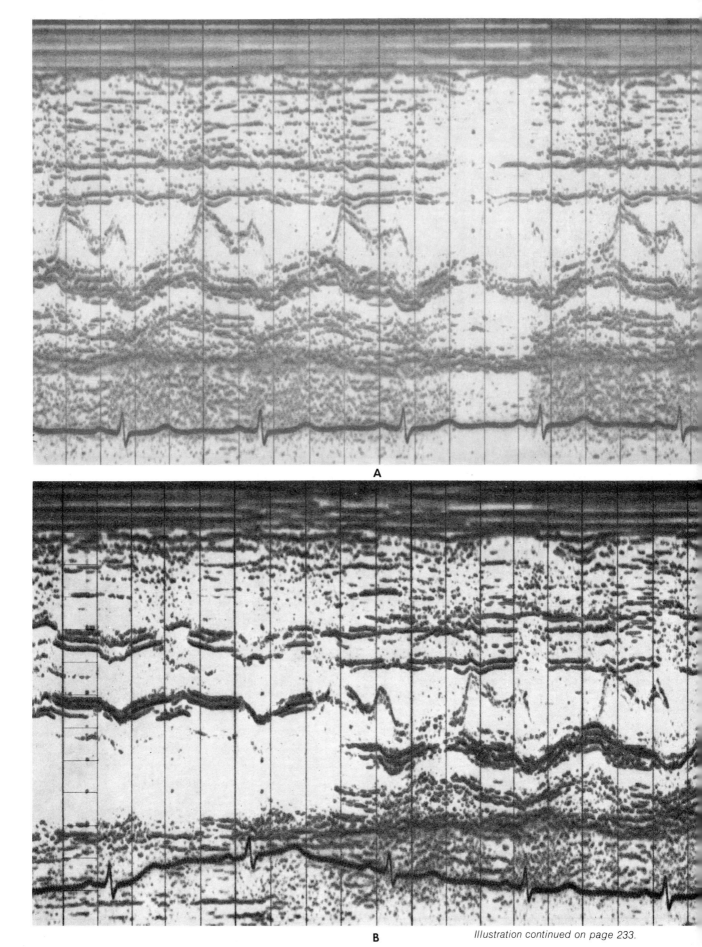

A

B

Illustration continued on page 233.

Figure 40C appears on the opposite page.

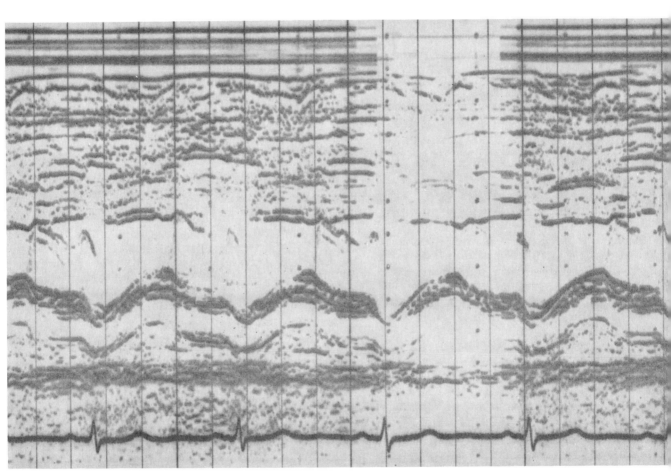

C

ANSWERS TO CASE 40
Calcified Mitral Annulus

MEASUREMENTS

cf	= 1.16	EDD	= 4.1 cm
Aorta	= 23 mm	ESD	= 3.1 cm
LA	= 4.2 cm	Ejection fraction	= 49%
D-E amplitude	= 16 mm	Percentage change	= 25%
D-E slope	= 300 mm/sec	IVS thickness	= 10 mm
E-F slope	= 55 mm/sec	IVS amplitude	= 1–2 mm
RV	= 2.8 cm	LVPW thickness	= 11 mm
		LVPW amplitude	= 9 mm

ANSWERS

1. Directly posterior to a thin, anterior mitral leaflet, a very echo-dense structure is observed that moves parallel to the endocardium of the posterior left ventricular wall. This band of echoes has the motion of a mitral annulus—i.e., slightly anteriorly in systole and posteriorly in diastole (Fig. 40–1). On M-mode scan from the aorta to the mitral valve, this echo-dense structure is seen to begin abruptly at about the level of the mid-left atrium anterior to the left atrial and left ventricular walls. This type of echo-dense structure is the characteristic echo finding in a calcified annulus fibrosis of the mitral valve.[70, 89] Calcification of the mitral annulus is thought to be a degenerative process, and although it may remain asymptomatic, it can be associated with significant mitral regurgitation, intraventricular con-

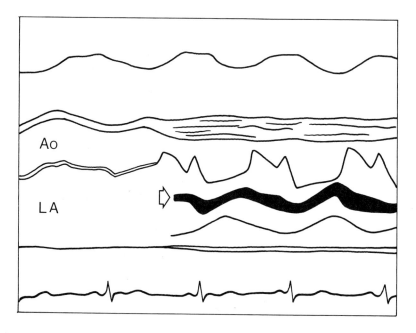

Figure 40–1 (Echo tracing *B*). Calcified mitral annulus. Note that on M-mode scan from the left atrium to the mitral valve that the echo-dense structure (*open arrow*) begins abruptly anterior to the left atrial wall and that it lies just anterior to and runs parallel with the left ventricular posterior wall.

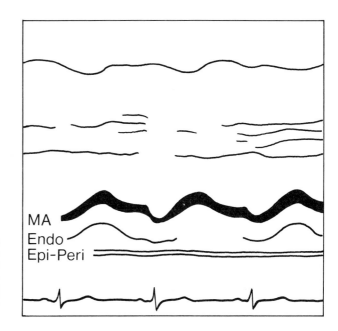

Figure 40–2 (Echo tracing C). Calcified mitral annulus with echo-dense structure lying anterior to the left ventricular posterior wall. The calcified mitral annulus (MA), the endocardium (ENDO), and the epicardial-pericardial interface (EPI—PERI) are identified. By properly identifying each structure, the mistaken diagnosis of posterior pericardial effusion can be avoided.

duction disturbances, and endocarditis. Echocardiography is far more sensitive than a plain chest x-ray in its detection and compares favorably with high intensity fluoroscopy. In the elderly lady shown in this case, calcification of the mitral annulus was suggested from the plain chest x-ray and confirmed with fluoroscopy.

The importance of this echo finding is that it is a cause for a murmur of mitral regurgitation (Table 16–1) and that it can closely simulate the echo pattern of a pericardial effusion. In fact, it is a very common cause of a false-positive reading of pericardial effusion (Table 34–1). On an echo tracing the echo-dense band of a calcified mitral annulus lies just anterior to and runs parallel with the endocardium of the left ventricular posterior wall. Often it can still be recorded when the transducer moves distal to the tip of the anterior leaflet to record the body of the left ventricle (Fig. 40–2). This echo appearance may closely mimic a pericardial effusion if the echo of the calcified annulus is mistaken for the endocardium, the endocardium for the epicardium, and the epicardium for the pericardium. Such a mistake can be avoided by careful adjustments of the gain and dampening controls to properly identify the endocardium just posterior to the calcified annulus and by demonstrating the abrupt termination of this echo-dense structure anterior to the left atrial wall on M-mode scanning. In a pericardial effusion, the true left ventricular posterior wall blends into the left atrial wall on M-mode scan from the left ventricle to the left atrium.

Why the echoes from a calcified mitral annulus are displayed just anterior to the left ventricular posterior wall is not completely clear. If, however, the left ventricular posterior wall is at a slightly greater distance from the transducer than the mitral annulus, the calcified annulus could be picked up by the lateral part of the echo beam, "verticalized" to the center of the beam and displayed on the echo tracing slightly anterior to the left ventricular free wall. A very dense structure is far more likely to be detected by the lateral part of the echo beam than is a less dense structure.

Even though a calcified mitral annulus often will obscure the posterior mitral leaflet, this entity should not be mistaken for rheumatic mitral disease—i.e., mitral stenosis—if the thin anterior mitral leaflet is noted anterior to the echo-dense mitral annulus.

2. (A) and (B). Both right ventricular and left atrial enlargement are documented on measurement as contributing to this patient's cardiomegaly. No echo-free space lies between the left ventricular wall and the pericardium, and thus there is no echo evidence of a pericardial effusion. The left ventricular cavity is not dilated, and the left ventricular free wall is not hypertrophied. Although the septum is not thickened, it has a markedly decreased amplitude of motion. The mildly reduced E-F slope may reflect loss of left ventricular compliance.

CASE 41

This 21-year-old asymptomatic ski instructor is referred for evaluation of systolic and diastolic murmurs detected on a routine physical examination.

MEASUREMENTS (Echo tracings A-C)   **Time lines = 200 msec**

cf	=	EDD	=
Ao	=	ESD	=
LA	=	IVS thickness	=
D-E amplitude	=	Percentage of septal thickening	=
E-F slope	=	LVPW thickness	=
RV	=	LVPW amplitude	=

QUESTIONS

1. What two abnormalities are illustrated on this echocardiogram?

2. Which of the following diagnoses would explain these two abnormalities? More than one may apply.
   (A) Patent ductus arteriosus
   (B) Atrial septal defect
   (C) Mitral valve prolapse
   (D) Anomalous pulmonary venous return
   (E) Ventricular septal defect
   (F) Septal infarction
   (G) Tricuspid regurgitation
   (H) Pulmonic insufficiency
   (I) Left bundle branch block

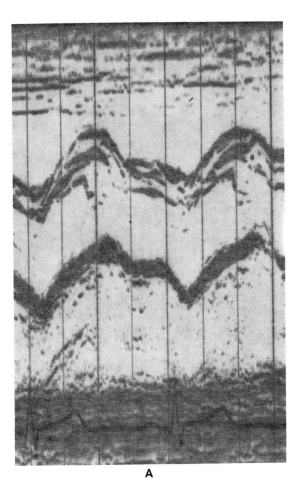

A

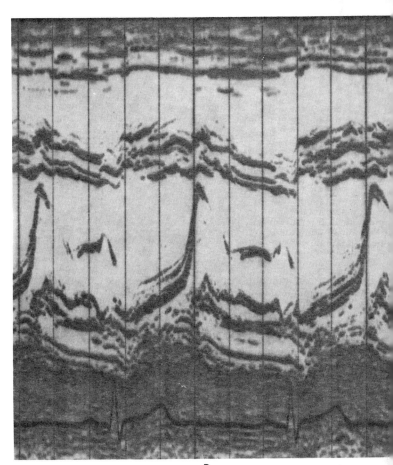

B

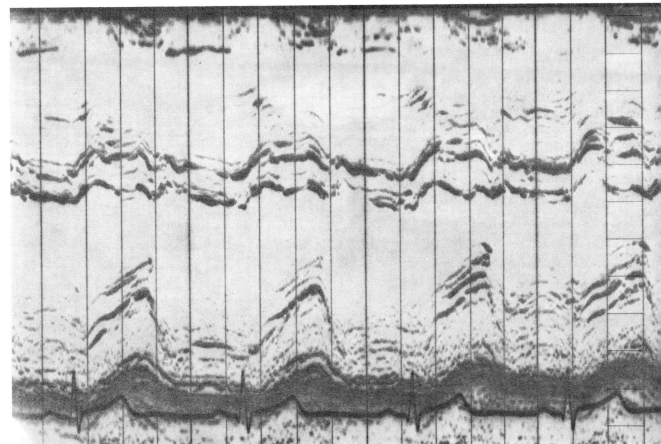

C

237

ANSWERS TO CASE 41
Atrial Septal Defect

MEASUREMENTS

cf	= 1.0	EDD	= 3.8
Ao	= 30 mm	ESD	= 2.5
LA	= 3.9 cm	IVS thickness	= 7 mm
D-E amplitude	= 27 mm	Percentage of septal thickening	= 50%
E-F slope	= 110 mm/sec	LVPW thickness	= 10 mm
RV	= 4.0 cm	LVPW amplitude	= 18 mm

ANSWERS

1. Right ventricular enlargement and abnormal motion of the interventricular septum are the two abnormalities present on this echocardiogram.

2. (B), (D), (G), and (H). As shown in Figure 41–1, there are several characteristic types of abnormal septal motion seen in echocardiography. Right ventricular enlargement and the type of abnormal septal motion present on this echocardiogram are the characteristic echo abnormalities found in states of significant right ventricular volume overload. Therefore, an atrial septal defect,[146, 209, 240-246] anomalous pulmonary venous drainage,[242, 245, 247] tricuspid regurgitation,[240] or pulmonic insufficiency[209] may produce these two abnormalities. Ventricular septal defects with right-to-left shunting are associated with volume overload of both the right and

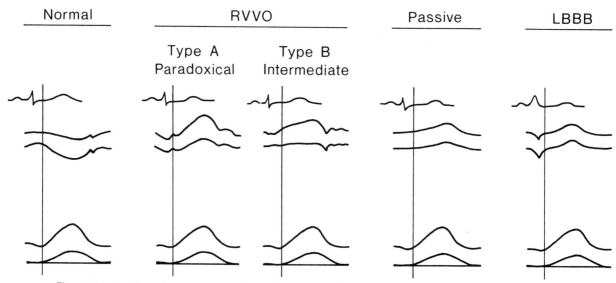

Normal	RVVO		Passive	LBBB
	Type A Paradoxical	Type B Intermediate		

Figure 41–1. Characteristic echocardiographic patterns of abnormal septal motion: the patterns in right ventricular volume overload (*RVVO*) showing active, paradoxic type A and intermediate type B septal motion; the passive paradoxic motion seen in coronary artery disease and cardiomyopathy, and the posterior septal beaking just after the QRS seen in left bundle branch block *(LBBB)*. After this posterior beaking, septal motion is usually paradoxic in LBBB, but it may be flat or even slightly posterior.

TABLE 41–1. Causes of Abnormal Septal Motion

1. Right ventricular volume overload (Cases 41, 42, 43; Table 2–2).
2. Left bundle branch block (Case 43).
3. Wolff-Parkinson-White Syndrome, Type B.[219a, 219b]
4. Coronary artery disease (Case 43).
5. Cardiomyopathy (Cases 32, 33).
6. Open heart surgery (Case 43).
7. Constrictive pericarditis.[210]
8. Absence of pericardium, congenital or acquired.[211]
9. Pericardial effusion (Cases 39, 42; Table 39–1).
10. Left ventricular volume overload (Cases 2, 11, 43; Table 2–2).

left ventricles and do not cause abnormal septal motion.[240] The other diseases listed in this question are either associated with left ventricular volume overload (patent ductus arteriosus and mitral valve prolapse), would not explain the right ventricular enlargement, or are associated with a different pattern of abnormal septal motion.

Two basic types of abnormal septal motion have been described in patients with right ventricular volume overload (Fig. 41–1).[146, 209, 240-242] Type A, in which septal motion is paradoxic or reversed, is recognized when both the septum and the left

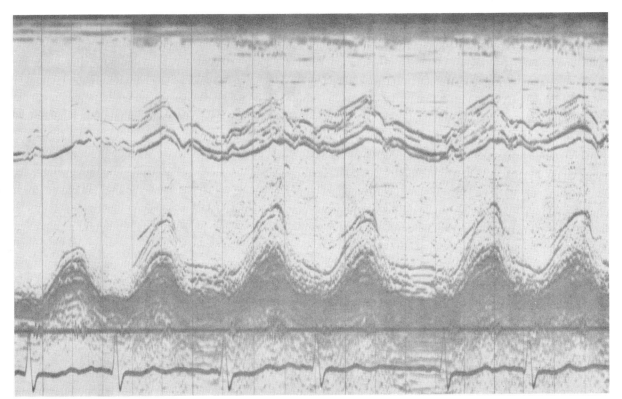

Figure 41–2. Echocardiogram in a patient with total anomalous pulmonary venous drainage. Note right ventricular enlargement and abnormal, paradoxic type A septal motion.

ventricular posterior wall move anteriorly toward the transducer during ventricular systole and posteriorly during diastole. This type of motion is the more common and is shown on echo tracing C of this patient with an atrial septal defect and in Figure 41–2 from a patient with total anomalous pulmonary drainage.

In type B septal motion, which has been described as intermediate between normal motion and type A, the left ventricular side of the septum is flattened with minimal or no movement during systole, and the right ventricular side of the septum moves anteriorly toward the transducer during part or all of systole. In this manner, normal septal systolic thickening is preserved despite abnormal septal motion. Initially, this type B motion was described only in terms of the left ventricular side of the septum, but Radtke and colleagues[246] have stressed the importance of looking at both sides of the septum, in order to appreciate that the right ventricular side moves abnormally toward the transducer even though the left side remains stationary.

Actually, in patients with right ventricular volume overload, there is a wide spectrum of septal motion from completely normal to truly paradoxic (type A). Normal septal motion tends to be associated with smaller left-to-right shunts,[209, 240-242, 244-246, 248] whereas truly paradoxic septal motion usually is observed with larger shunts and probably represents the other end of the spectrum.[240, 242, 245, 246]

Septal motion should be evaluated from tracings recorded at the level of the chordae tendineae below the mitral valve. In normal subjects, on M-mode scan from the aorta toward the left ventricular apex, the superior portion of the septum can be observed to move anteriorly during systole along with the aortic root. As the scan continues inferiorly below the mitral valve to the level of the chordae tendineae, the normal septum moves posteriorly toward the left ventricular posterior wall during systole. Multicrystal, cross-sectional echocardiography in normal subjects has established that there is a pivot point at the junction of the upper one-third and the lower two-thirds of the septum.[209] Above this point, which is located in the plane of the mitral valve, the septum moves anteriorly with the aortic root during systole, whereas below this point it has appropriate posterior systolic motion. Consequently, at the level of the mitral valve, the septum in normal subjects may have either anterior, posterior, variable, or flat motion. Accurate assessment of septal motion, therefore, can only be made at the level of the chordae tendineae below the mitral valve. An exception to this rule is that in young children septal motion is evaluated at the level of the posterior mitral leaflet because the mitral valve lies relatively lower in the ventricle.[3]

With right ventricular volume overload, this septal pivot point shifts to varying degrees inferiorly along the septum, causing a larger area of the septum to move abnormally.[209] This concept of the normal pivot point shifting inferiorly explains the variable spectrum of septal abnormalities observed in patients with atrial septal defects. Pure paradoxic type A septal motion occurs when this pivot point is located low in the septum; intermediate type B motion is seen with less inferior shift of this point. Normal septal motion, which occasionally occurs in atrial septal defects, is recorded if the pivot point does not move below the level of the mitral valve.

The sensitivity of the echo detection of secundum atrial septal defects and sinus venous defects by abnormal septal motion has been reported by several authors and is summarized in Table 41–2. It is apparent that approximately 12 per cent of patients with these defects will have normal septal motion, even at the level of the chordae tendineae. Other workers have reported an even higher incidence of normal septal motion in patients with right ventricular volume overload.[209] Therefore, normal septal motion does not exclude an atrial septal defect. The magnitude of the left-to-right shunt is a factor in determining the pattern of septal motion, although the amount of shunting cannot be accurately predicted from the type of septal mo-

TABLE 41–2. Septal (IVS) Motion in Secundum Atrial Septal Defects or
Sinus Venosus Defects

	Total Patients	*Abnormal IVS Motion*	*Normal IVS Motion*	*Percentage of Abnormal Septal Motion*	*Percentage of Normal Sepal Motion*
Diamond[240]	33	31	2	94	6
Meyer[241]	17	16	1	94	6
Kerber[245]	17	13	4	76	24
Radtke[246]	120	104	16	87	13
TOTALS	187	164	23	88	12

tion. Large left-to-right shunts usually are associated with paradoxic type A motion. Patients with atrial septal defects and normal septal motion tend to have smaller left-to-right shunts with pulmonic-to-systemic flow ratios of less than 2:1 (Table 41–3).[240–242, 245, 246, 248] Although this is not invariably true, the diagnostic accuracy of echo is certainly decreased in patients with smaller shunts.

Other factors may produce normal septal motion, even in the presence of a large atrial septal defect (Table 41–3). As might be expected, patients with balanced atrial shunts in whom there is no right ventricular volume overload have normal septal motion.[240] Mitral regurgitation, as might occur with a cleft mitral valve in an ostium primum defect or with mitral prolapse, may be associated with enough left ventricular volume overload to normalize septal motion even in patients with large atrial septal defects.[242] Pericardial effusions associated with excessive motion of the heart as a whole also may normalize abnormal septal motion.

Whereas normal septal motion may be present in a significant although small number of patients with secundum atrial septal defects, right ventricular enlargement is detected in virtually all these patients. Using the upper limits of the normal right ventricular index as 1.2 cm/m^2, 97 per cent of the patients reported in the four articles summarized in Table 41–2 had right ventricular enlargement.[240, 241, 245, 246] In the six patients reported in these series with a normal right ventricular index, the calculated pulmonic-to-systemic flow ratio was 1.1, 1.2, 1.6, 1.8, 2.4, and 2.8. However, no correlation exists between the size of the right ventricle and the magnitude of the left-to-right shunt. Patients with large shunts may have only minimal right ventricular enlargement, whereas patients with small shunts may show very prominent right ventricular dilatation.[240, 246]

The cause of abnormal septal motion in right ventricular volume overload states is unclear. Diamond and colleagues[240] suggested that abnormal septal motion results from right ventricular stroke volume exceeding left ventricular stroke volume, with the result that the septum functions primarily as a right ventricular structure and moves anteriorly during systole. Tajik and colleagues[242] suggested that the magnitude of the left-to-right shunt was a factor in determining the echocardiographic ab-

TABLE 41–3. Causes of Normal Septal Motion in Atrial Septal Defect

1. Small left-to-right shunt.
2. Balanced shunt.
3. Left ventricular volume overload (i.e., mitral regurgitation).
4. Pericardial effusion.

normalities seen in atrial septal defect, and these observations have been supported by experimental animal studies.[245] However, these factors cannot be the *only* determinants of abnormal septal motion in atrial septal defects. In a substantial portion of cases, surgical correction of the atrial defect does not change the abnormal septal motion.[241, 242, 245, 246] In fact, persistence of abnormal septal motion and right ventricular enlargement postoperatively should not be taken as evidence of residual shunt. Meyer[241] suggested that the mechanism for reversal of septal motion in atrial septal defects is that, as the dilated right ventricle ejects a larger volume of blood during systole, anterior movement of the entire heart exceeds the normal posterior motion of the septum, resulting in a net anterior septal motion. Using cross-sectional echocardiography, Weyman[250a] recently proposed that abnormal septal motion seen in right ventricular volume overload primarily results from a change in the diastolic shape of the left ventricle. As the right ventricle enlarges, the septum becomes concave toward the right ventricle and convex toward the left ventricle. Thus, when the left ventricular walls begin to contract and move inward, the septum is obliged to move anteriorly. He stressed that recorded septal motion results from a complex interplay of this change in diastolic shape of the left ventricle and the motion of the entire heart.

At cardiac catheterization in the young man shown in this case, an atrial septal defect with a pulmonic-to-systemic flow ratio of 4:1 was documented. The systolic pressures in the right ventricle and pulmonary artery were at the upper limits of normal. Surgical correction is planned.

CASE 42

This 28-year-old forest ranger, previously in good health, has experienced pleuritic chest pains, dyspnea, orthopnea, increasing abdominal girth, and weight gain for four weeks. He is admitted to the hospital with prominent cardiomegaly on x-ray, markedly increased jugular venous pressure, and a blood pressure of 70/50. On examination a parasternal heave, systolic and diastolic rubs, and a grade 2/6 basal systolic ejection murmur are present. S2 appears single. His liver is tender and enlarged, and his skin is cold and clammy.

Echo tracings *A*, *B*, and *C* are obtained on admission. The patient undergoes a therapeutic procedure, after which his cardiovascular status improves and echo tracing *D* is obtained.

MEASUREMENTS (Echo tracings *A-D*. Make measurements on both tracings *C* and
D where applicable.)   Time lines = 200 msec

cf	=		EDD	=
Ao	=		ESD	=
LA	=		Percentage of systolic septal thickening	=
RV	=			

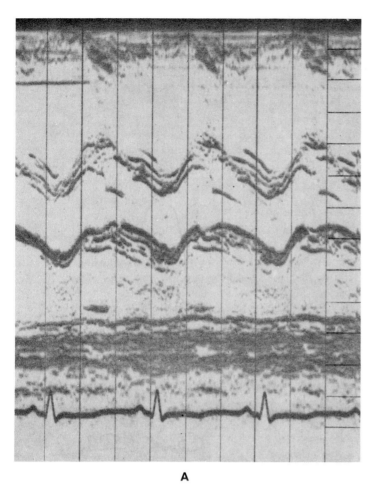

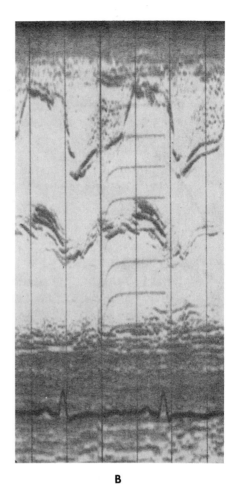

A

B

Illustration continued on the following page.

QUESTIONS

1. This young man probably had which of the following on admission? More than one diagnosis may apply.

   (A) Congenital heart disease
   (B) Endocarditis
   (C) Cardiac tamponade
   (D) Mitral prolapse
   (E) Truncus Arteriosus
   (F) Aortic root dissection

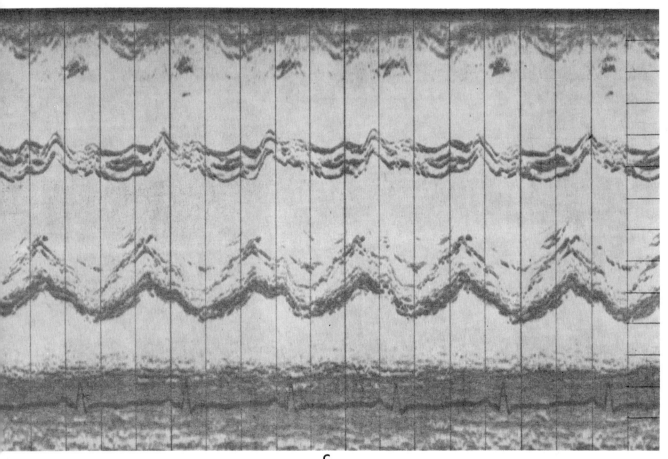

C

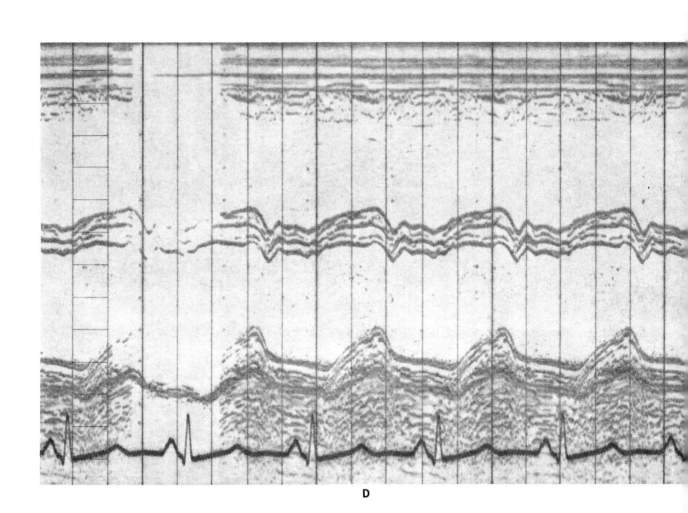

D

ANSWERS TO CASE 42
Atrial Septal Defect
Cardiac Tamponade

MEASUREMENTS

	Echo A to C	*Tracings* D			*Echo* A to C	*Tracings* D
cf =	1.20	1.17	EDD =		3.8 cm	3.6 cm
Ao =	29 mm		ESD =		2.2 cm	2.8 cm
LA =	3.0 cm		Percentage of systolic = septal thickening		35%	33%
RV =	3.6 cm	4.1 cm				

ANSWERS

1. (A) and (C). On echo tracing C, a large echo-free space is present posterior to the epicardium of the left ventricular free wall with the pericardium remaining flat throughout the cardiac cycle. These findings indicate a large pericardial effusion (estimated volume = 670 cc)[1, 185-195] and, in the clinical setting of cardiomegaly, hypotension, and grossly elevated venous pressure, suggest cardiac tamponade. This diagnosis is confirmed by the subsequent clinical course. As 1050 cc of straw-colored fluid were removed by percutaneous pericardiocentesis, the patient's blood pressure rose to 110/80, his venous pressure fell, and his dyspnea improved. Echo tracing D, done within one hour of this procedure, shows loss of the posterior echo-free space.

   This series of echoes is interesting from several standpoints. Despite a pericardial effusion large enough to produce cardiac tamponade, no anterior echo-free space is present. Even though tamponade undoubtedly was present, the heart remains essentially stationary without exaggerated motion (Table 39–1), and the right ventricle is significantly enlarged. The cause of this right ventricular enlargement is discussed below. These findings indicate that a large pericardial effusion is not invariably associated with an anterior echo-free space and that cardiac tamponade can exist even in the presence of significant right ventricular dilatation.

   In addition, motion of the interventricular septum is abnormal. On echo tracing D, after the pericardiocentesis, the left side of the septum is flat during systole, whereas the right side actively moves anteriorly toward the transducer. This pattern of septal motion is the typical type B abnormal septal motion seen in right ventricular volume overload (Fig. 41–1). In combination with marked right ventricular enlargement, it suggests that this young man has congenital heart disease—i.e., an atrial septal defect or anomalous pulmonary venous drainage.[240-247] However, it is noteworthy on tracing C, in the presence of a large pericardial effusion, that septal motion is more nearly normal than immediately after removal of the pericardial fluid. During systole, the right side of the septum on tracing C does not move anteriorly, and the left side of the septum even has a slight posterior motion. The septal notch seen just after the systolic peak of the posterior left ventricular wall is present on both tracings C and D. The basic difference between the septal motion on these two tracings is that on tracing D the septum moves anteriorly during systole, whereas this motion is abolished in the presence of pericardial effusion. Thus, abnormal septal motion secondary to a large atrial septal defect was normalized during cardiac tamponade (Table 41–3). There are several theoretical explanations for this observation. If excess anterior systolic motion of the entire heart is responsible for the abnormal septal motion in right ventricular volume overload, as Meyer and colleagues[241] proposed, and if anterior motion of the heart is dampened in tamponade, septal motion may become normal. Abnormal anterior systolic motion of the septum would also be normalized by excess posterior swinging of the heart with each systole.

These echoes again illustrate that motion of all intracardiac structures relative to the transducer can be altered in the presence of a large pericardial effusion. They emphasize the hazards of making echocardiographic diagnoses in the presence of large pericardial effusions and suggest the need for repeat echo evaluation following resolution of such effusions.

An atrial septal defect with a pulmonic-to-systemic flow ratio of 3:1 was documented at cardiac catheterization done three months after the patient recovered from this episode of idiopathic pericarditis and tamponade. The right ventricular and pulmonary artery pressures were normal. A secundum atrial septal defect was found at the time of surgery.

Right ventricular enlargement and abnormal septal motion are the echo findings in secundum atrial septal defects and in sinus venosus defects. The echo findings in ostium primum and the other manifestations of endocardial cushion defects have been described[251–257] and will be discussed in a later case.

CASE 43

The following six echocardiograms (echo tracings *A-F*) were obtained on patients referred for evaluation of left ventricular function. Identify the abnormalities on each of the echo tracings and then match each echo with the most appropriate case history. The echo tracings should only be used once.

CASE HISTORIES

I. A 55-year-old surgeon with a history of a large antero-septal myocardial infarction eight weeks ago wishes to resume his busy practice and his avocations of tennis and hunting. His heart size is within normal limits on x-ray.

II. A 48-year-old stock broker continues to experience dyspnea with exertion, fatigue, and one-pillow orthopnea three weeks after aortic valve replacement for stenosis and insufficiency. On examination, the prosthetic sounds are intact, but a grade 3/6 murmur of aortic regurgitation has recurred along the left sternal border. The degree of preoperative cardiomegaly has increased on x-ray.

III. A 62-year-old musician with a history of a heart attack three years ago is admitted to the coronary care unit with hypotension and pulmonary edema. One week ago, he was started on a low dose of propranolol for continuing, stable exertional angina.

IV. A 45-year-old disk jockey complains of anginal-type chest pain associated with mild breathlessness on climbing stairs. He has other episodes of more marked dyspnea, but without chest pain, with jogging and sexual intercourse. During a recent treadmill exercise test, he completed Stage III (heart rate = 168/minute) and developed mild chest discomfort and moderate dyspnea. A left bundle branch block pattern occurred during Stage I of the treadmill test and persisted until recovery, when it disappeared.

V. A 55-year-old truck driver with angina and significant congestive heart failure has a large, discrete, left ventricular apical aneurysm on cineangiography. Cardiac index = 1.8 L/min.

VI. A 48-year-old research librarian with pulmonary hypertension develops increasing signs of right-sided heart failure. With an enlarging heart evident on chest x-ray, an echocardiogram is ordered to evaluate left ventricular function.

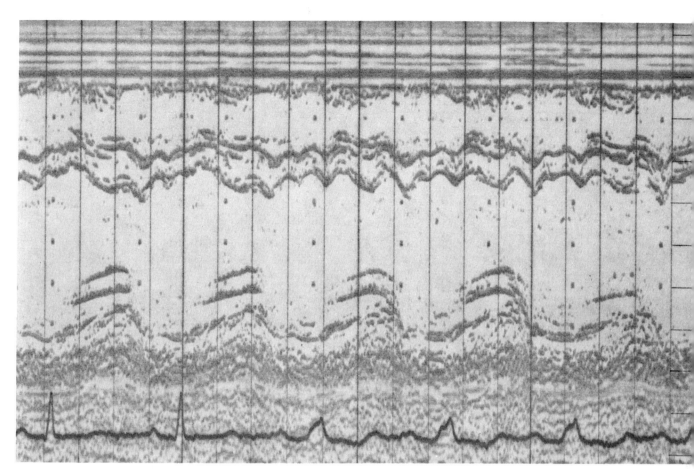

A

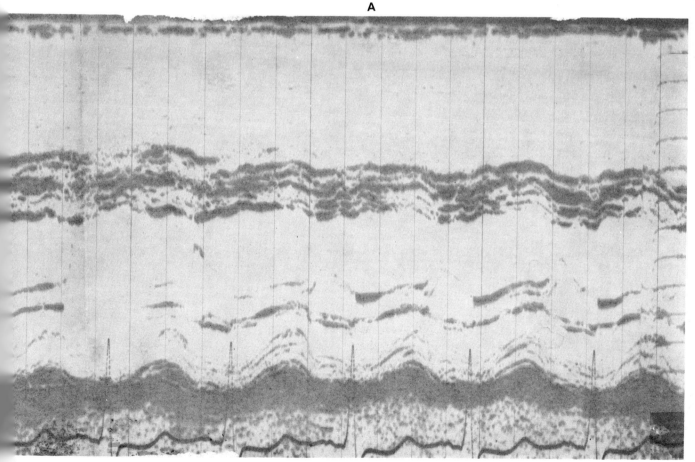

B

249

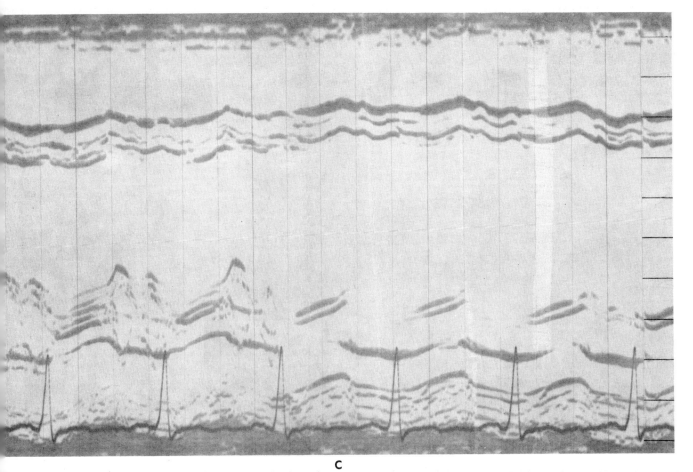

C

250   D

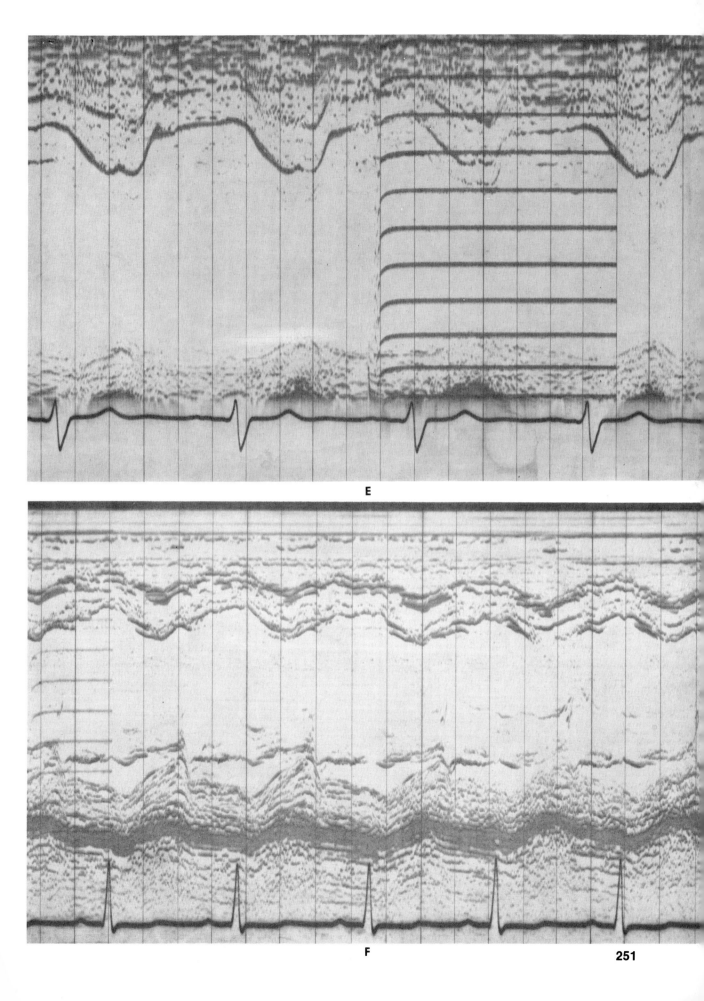

E

F

251

ANSWERS TO CASE 43

ANSWERS

I. Anteroseptal Myocardial Infarction. (D) Flat septum with compensatory increase in LVPW amplitude.

The interventricular septum in this echocardiogram has markedly diminished and almost flattened amplitude of motion, while the left ventricular wall shows an exaggerated amplitude. Localized or isolated reduction of septal motion has been reported to suggest coronary artery disease and to occur in patients with significant obstructive lesions of the left anterior descending coronary artery, even in the absence of myocardial infarction.[171, 171a] Thus, echo tracing *D*, with normal right and left ventricular dimensions, is most compatible with the patient in Case I, who had an anteroseptal infarction but who retains a normal-sized heart on x-ray. Of course, severe lesions of the left anterior descending coronary artery may also occur with completely normal septal motion.

On this echo, the increased amplitude of the left ventricular posterior wall results in a normal calculated ejection fraction and percentage change of the minor diameter, despite the flattened interventricular septum. This type of exaggerated motion of one left ventricular wall with localized disease of another wall illustrates the potential inaccuracy of using echocardiography to evaluate left ventricular function in patients with coronary artery disease who have areas of left ventricular dyssynergy.[148, 155, 168-170] Basic to evaluating myocardial function with echo is the assumption that the recorded motion of the septum and left ventricular posterior wall is representative of all left ventricular walls. This assumption is reasonably valid in the symmetrically contracting ventricle, such as occurs normally and in valvular, generalized myopathic, and congenital heart disease. However, when there is localized myocardial disease, as commonly occurs in coronary disease, these two walls may not be representative of the entire ventricle. Thus, calculations based on these walls—such as volumes, ejection fraction, percentage shortening of the minor diameter, and velocity of circumferential fiber shortening—may not accurately reflect over-all cardiac function. For example, in a patient with an infarction of the left ventricular apex and a large apical aneurysm, the septum and left ventricular posterior wall may continue to move normally. In fact, they may demonstrate compensatory increase in motion, as seen in this patient's posterior wall. In either case, the standard echo, which reports the left ventricle just inferior to the tip of the mitral valve, may overestimate left ventricular function. On the other hand, if there is localized disease of either the proximal septum or left ventricular posterior wall not extensive enough to compromise cardiac output, echocardiography may grossly underestimate over-all left ventricular function. Such considerations illustrate potential limitations of the "ice pick" view of the heart provided by M-mode echocardiography.

Technical Hints. Several echocardiographic techniques have been proposed for examining different parts of the left ventricle in patients with coronary artery disease.[164]

1. By tilting the transducer from its usual position along the left sternal border toward the apex, an M-mode scan of more areas of the left ventricular free wall and of the septum may be obtained.[171]

2. Recording from a lower intercostal space than is usual may show other areas of these walls.
3. Moving the transducer 1 to 2 cm to the left of the sternum so that it does not lie over the interventricular septum has been reported to be a useful technique for recording the anterior wall of the left ventricle.[172]
4. In addition, the left ventricle can be examined with the transducer in the subxiphoid area.[173] With this technique, the transducer is angled superiorly from below the diaphragm to record other, more distal areas of the septum and the posterior lateral wall of the left ventricle. This subxiphoid approach is an extremely useful technique in patients who are difficult to record through the chest because of emphysema or a thick chest cavity.
5. Another technique that is useful in examining the left ventricle is to record the echo at a paper speed of 10 or 25 mm/sec rather than at 50 mm/sec as an M-mode scan is made from the aorta to the left ventricular apex.[164, 174] This technique has been called "condensed" M-mode scanning[174] and is useful in obtaining an appreciation of the over-all shape and function of the left ventricle. This condensed technique may be done from more than one intercostal space and from the subxiphoid area in order to visualize different areas of the left ventricle.

II. Paraprosthetic Aortic Regurgitation. (E) Increased septal amplitude and left ventricular cavity dilatation.

These abnormalities shown on echo tracing E suggest left ventricular volume overload and are most compatible with Case History II of a patient with cardiomegaly and the recurrence of aortic regurgitation after aortic valve replacement. Abnormal septal motion of either a true paradoxic or hypokinetic type is the usual pattern immediately after aortic and, to a lesser extent, mitral valve replacement.[212] This abnormality occurs regularly, even in the absence of conduction disturbances such as left bundle branch block. The explanation for this postoperative abnormal septal motion is not completely clear. Some patients have return of normal septal motion during the first several postoperative months, but the finding of exaggerated septal motion after aortic valve replacement suggests a cause of left ventricular volume overload, such as paraprosthetic aortic regurgitation. Miller[213] and Brodie[214] have reported that patients with paravalvular regurgitation have normal or increased septal motion similar to that shown by this patient. In fact, Brodie has stated that hypokinetic or paradoxic septal motion makes significant paravalvular regurgitation unlikely.[214]

Significant localized paraprosthetic aortic regurgitation was documented on cineangiography in this patient. The septum, which was well visualized on the angiogram, was noted to be extremely active.

III. Heart Failure and Hypotension After Propranolol Therapy. (C) Marked left ventricular cavity dilatation and dysfunction with passive septal motion.

Of the echo tracings shown, tracing C is the left ventricle most likely to develop marked failure as a result of the negative inotropic effect of propranolol. The EDD is significantly increased, the septum shows a passive type of paradoxic motion, and the echo of the mitral valve suggests left ventricular dilatation and dysfunction with a "double-diamond" configuration and increased distance between the E point and septum (Cases 32 and 33).[70] Echocardiographic evaluation of left ventricular size and function prior to initiating propranolol therapy may aid in identifying those patients with such compromised myocardial function who are at increased risk of developing significant cardiac failure when using this drug. Propranolol has been demonstrated by echocardiography to increase left ventricular end-diastolic volume and to decrease left ventricular ejection fraction in patients with stable angina.[182] A similar study has shown an increase in the left ventricular end-diastolic dimension produced by propranolol in patients with mitral prolapse.[182a]

The interventricular septum on echo tracing C has paradoxic motion toward the transducer during systole, but note that its motion is of a completely passive nature, as compared to the active type of abnormal septal motion seen with right ventricular volume overload (Fig. 41–1).[171, 215] In these volume overload states, the septum actively thickens during systole, even though it moves toward the transducer or remains predominantly flat. With passive paradoxic motion, septal thickness does not change significantly during systole and the septum appears to be pushed toward the transducer, away from the contracting posterior left ventricular wall. This lack of change will be reflected in a low value for percentage of septal thickening. Such passive septal motion occurs in coronary artery disease with severe obstructive disease of the left anterior descending coronary artery, following acute septal myocardial infarctions, with septal dyskinesia and aneurysms, and in cardiomyopathy.[2, 171, 216] It must be distinguished from abnormal septal motion with active systolic thickening, because it does not suggest right ventricular volume overload.

IV. Rate Dependent Left Bundle Branch Block. (A) Development of posterior "beaking" of the septum just after the QRS.

The typical septal abnormality of left bundle branch block begins with the third cardiac cycle on echo tracing A, as the patient develops a rate-related left bundle branch block (Fig. 41–1).[217-219] With the development of this conduction abnormality, the left side of the septum characteristically shows a very rapid posterior motion within approximately 50 msec of the QRS prior to the beginning of the contraction

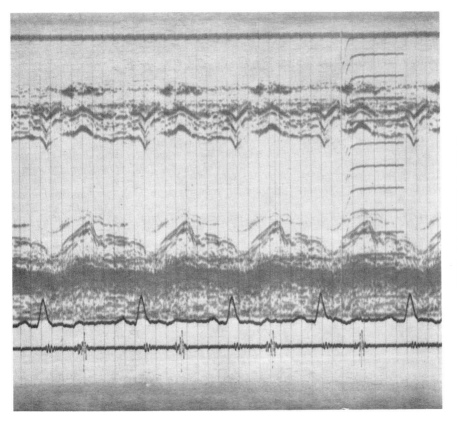

Figure 43–1. Abnormal septal motion typical of left bundle branch block with very rapid posterior motion of the septum occurring just after the QRS and before contraction of the left ventricular posterior wall. Following this early contraction, the septum moves anteriorly toward the transducer during systole in a paradoxic manner. This patient also had a rate-dependent left bundle branch block.

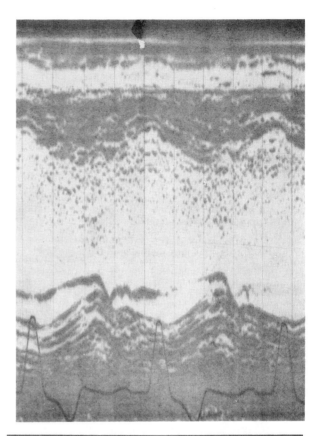

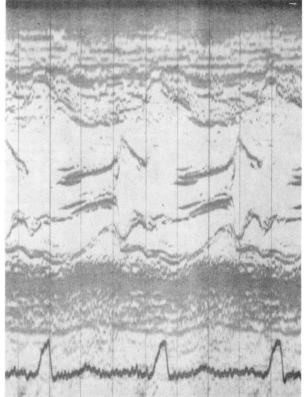

Figure 43–2. Echocardiograms from two patients with the typical ECG pattern of left bundle branch block who have normal septal motion. Both patients have systemic hypertension.

of the left ventricular posterior wall. This sharp posterior "beaking" is the primary feature that distinguishes the septal motion of left bundle branch block from other types of abnormal septal motion.[217] Following this posterior motion, the septum usually moves anteriorly toward the transducer, as the left ventricular posterior wall contracts. This typical paradoxic motion following the posterior "beaking" is shown in Figure 43–1 from another patient, who also has a rate-related left bundle branch block. However, the motion of the septum after the posterior "beaking" is variable in left bundle branch block. It may be flat[218, 219] or it may even have some posterior motion, as on echo tracing *F* from this case.

Septal activation prior to contraction of the left ventricle has been suggested as the mechanism of the typical abnormal septal motion in left bundle branch block.[217-219] With initial septal activation from right-to-left instead of from the usual left-to-right, the septum contracts and moves sharply posteriorly, while the rest of the left ventricle is quiescent. When the rest of the left ventricle does contract, the septum is relaxed and is pushed anteriorly away from the posterior left ventricular wall.[218]

Some patients with typical left bundle branch block have completely normal septal motion, as shown in Figure 43–2.[218, 219] These patients probably have a left bundle branch block pattern on the basis of delayed conduction in the distal left Purkinje system rather than in the bundle branch itself. Right bundle branch block is not associated with abnormal septal motion.

Patients with Wolff-Parkinson-White syndrome who have pre-excitation of the anterior or lateral wall of the right ventricle (Type B pre-excitation) have been reported to have abnormal septal motion during anomalous conduction that is very similar to that occurring in left bundle branch block.[219a, 219b] Immediately after the delta wave on the electrocardiogram, the septum in these patients may move abruptly posteriorly.[219a] It then moves anteriorly during systole along with the left ventricular free wall in a truly paradoxic manner.

V. Left Ventricular Apical Aneurysm. (F) Normal septum and posterior left ventricular wall.

Echo tracing *F* is consistent with a discrete left ventricular apical aneurysm large enough to compromise cardiac output, even though the motion of the septum and posterior wall is within normal limits and the minor left ventricular diameter is only slightly increased. By recording the usual "ice pick" view of the septum and basalar portions of the left ventricular free wall, the echo in this case completely misses the presence of the apical aneurysm. Consequently, because the septum and posterior wall are not representative of all cardiac walls, cardiac function is grossly overestimated. The aneurysm might have been detected if the techniques of scanning toward the apex, recording from a lower intercostal space or from the subxiphoid area, had been used.[171-174] However, this case serves as a dramatic example of the limitation of standard echo techniques in coronary artery disease, especially in reference to not detecting abnormalities of the anterior apical wall.

VI. Pulmonary Hypertension. (B) RV enlargement, asymmetric septal hypertrophy, and abnormal IVS motion.

Marked right ventricular enlargement and asymmetric septal hypertrophy shown on echo tracing *B* suggest pulmonary hypertension and are most compatible with Case History VI. In addition, the septal motion is abnormal, moving paradoxically toward the transducer during systole and away in diastole. With right ventricular enlargement, this abnormal septal motion suggests a cause of right ventricular volume overload, i.e., tricuspid regurgitation, pulmonic insufficiency, atrial septal defect, or anomalous pulmonary venous drainage.

At cardiac catheterization, this patient was shown to have an atrial septal defect with left-to-right shunting and severe pulmonary hypertension.

CASE 44

This 39-year-old hospital administrator who is experiencing increasing dyspnea on exertion is sent for an echocardiogram to exclude an atrial septal defect, pulmonic stenosis, or any mitral valve disease. The patient has known of heart disease and an enlarged heart since age 13, when a cardiac catheterization, the details of which are not available, was performed. A parasternal lift, a grade 2/6 systolic ejection murmur along the left sternal border, and clubbing without cyanosis are present.

MEASUREMENTS   (Echo tracings *A-F*)   **Time lines = 200 msec**

cf	=	IVS thickness	=
Ao leaflet opening	=	IVS amplitude	=
LA	=	LVPW thickness	=
E-F slope	=	LVPW amplitude	=
D-E amplitude	=		
RV	=		
EDD	=		

QUESTIONS

1. Which of the following abnormalities are present on this echocardiogram?

   (A) Asymmetric septal hypertrophy
   (B) Abnormal septal motion
   (C) Abnormal tricuspid valve
   (D) Right ventricular enlargement
   (E) Small left ventricular cavity
   (F) Pansystolic mitral bowing
   (G) Systolic anterior mitral motion
   (H) Left ventricular hypertrophy
    (I) Left atrial enlargement
    (J) Bicuspid aortic valve
   (K) Partial midsystolic closure of the pulmonic valve

2. Which of the following diagnoses is (are) suggested by these observations?

   (A) Ebstein's anomaly
   (B) Mitral valve prolapse
   (C) Right ventricular volume overload (atrial septal defect, tricuspid insufficiency)
   (D) Hypertrophic subaortic stenosis
   (E) Pulmonic stenosis
   (F) Pulmonary hypertension

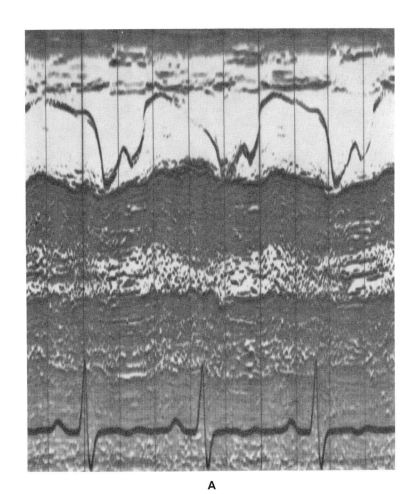

A

B

259

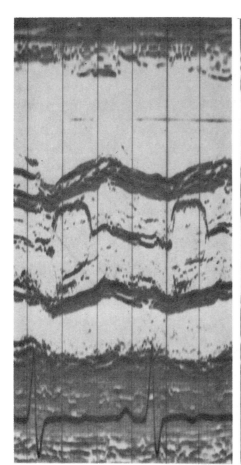
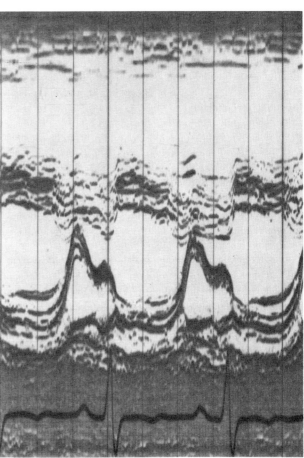

C   D

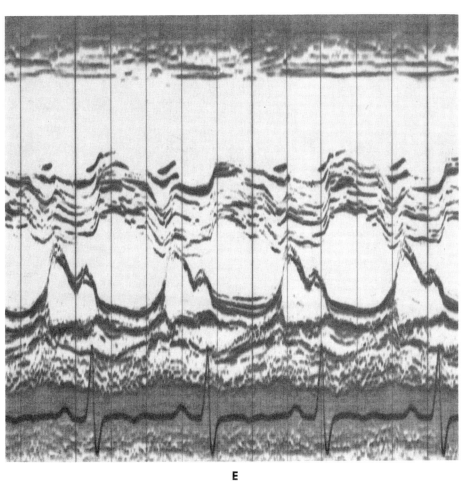

E

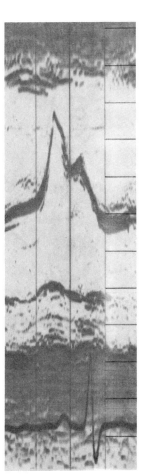

F

ANSWERS TO CASE 44
Primary Pulmonary Hypertension

MEASUREMENTS (Echo tracings A-F)   **Time lines = 200 msec**

cf	= 1.02	IVS thickness	= 15 mm
Ao leaflet opening	= 1.8 cm	IVS amplitude	= 10–13 mm
LA	= 2.0 cm	LVPW thickness	= 9–10 mm
E-F slope	= 110–140 mm/sec	LVPW amplitude	= 7 mm
D-E amplitude	= 21 mm	e-f slope of	
		pulmonic valve	= 20 mm/sec
RV	= 3.3 cm	a wave of	
		pulmonic valve	= < 2 mm
EDD	= 3.7 cm		

ANSWERS

1. (A), (B), (D), (F), (K); 2. (B), (C), and (F).

As listed in Table 44-1, the echocardiographic observations in pulmonary hypertension fall into two categories: (1) certain abnormal changes in the echo of the pulmonic valve and (2) certain other associated abnormalities, such as right ventricular dilatation, abnormal septal motion, and asymmetric septal hypertrophy.[1,2, 220-224] The echo of the normal pulmonic valve and the changes that occur in it with pulmonary hypertension are discussed below. However, if the pulmonic valve is not recorded, right ventricular dilatation and asymmetric septal hypertrophy (ASH) may be the only echo hints of pulmonary hypertension. In fact, when ASH occurs with right ventricular dilatation, it suggests pulmonary hypertension. These two abnormalities are the echo findings in primary pulmonary hypertension. Asymmetric septal hypertrophy with ratios of septal thickness/LVPW thickness of greater than 1.3 results from the right ventricular hypertrophy associated with pulmonary hyperten-

TABLE 44-1. Echocardiographic Findings in Pulmonary Hypertension

Pulmonic Valve[221]

1. "a wave" depth = 0 to 2 mm   (normal = 2–7 mm)
2. e-f slope   = −9 to +30 mm/sec (normal = 6–115 mm/sec)
3. Partial midsystolic closure or systolic notch

Associated Findings	*Diagnoses Simulated*	*How Differentiate*
1. RV dilatation 2. Abnormal septal motion	Atrial septal defect	Cardiac catheterization

3. Asymmetric septal
  hypertrophy (ASH)
 	
4. Small LV cavity
	Hypertrophic subaortic
	stenosis
		RV dilatation
		Absent mitral systolic
		  anterior motion (SAM)

5. Reduced E-F slope of
  mitral valve
	Mitral stenosis	Normal mitral density
		Normal motion of the
		  posterior mitral leaflet

sion. It is differentiated from the septal hypertrophy found in hypertrophic subaortic stenosis by the presence of right ventricular dilatation and by the absence of systolic anterior motion of the mitral valve.

Abnormal motion of the interventricular septum, either of type A or B, can also be associated with pulmonary hypertension. Because septal motion is normal in patients with only a right ventricular pressure overload,[1, 240] such abnormal septal motion combined with right ventricular dilatation suggests an associated cause of right ventricular volume overload—i.e., tricuspid regurgitation, pulmonic insufficiency, or an atrial septal defect. However, the echocardiographic picture of primary pulmonary hypertension with secondary tricuspid or pulmonic regurgitation may be very difficult to differentiate from an atrial septal defect with secondary pulmonary hypertension. In both cases, there may be right ventricular dilatation, abnormal septal motion, and asymmetric septal hypertrophy. The echo of the pulmonic valve in such cases would be consistent with pulmonary hypertension. Differentiation between such similar abnormalities requires cardiac catheterization.

A small left ventricular minor dimension may also be recorded in pulmonary hypertension. The reduced cardiac output and stroke volume found in these patients may be related to this finding. In addition, the shape and orientation of the left ventricle may be so altered by the hypertrophied, dilated right ventricle that an abnormally small left ventricular dimension is detected echocardiographically.

Reduction in the E-F slope of the anterior mitral leaflet is also sometimes recorded. This decreased diastolic slope may result from a reduced rate of left ventricular filling secondary to distortion of the left ventricular geometry or to alteration in the actual diastolic compliance of the interventricular septum.[223] In some patients with pulmonary hypertension and a low E-F slope, the anterior leaflet comes in direct contact with the septum during the entire initial part of diastole. In these patients, an abnormally small left ventricular minor diameter that mechanically restricts mitral valve motion may be responsible for the low mitral E-F slope.[220] Mitral stenosis can be excluded in such cases by identifying a normal echo density of the mitral valve and normal motion of the posterior mitral leaflet.

On echo tracing *B* from this case, asymmetric septal hypertrophy (IVS thickness/LVPW thickness ratio = 1.5 to 1.7) and right ventricular dilatation suggest pulmonary hypertension. In addition, septal motion is abnormal. It is not typical type A or type B abnormal motion in that the left side of the septum moves posteriorly away from the transducer as the left ventricular wall moves anteriorly during systole.[240] However, there is abrupt, prominent anterior motion of the septum within 50 msec of the R wave on the electrocardiogram before the septum moves posteriorly. Thus, there is no net posterior motion of the left side of the septum from end-diastole to end-systole.[220, 246] This type of prominent anterior motion of the septum in early systole may be the only septal abnormality seen in some patients with right ventricular volume overload. In combination with right ventricular dilatation, this abnormal septal motion suggests a cause of right ventricular volume overload such as tricuspid regurgitation, pulmonic insufficiency, or atrial septal defect in the patient shown in this case.

On echo tracings *D* and *E*, the systolic motion of the mitral valve is abnormal, with gradual bowing of the C-D segment posterior to an imaginary line connecting the C and the D points. This pattern suggests pansystolic mitral prolapse. Goodman and colleagues[220] reported similar findings of prolapse in four of nine patients with primary pulmonary hypertension in whom there was no evidence of the midsystolic click, late systolic murmur syndrome. They postulated that this finding may be evidence of a connective tissue disorder involving the mitral valve in these patients. It could also be postulated that right ventricular dilatation changes the orientation of

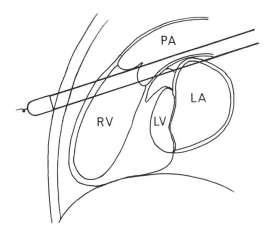

Figure 44–1. Anatomic relationship of the pulmonary artery (*PA*) and the pulmonic valve to the transducer and echo beam. Note that the pulmonic valve is recorded from below and that only one cusp is usually seen. When the valve opens, this cusp moves away from the transducer.

the mitral valve so that it moves primarily away from the transducer during systole. This change could result in an echo pattern of pansystolic mitral prolapse similar to the false mitral prolapse recorded with inferior angulation of the transducer.

Understanding the echo of the pulmonic valve is facilitated by an appreciation of the relationship of the echo beam to the pulmonary artery and its valve (Fig. 44–1). The transducer is aimed very superiorly to record the pulmonic valve, with the result that its beam usually passes obliquely through the vertical axis of the main pulmonary artery and records the pulmonic valve from below. Because of this orientation of the pulmonary artery and valve, only a posterior pulmonic cusp is usually recorded (Fig. 44–2). During diastole, this cusp is visualized as an anteriorly located echo, whereas, when the pulmonic valve opens, the cusp moves sharply away from the transducer and is recorded as a posteriorly moving echo. In the rare instances in which anterior pulmonic cusp is also recorded, it is seen to move anteriorly toward the transducer during ventricular systole (Fig. 44–3). Normally during atrial systole, as blood flows into the right ventricle, the right ventricular end-diastolic pressure is increased and may momentarily slightly exceed a normal pul-

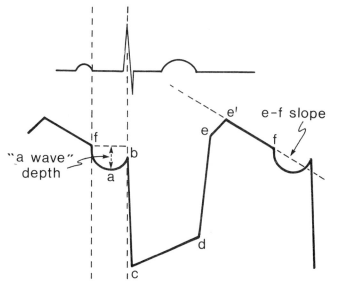

Figure 44–2. Illustration of the normal echo pattern of the posterior pulmonic cusp in diastole and systole. Relationship of this pattern to the electrocardiogram and the measurement of the depth of the "a wave" and the e-f slope are shown.

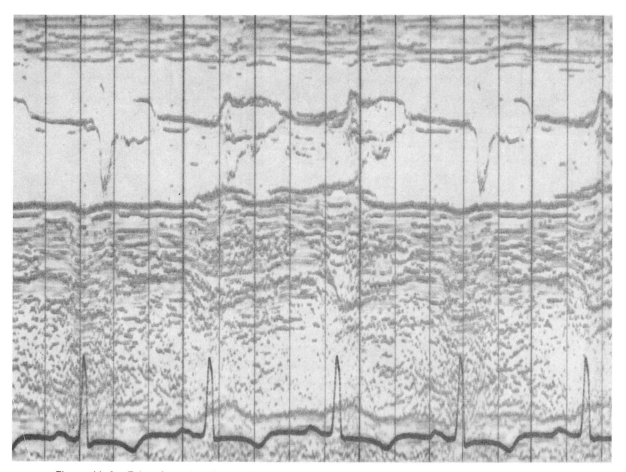

Figure 44–3. Echo of a pulmonic valve from a patient with pulmonary hypertension in whom two pulmonic cusps were recorded. Note the prominent partial midsystolic closure of the posterior cusp, the flat e-f slope and the absent "a wave."

monary artery end-diastolic pressure. As a result, the pulmonic cusps are slightly elevated. This elevation or doming of the pulmonic valve is represented on the echo as a posterior motion, the "a wave," beginning just after the P wave of the electrocardiogram and prior to the opening of the pulmonic valve with ventricular systole. In normal subjects, the depth of this "a wave" varies with respiration, with its maximal depth occurring during inspiration as the amount of venous return to the right side of the heart increases.

Lettering of the systolic and diastolic portions of the pulmonic valve echo has been proposed to facilitate discussion and examination.[221, 225] These lower case letters, which are temporally similar to those used to describe mitral valve motion, are illustrated in Figure 44–2. The "a wave," which begins just after the P wave of the electrocardiogram, represents the slight doming of the pulmonic valve that occurs as a result of right atrial systole ejecting blood into the right ventricle. Point b represents the position of the cusp at the beginning of ventricular systole. In normal subjects, particularly when the "a wave" is deep during inspiration or the PR interval is short, the cusp may not have time to return to the base line before it opens. After the onset of ventricular systole, the pulmonic cusp echo moves rapidly posteriorly and reaches its fully opened position at point c. A pulmonic ejection click would be coincident with this c point. The c-d portion, which may normally have some high-frequency vibration, rises slightly anteriorly throughout systole. It is followed by rapid closure of the cusp at the e point. During diastole, the cusp gradually moves posteriorly to point f, which immediately precedes the onset of the "a wave." Sometimes after closure of the pulmonic valve at point e, the cusp continues to move anteriorly to point e' before moving posteriorly to point f.

Several measurements useful in the diagnosis of pulmonary hypertension and pulmonic stenosis can be made from the pulmonic valve echogram.[2, 221, 225-227] The depth of the "a wave" is measured from where the slope of the diastolic portion of the pulmonic valve echo abruptly changes just following the P wave of the ECG to where the "a wave" reaches its maximum depth. Because the "a wave" depth normally increases with inspiration and decreases with expiration, the maximum depth recorded during the inspiratory phase of quiet respiration should be measured. Deep inspiration should be avoided, as it may falsely exaggerate this measurement. The e-f slope of the pulmonic valve is measured in millimeters/second from the most anterior position of the cusp at the beginning of diastole (point e or e') to the position of the cusp at the onset of atrial contraction (point f). If the e-f slope changes in mid-diastole, before the beginning of the "a wave," the initial rapid slope just after the most anterior position of the cusp should be measured.

In pulmonary hypertension, the echo abnormalities of the pulmonary valve usually are (1) an absent "a wave," (2) a flattened e-f slope, and (3) partial midsystolic closure or systolic notch of the posterior pulmonic cusp (Table 44-1).[2, 220-222, 224, 227] As discussed above, the "a wave" is a reflection of doming of the pulmonic valve, when right ventricular end-diastolic pressure briefly exceeds pulmonary artery end-diastolic pressure as a result of atrial systole. However, in pulmonary hypertension, pulmonary artery end-diastolic pressure usually is well above right ventricular end-diastolic pressure. The pulmonic valve is under pressure, tense, and essentially stationary. Consequently, the "a wave" of the pulmonic valve echo usually is abolished or markedly dampened. The level of pulmonary hypertension at which these changes occur has not been firmly established, although Gramiak[2] has reported that the "a wave" is abolished when the mean pulmonary artery pressure exceeds 50 mm Hg, and that its amplitude is reduced under 2 mm when the mean pulmonary artery pressure ranges between 20 and 40 mm Hg. However, the presence of right ventricular failure can alter these findings.[2, 221] If right ventricular end-diastolic pressure is significantly increased, it may exceed an elevated pulmonary artery end-diastolic pressure as the result of atrial systole. Thus, a normal "a wave" of the pulmonic valve echogram can occur in pulmonary hypertension if right ventricular failure also is present. In addition, the presence of a pericardial effusion of moderate or large size can spuriously increase the "a wave" of the pulmonic valve secondary to excess motion of the entire heart.

Although a flat e-f slope usually occurs in pulmonary hypertension, this finding is generally less useful. The large overlap of the normal values and those found in pulmonary hypertension for this slope is evident from Table 44-1. In fact, a flat e-f slope occasionally may be recorded in normal individuals. Consequently, pulmonary hypertension should not be suggested from the echo solely on the basis of a flat or reduced e-f slope. On the other hand, Weyman and co-workers[221] have reported that a negative e-f slope only occurs in patients with pulmonary hypertension.

Partial midsystolic closure of the pulmonary valve or an abrupt notch occurring on the systolic c-d portion of the pulmonic valve echo has been reported as a reliable finding in pulmonary hypertension.[221] The explanation for this systolic notch is unclear, but it may be related to alterations in pulmonary artery flow secondary to loss of capacity of the pulmonary bed or to elevation in pulmonary resistance. Various echo patterns of the posterior pulmonic cusp during systole may be seen in pulmonary hypertension (Fig. 44-4). Partial midsystolic closure of the c-d segment of the pulmonic valve can be recorded as either a smooth or irregularly vibrating notch that is followed by reopening. On the other hand, the posterior cusp may partially close in midsystole and not move posteriorly again prior to complete closure.

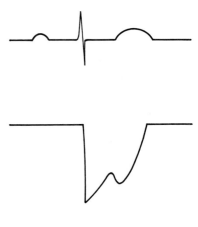

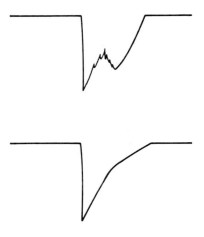

Figure 44–4. Patterns of the partial midsystolic closure or systolic notch of the pulmonic valve seen in pulmonary hypertension.

These types of notching must be distinguished from the fine, high-frequency vibration that may be seen on the pulmonic valve echo in normal patients.

Other abnormalities of the pulmonary valve echogram have been found in pulmonary hypertension. Gramiak[2] reported that the maximal opening slope of the pulmonic valve exceeds 350 mm/sec in pulmonary hypertension. Hirschfeld and co-workers[228] reported that determination of right ventricular systolic time intervals from the pulmonic valve echogram was useful in evaluating the pulmonary vascular bed in a selected group of patients with congenital heart disease.

The pulmonic valve echo from the patient in this case is shown on echo tracing A. A dampened "a wave," less than 2 mm, and a typical midsystolic notch of the C-D segment of the pulmonic valve are shown. These findings support enlargement of the right ventricle and asymmetric septal hypertrophy in suggesting pulmonary hypertension in this patient. Note that the e-f slope of the pulmonic valve is within normal limits, although it does fall within the range reported to occur in pulmonary hypertension.[221]

At a recent cardiac catheterization, moderately severe primary pulmonary hypertension was documented in this man. The pulmonary artery pressure was 74/30, with a mean of 44 mm Hg; the right ventricular pressure was 74/12; and the mean right atrial pressure was 13 mm Hg, with a prominent "v" wave. The cardiac index was within normal limits at 2.4 L/min. No intracardiac shunting was present, as evidenced by the absence of oxygen step-ups, normal hydrogen appearance times, and normal dye dilution curves.

As discussed above, this case illustrates the similarity of the echocardiograms in primary pulmonary hypertension with tricuspid or pulmonic regurgitation and an atrial septal defect with secondary pulmonary hypertension. Only cardiac catheterization can reliably make this distinction.

CASE 45

This 52-year-old union leader with a history of emphysema is admitted to the Pulmonary Intensive Care Unit with severe dyspnea, hypotension, and hypoxia. He is promptly intubated and treated for pulmonary edema. Increased venous pressure, cyanosis, weak carotid pulses, and a blood pressure of 80/60 are present. S1 is normal, S2 is very soft and single, and a grade 2/6 systolic ejection murmur is heard along the left sternal border. With cardiomegaly evident on his chest x-ray, an echocardiogram is ordered to exclude a pericardial effusion and assess valvular disease.

MEASUREMENTS (Echo tracings *A-B*)   **Time lines = 200 msec**

Make all appropriate measurements.

QUESTION

Which of the following diagnoses is (are) suggested by this echocardiogram? For each diagnosis selected, list at least three abnormal echo observations that are present on this tracing and that support the diagnosis.

- (A) Aortic root dissection
- (B) Aortic stenosis
- (C) Mitral stenosis
- (D) Tricuspid stenosis
- (E) Endocarditis
- (F) Prosthetic valve dysfunction
- (G) Intracardiac tumor
- (H) Pulmonary hypertension
- (I) Pericardial effusion
- (J) Congenital heart disease

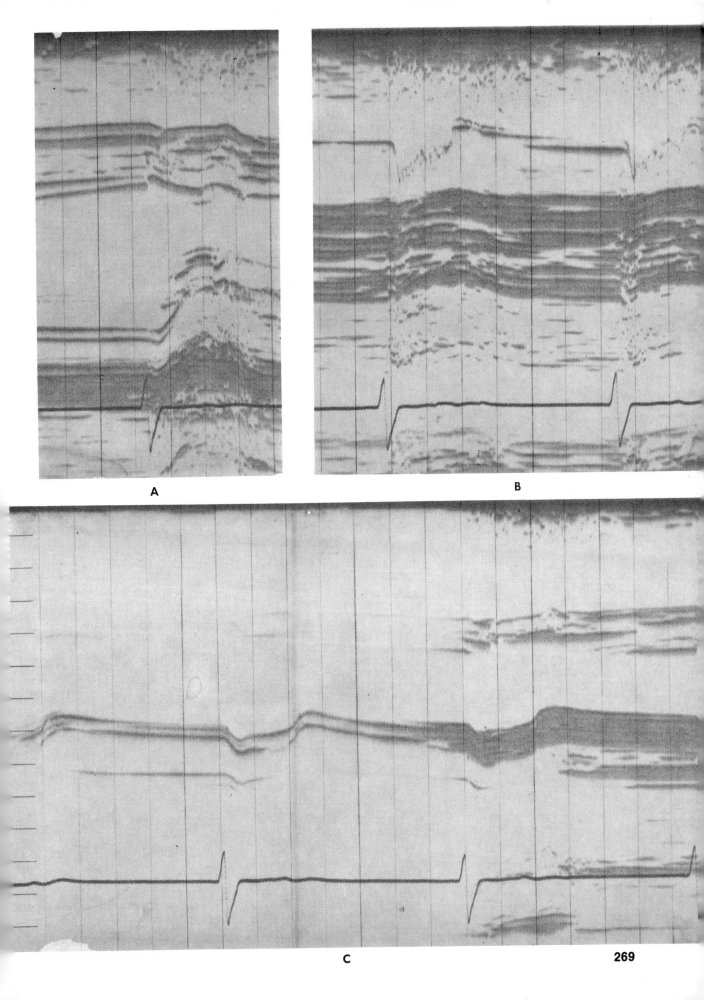

A

B

C

ANSWERS TO CASE 45
Mitral Stenosis, Severe
Pulmonary Hypertension

MEASUREMENTS

cf	= 1.16	LVPW thickness	= 11 mm
E-F slope	= 5 mm/sec	LVPW amplitude	= 16 mm
C-E amplitude	= 8 mm	IVS thickness/LVPW thickness	= 1.5
D-E amplitude	= 5 mm	EDD	= 4.6
RV	= 2.6 cm	ESD	= 2.9
IVS thickness	= 17 mm	Ejection fraction	= 68%
IVS amplitude	= 4 mm	Percentage change	= 37%
		e-f slope of pulmonic valve	= 5–10 mm/sec

ANSWER

(C) and (H).

The diagnosis of severe mitral stenosis is evident from echo tracing C, which shows a markedly echo-dense mitral valve with a very reduced E-F slope and opening amplitude of the anterior leaflet (Tables 8–1, 8–2).[42-47] The mitral valve has such increased echo density that the anterior leaflet is well seen, even when the reject control is increased to completely abolish the septum and posterior cardiac wall. Conglomerate mitral echoes are recorded when the septum is seen.[61] An absent mitral A wave, of course, is expected in atrial fibrillation.

Pulmonary hypertension is also suggested by the asymmetric septal hypertrophy and right ventricular dilatation shown on echo tracing A and by the pattern of the pulmonic valve on tracing B (Table 44–1).[220-224] The e-f slope of this pulmonic valve is very reduced, and its c-d segment shows partial midsystolic closure. Again, the absence of an "a wave" is expected in atrial fibrillation and, in this case, cannot be used to support the diagnosis of pulmonary hypertension.

Both severe mitral stenosis and severe pulmonary hypertension were documented at cardiac catheterization.

Technical Hints. Several methods have been described for recording the pulmonic valve, which is located superior and anterior to the mitral valve, and superior, leftward, and more anterior than the aortic valve (Fig. 45–1).

1. In one approach described by Gramiak,[2, 229] the aortic valve is first identified. Then the echo beam is aimed through the supravalvular portion of the aortic root either by angling the transducer cephalad or by moving the transducer one interspace higher. From this higher location, the beam is gradually angled in a lateral cephalad direction toward the patient's left shoulder. As the parallel walls of the aorta disappear, the pulmonary artery becomes visible as another echo-free space more anterior than the aorta. With small adjustments of the angle of the transducer and the gain settings, the pulmonary valve cusps can be recorded as thin echoes moving within the pulmonary artery. The posterior boundary of the pulmonary artery is recorded as a wide band of dense echoes just posterior to the pulmonic valve. These echo densities are thought to be the right ventricular outflow tract.

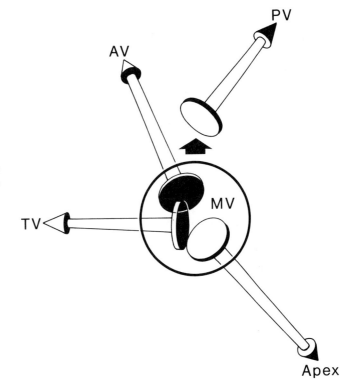

Figure 45–1. Transducer positions in reference to the mitral valve (*MV*), aortic valve (*AV*), tricuspid valve (*TV*), pulmonic valve (*PV*), and cardiac apex.

2. Another method of recording the pulmonic valve is to first visualize the mitral valve.[221, 225, 227] Then, either from the same interspace or more commonly from one interspace higher, the transducer is angled superiorly toward the patient's throat, but not as medially as when a scan is made to the aorta. As the echo beam moves superiorly, first a dense band of echoes and then a more anterior echo-free space is visualized. Within this echo-free pulmonary artery, the thin pulmonary valve cusps can be recorded with slight adjustments of the transducer and gain settings.

Examples of the pulmonic valve echo in pulmonary hypertension have been shown in previous cases. In Case 7, on echo tracing *E*, the posterior pulmonic cusp has no "a wave," even in the presence of sinus rhythm. There is partial midsystolic closure, and the e-f slope is flattened. In Case 33, on echo tracing *B*, the pulmonic cusp has no "a wave" following the P wave of the electrocardiogram. The e-f slope, however, is within the normal range, and a midsystolic notch is not clearly recorded.

CASE 46

A 32-year-old graduate student who had a cardiac operation 20 years ago is found to have a grade 3/6 systolic ejection murmur at the base of the heart and a grade 3/6 blowing early diastolic murmur along the left sternal border. The following echocardiogram is obtained.

MEASUREMENTS   (Echo tracings *A-D*)   **Time lines = 200 msec**

Make all appropriate measurements.

QUESTIONS

1. What abnormality of the pulmonic valve echo is demonstrated? What hemodynamic abnormality could cause this pattern?

2. Which of the following diagnoses explain this echocardiogram?

   (A) Pulmonary hypertension
   (B) Pulmonic insufficiency
   (C) Pulmonic stenosis
   (D) Aortic insufficiency

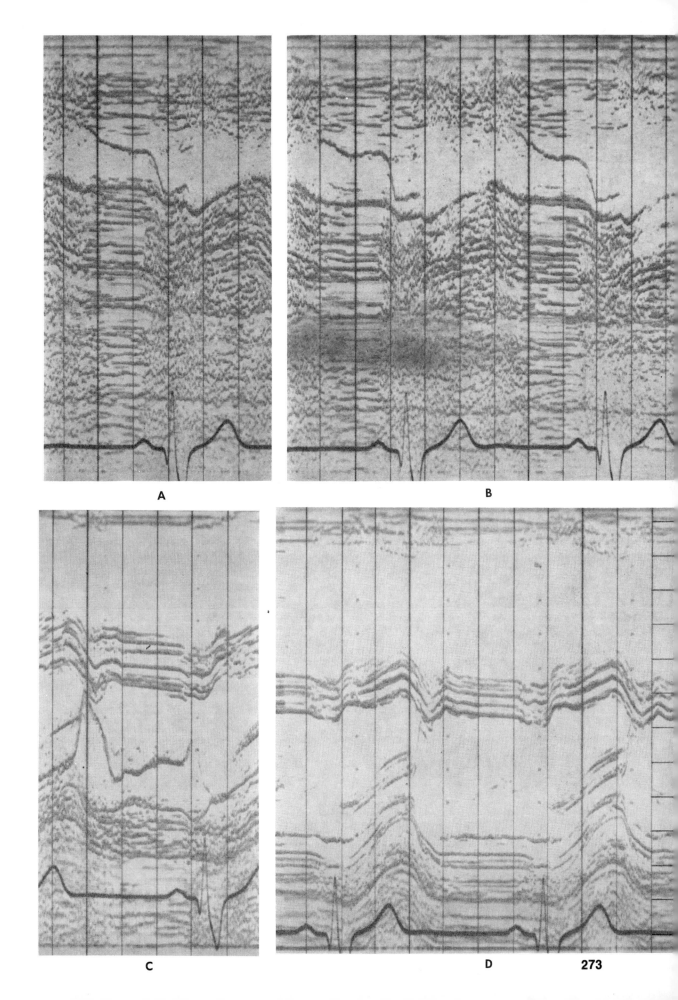

A

B

C

D

ANSWERS TO CASE 46
Valvular Pulmonic Stenosis

MEASUREMENTS

cf	= 1.10	EDD	= 4.1 cm
E-F slope	= 130 mm/sec	ESD	= 3.4 cm
D-E amplitude	= 20 mm	IVS thickness	= 11 mm
RV	= 4.1 cm	LVPW amplitude	= 17 mm

ANSWERS

1. See discussion below. 2. (B) and (C).

Careful examination of the pulmonic valve echo on tracings *A* and *B* shows that the posterior cusp appears to open completely just after the P wave of the electrocar-

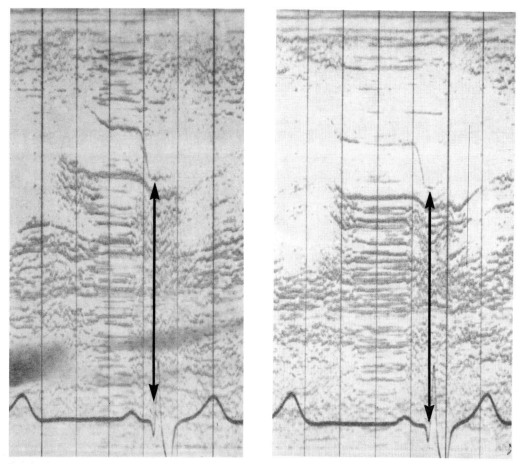

Figure 46–1. Valvular pulmonic stenosis, severe, with opening or doming of the posterior pulmonic cusp to the completely open position after right atrial contraction, but prior to right ventricular systole. The solid vertical arrow marks the Q wave on the electrocardiogram.

VALVULAR PULMONIC STENOSIS

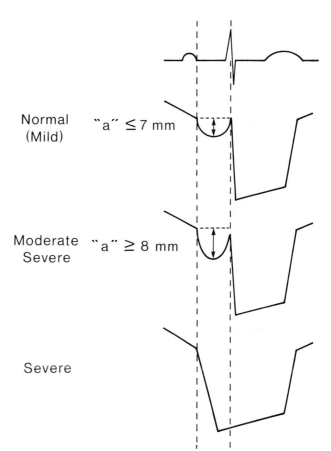

Normal (Mild) "a" ≤ 7 mm

Moderate Severe "a" ≥ 8 mm

Severe

Figure 46–2. Echo patterns of the posterior pulmonic cusp in valvular pulmonic stenosis.[225] See text for discussion.

diogram, but prior to the beginning of the QRS (Fig. 46–1). This abnormal pattern of an exaggerated posterior motion of the pulmonic valve echo just following the P wave of the ECG, i.e., an increased "a wave" depth, is the characteristic echo finding in significant valvular pulmonic stenosis. In moderate or severe pulmonic stenosis, with right ventricular hypertrophy and decreased right ventricular compliance, forceful right atrial contraction often generates a prominent increase in the right ventricular end-diastolic pressure. With a normal or low pulmonary artery diastolic pressure, a significant end-diastolic gradient may thus be created across the valve as the result of right atrial systole. This gradient may produce an exaggerated presystolic opening or doming of a mobile and stenotic pulmonary valve. Weyman and colleagues[225] found that this opening or doming motion in pulmonic stenosis is reflected in the echocardiogram as an increased depth of the "a wave" of the posterior pulmonic cusp (Fig. 46–2). In their patients with pulmonic valvular gradients of 50 to 142 mm Hg, the maximum "a wave" depth ranged from 8 to 13 mm. Normal "a wave" depth ranged from 0 to 7 mm. When the posterior pulmonic cusp did not return to the closed position before ventricular systole and the "a wave" depth was increased, the pulmonic gradient exceeded 65 mm Hg. In two of their patients with severe pulmonic stenosis, atrial systole caused full opening or doming of the valve prior to the onset of ventricular systole, similar to the patient shown in this case. In their study, patients with pulmonic gradients of less than 50 mm Hg, and patients with only increased pulmonary blood flow secondary to left-to-right shunting (atrial septal defect, anomalous pulmonary venous return) had a normal depth of the pulmonic "a wave."

It must be emphasized that this increased "a wave" of the pulmonic valve echo is not specific for a structural abnormality of the pulmonary valve, but rather reflects an end-diastolic pressure gradient across the pulmonary valve. This dependence on certain hemodynamic conditions may explain why some cases of even significant pulmonic stenosis have normal "a waves."[3] If pulmonary hypertension and valvular pulmonic stenosis coexist, the pattern of the pulmonic valve will depend on the relative magnitude of these two abnormalities. If both infundibular and valvular pulmonic stenosis are present, the characteristic sign of pulmonic stenosis may also be altered.

In addition, various other factors besides valvular pulmonic stenosis may increase the depth of the "a wave." (Table 46–1). Bradycardia, as is present in the pa-

TABLE 46–1.   Causes of Increased Depth of Pulmonic Valve "a Wave"

1. Valvular Pulmonic Stenosis
2. Bradycardia
3. Right Ventricular Failure
4. Exaggerated Inspiration

tient in this case, allows more time for right ventricular filling and for the pulmonary artery diastolic pressure to fall. Consequently, right ventricular diastolic pressure may exceed pulmonary artery diastolic pressure more than it would at a faster heart rate, resulting in increased depth of the pulmonic "a wave."[225a] An increased right ventricular end-diastolic pressure may also increase the end-diastolic gradient across the pulmonary valve and result in an exaggerated depth of the pulmonic "a wave." During deep inspiration in normal persons the "a wave" may increase abnormally. These observations emphasize that all the echo patterns observed in the pulmonic valve in pulmonary hypertension or stenosis do not represent anatomic abnormalities, but rather depend on and reflect certain hemodynamic conditions.

Right ventricular volume overload with marked right ventricular dilatation and abnormal, paradoxic type A septal motion is present on echo tracing *D*. Of the choices given in Question 2, pulmonic insufficiency accompanying valvular pulmonic stenosis is the most likely cause of this abnormal septal motion.

Twenty years prior to this echocardiogram, this patient had a pulmonic valvotomy for significant valvular pulmonic stenosis with a gradient of 85 mm Hg. An atrial septal defect was not demonstrated. When seen at the time of this echo, the patient was asymptomatic but had the physical findings of pulmonic stenosis and insufficiency associated with a mild right ventricular lift. He has not had a repeat cardiac catheterization.

CASE 47

This 16-month-old boy is referred for evaluation of a left parasternal systolic murmur that has been increasing in intensity since his birth.

MEASUREMENTS   (Echo tracing A)   **Time lines = 200 msec**

cf	=		RV	=	˙(0.3–1.5 cm)*
Ao	=	(7–17 mm)*	EDD	=	(1.3–3.2 cm)*
Ao valve opening	=	(0.5–1.2 cm)*	ESD	=	
LA	=	(0.7–2.3 cm)*			

*Normal values for children based on weight (0–25 lbs).[1, 3]

QUESTIONS

1. Which of the following observations are shown on this echocardiogram? More than one may apply.

   (A) Mitral-semilunar displacement
   (B) Overriding aorta
   (C) Septal "drop-out"
   (D) Simultaneously recorded semilunar valves
   (E) Right ventricular volume overload

2. This echocardiogram is most consistent with which of the following diagnoses?

   (A) Atrial septal defect
   (B) Ventricular septal defect
   (C) Tetralogy of Fallot
   (D) Double outlet right ventricle
   (E) Transposition of the great vessels

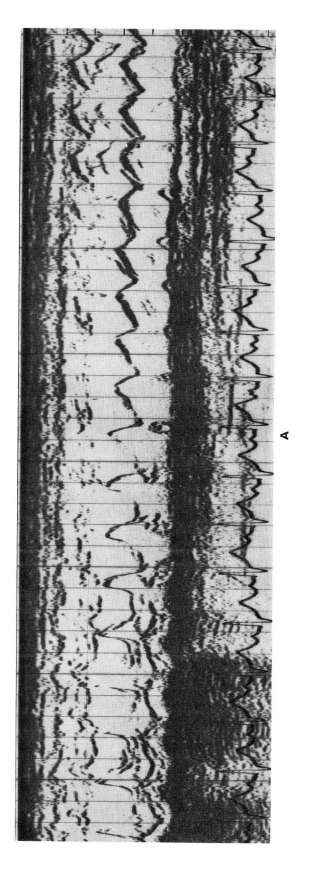

ANSWERS TO CASE 47
Ventricular Septal Defect

MEASUREMENTS

cf	= 1.29	RV	= 0.6 cm (0.3–1.5 cm)*
Ao	= 18 mm (7–17 mm)*	EDD	= 2.6 cm (1.3–3.2 cm)*
Ao valve opening	= 1.0 cm (0.5–1.2 cm)*	ESD	= 1.7 cm
LA	= 1.8 cm (0.7–2.3 cm)*		

*Normal values for children based on weight (0–25 lbs).[1, 3]

ANSWERS

1. (C). 2. (B).

On the M-mode scan from the left ventricle to the aorta, shown on this echo tracing, a "drop-out" or absence of septal echoes is observed between the interventricular septum on the left and the anterior wall of the aorta on the right. The septum and anterior aortic wall are at approximately equal distances from the transducer without evidence of abrupt displacement or of aortic overriding. Such observations are the characteristic findings of a large, uncomplicated ventricular septal defect located high in the membranous septum.[1-4, 233, 267]

Both the size and the location of a ventricular septal defect may limit its detection by M-mode echocardiography. For example, small ventricular septal defects cannot be reliably detected. As illustrated in Figure 47–1, the defect must be larger than the effective width of the echo beam at the level of the septum in order to record "drop-out" or absence of echoes on M-mode scan. With ventricular septal defects smaller than this beam width, echoes will be continuously returning to the transducer, and the characteristic "drop-out" will not be recorded. Ventricular septal defects that course obliquely through the septum with overlapping edges will not be detected for similar reasons. Figure 47–1 also illustrates that if a ventricular septal defect is recorded, the length of the "drop-out" of echoes is proportional to the speed of the M-mode scan, as well as to the size of the ventricular defect. For a ventricular septal defect of a given size, a longer area of echo "drop-out" will be recorded the more slowly the transducer is moved.

The location of the ventricular septal defect may also limit its detection by echo. Fortunately, most large, congenital ventricular septal defects occur immediately below the aortic valve in a portion of the septum readily visualized by M-mode echocardiography. However, defects in the muscular portion of the septum that are located more toward the cardiac apex, such as those that occur with ventricular septal rupture after a myocardial infarction, are not reliably visualized by single-crystal echocardiography. Ventricular septal defects that are located posteriorly in the membranous septum also may not be demonstrated.[267] Thus, echocardiography reliably detects only large, high ventricular septal defects.

Occasionally, even when the ventricular septum is intact, a "drop-out" of septal echoes is recorded. This false pattern of a ventricular septal defect probably occurs when septal angulation or rotation during contraction moves the septum so that it is not perpendicular to the echo beam throughout the cardiac cycle. To avoid this source of error, a "drop-out" of septal echoes should be convincingly recorded on multiple M-mode scans before the diagnosis of ventricular septal defect is made.

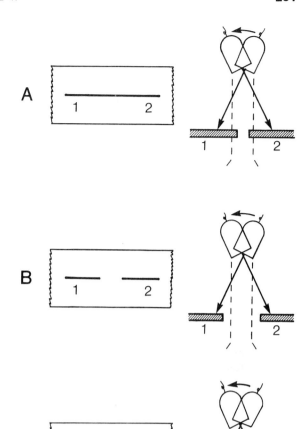

Figure 47–1. Illustration of how both the size of a ventricular septal defect (VSD) and the speed of the M-mode scan influence the echogram. If the VSD is smaller than the effective width of the echo beam, echoes will continuously return to the transducer and no "drop-out" will be recorded (A). For a VSD of a given size that is large enough to be detected, a slow M-mode scan (C) will record a longer area of "drop-out" than a faster scan (B).

Motion of the interventricular septum during systole is appropriately timed in ventricular septal defects, despite the left-to-right shunt.[240] A lack of disproportion between right and left ventricular stroke volume has been proposed as an explanation for this normal septal motion.

Dilatation of the right ventricle, left atrium, and left ventricle may accompany ventricular septal defects with large left-to-right shunts.[3, 240, 269] The amount of left-to-right shunting has been reported to correlate well with left atrial dimensional index[269] and with the left atrial/aortic root ratio.[269a, 292] Patients with shunt flow equal to or greater than 2:1 had left atrial dimensional indices in excess of 3 cm/m^2.[269] In fact, serial measurement of left atrial size by echo has been said to be useful in following patients with ventricular septal defects.[3]

Ventricular septal defects with left-to-right shunting may also cause left ventricular volume overload, characterized by exaggerated septal and left ventricular free wall motion and by left ventricular dilatation (Table 2–2). This pattern may be associated with increased values of the velocity of circumferential fiber shortening (Vcf) in patients with large left-to-right shunts. If the left-to-right shunt is large and cardiac function is normal, the Vcf also has been reported to reflect the shunt size.[3]

Aneurysms of the membranous septum, as occur in patients with small ventricular septal defects, may be detected by echocardiography.[268, 268a, 268b] These aneurysms are recorded as thin, sharply moving echoes protruding from the right side of the septum into the right ventricular outflow tract during systole. This pattern is similar to that reported with herniation of a right sinus of Valsalva aneurysm through a supracrystal ventricular septal defect into the right ventricular outflow tract.[268c]

In this young patient, a ventricular septal defect was demonstrated by oxygen step-up in the right ventricle and by angiography. The calculated pulmonic-to-systemic flow ratio was 2.3:1. Infundibular pulmonic stenosis was also present, with equilibration of right ventricular and systemic systolic pressures. There was no evidence for right-to-left shunting.

CASE 48

This 26-year-old bookstore clerk who had a heart operation as a child has noted increasingly frequent episodes of lightheadedness and excess fatigue with exertion, such as riding his bicycle. An associate observed that he was "blue" during one such episode. On physical examination, a harsh systolic murmur along the left sternal border and a continuous murmur at the base are detected.

MEASUREMENTS   (Echo tracings A-C)   **Time lines = 200 msec**

Make the appropriate measurements.

QUESTIONS

1. Which of the following observations are shown on this echocardiogram? More than one may apply.

    (A) Dilated aortic root
    (B) Left atrial enlargement
    (C) Right ventricular dilatation
    (D) Left ventricular dilatation
    (E) Abrupt posterior displacement of the septum
    (F) Simultaneously recorded semilunar valves

2. This echocardiogram is suggestive of which one of the following diagnoses?

    (A) Atrial septal defect
    (B) Ventricular septal defect
    (C) Tetralogy of Fallot
    (D) Truncus arteriosus
    (E) Transposition of the great vessels

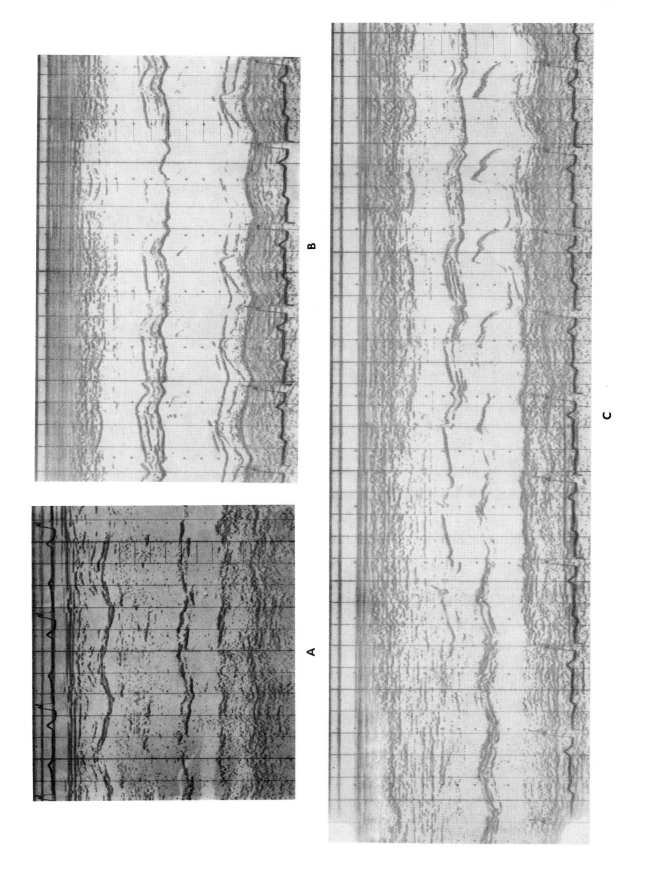

ANSWERS TO CASE 48
Tetralogy of Fallot

MEASUREMENTS

cf	= 2.38	IVS thickness	= 12 mm
Ao	= 52 mm	LVPW thickness	= 10 mm
LA	= 2.6 cm	LVPW amplitude	= 12 mm
RV	= 3.3 cm		
EDD	= 4.3 cm		
ESD	= 3.3 cm		

ANSWERS

1. (A), (C), and (E). 2. (C) and (D).

The aortic root shown on this echo tracing is significantly dilated. On M-mode scan from this great vessel inferolaterally to the mitral valve and interventricular septum, an abrupt and significant posterior displacement of the septum from the level of the anterior aortic wall is demonstrated. The mitral valve echoes appear to be continuous with the posterior aortic wall and do not show abrupt posterior displacement. These observations of a dilated, overriding aortic root with abrupt posterior displacement of the septum and with a normal relationship between the mitral valve and the aorta are the characteristic echo findings in tetralogy of Fallot (Table 48–1).[2, 272, 274] Right ventricular dilatation and hypertrophy of the interventricular septum and anterior right ventricular wall also may be seen. Another case of tetralogy of Fallot, illustrated in Figure 48–1, also shows a dilated aortic root with abrupt posterior displacement of the septum.

Similar echo findings may be observed in truncus arteriosus.[2, 273-275] In Figure 48–2, from a patient with a proved truncus, a dilated, overriding anterior great vessel with abrupt posterior displacement of the septum is observed. The single semilunar valve is seen within this truncal vessel. Unless a pulmonic valve is recorded in a tetralogy, the differentiation between these two entities cannot be made by single-crystal echocardiography. However, because the pulmonic valve often can be difficult to record in tetralogy of Fallot, one should not assume that an overriding great artery is a truncus arteriosus just because a pulmonic valve cannot be recorded.

A dilated overriding aortic root may also occur in double outlet right ventricle. When both great vessels arise from the right ventricle, both semilunar valves are

TABLE 48–1. Echocardiographic Findings in Tetralogy of Fallot
(and Truncus Arteriosus)*

1. Dilated aortic (truncal) root.
2. Abrupt aortic (truncal)–septal displacement ("overriding aorta").
3. Lack of mitral–semilunar displacement.
4. Possible right ventricular dilatation.
5. Possible hypertrophy of septum and/or anterior right ventricular wall.

*Can be excluded only if pulmonic valve recorded.

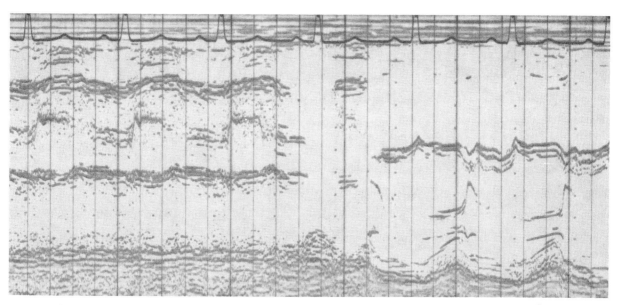

Figure 48–1. Tetralogy of Fallot in an 18-year-old girl with a dilated overriding aorta. A high transducer position, used to record the anterior aortic wall, contributes to the degree of abrupt posterior septal displacement and to the apparent posterior mitral displacement.

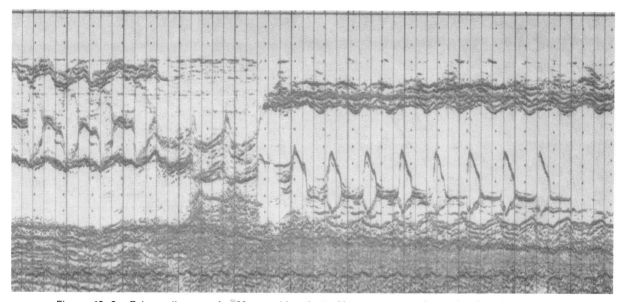

Figure 48–2. Echocardiogram of a 23-year-old patient with a truncus arteriosus showing abrupt truncal-septal displacement with the common semilunar valve opening within the dilated truncal root. (Paper speed = 25 mm/sec).

TABLE 48–2. Causes of Aortic (Truncal) Overriding Detected
by Echocardiography

1. Tetralogy of Fallot.
2. Truncus arteriosus.
3. Double outlet right ventricle.
4. High transducer position.
5. Dilated aortic root.
6. Right ventricular dilatation.

usually located in the same horizontal plane, and fibromuscular tissue separates these valves from the mitral valve. This anatomic discontinuity leads to the echo finding of abrupt, posterior displacement of the mitral valve from the plane of the posterior aortic wall. Because this mitral-semilunar displacement usually is not seen with tetralogy of Fallot, it is a key to the echocardiographic, as well as angiographic, differentiation of tetralogy and double outlet right ventricle.[276] However, the criteria for the detection of mitral-semilunar displacement by single-crystal echocardiography are not well defined.[278-280] A double outlet right ventricle is not always present when abrupt posterior displacement of the mitral valve is demonstrated on

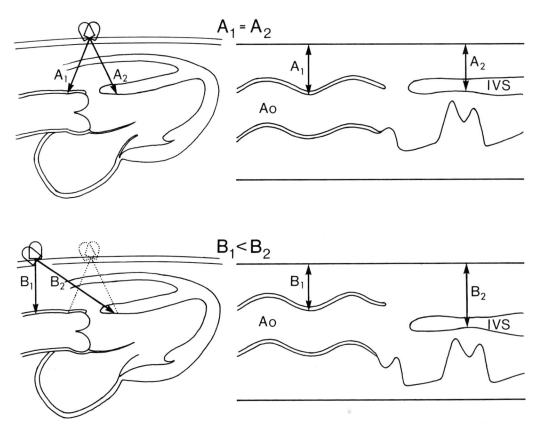

Figure 48–3. Illustration of the effect of transducer position on the relationship of the anterior aortic wall and septum in an uncomplicated ventricular septal defect (VSD). When the aortic wall and the septum are at equal distances from the transducer ($A_1 = A_2$), these structures are recorded with M-mode scan as if they were at the same level. However, when the transducer is located higher on the chest wall so that it is closer to the aorta than the septum ($B_1 < B_2$), an overriding aortic root with abrupt posterior septal displacement may be recorded on the echocardiogram.

echo. Left ventricular dilatation may produce the echo picture of mitral-semilunar displacement when no true anatomic discontinuity exists. In such cases, as is well illustrated in Case 33, a very carefully performed, slow sweep from the aorta to the mitral valve usually will reveal continuity. Too high a transducer position may have a similar effect of producing mitral-semilunar displacement in the absence of anatomic discontinuity.

The detection of an overriding aorta with abrupt posterior displacement of the septum by echo may present several problems. First, if the anterior wall of the aorta is obscured, as it often is with a dilated aorta, the diastolic closure line of the semilunar valve may be mistakenly identified as this wall. This results in failing to detect either the dilated aorta or abrupt posterior septal displacement. Such an error can be avoided by carefully establishing the width of the aorta and by recording the full systolic excursion of the aortic valve.

A second problem in the echo detection of an overriding aorta is that several conditions other than congenital heart disease may produce this echo picture (Table 48–2). As illustrated in Figure 48–3, the transducer position on the chest wall can influence the relationship of the aorta and septum as recorded with an M-mode scan.[278] If the transducer is an equal distance from the anterior aortic wall and the septum ($A_1 = A_2$), these structures will be recorded as if they were at the same level. However, if the transducer is located too high on the chest wall, it will be closer to the anterior aortic wall than the septum ($B_1 < B_2$). The aorta may then be recorded as "overriding the septum" with abrupt posterior septal displacement, whereas anatomically these structures are on the same level. Conversely, too low a transducer position may fail to record true anatomic aortic overriding.

A markedly dilated aortic root, as may occur in Marfan's syndrome or chronic aortic insufficiency, can also result in an echo picture of an enlarged overriding aorta similar to that seen in tetralogy (Fig. 48–4). Such an aortic root may bulge prominently anterior to the septum so that part of the anterior aortic wall is parallel to the echo beam (*open arrow*, Fig. 48–4). This segment of aorta may not be detected, because it will not reflect echoes back to the transducer. On M-mode scan, a dilated aorta with abrupt posterior displacement of the septum will be recorded. Marked right ventricular enlargement also may produce the echo picture of an overriding aorta by actually displacing the septum posteriorly.

French and Popp[278] have attempted to define what represents a significant degree of aortic or truncal overriding as opposed to that which may be secondary to transducer position in patients with truncus arteriosus and double outlet right ven-

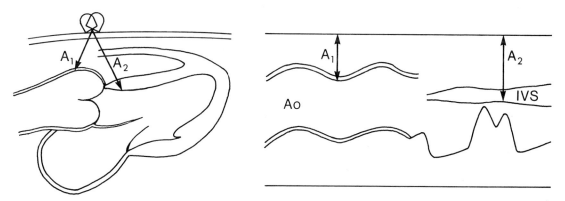

Figure 48–4.   Illustration of the effect of a markedly dilated aorta on the relationship of the anterior aortic wall and the septum. The aortic wall is closer to the transducer than is the septum, and on M-mode sweep from A_1 to A_2 abrupt posterior displacement of the septum is recorded.

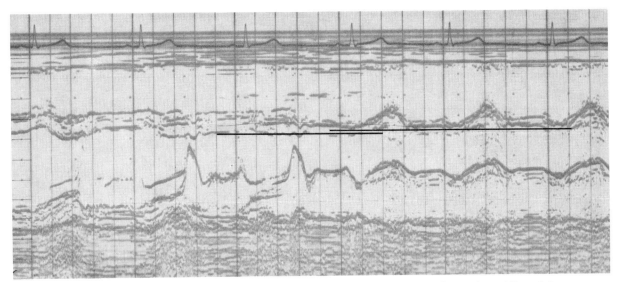

Figure 48–5. M-mode scan from the mitral valve to the aorta in a normal subject. The horizontal lines define the plane of the left ventricular side of the septum and the anterior aortic wall at end-diastole for determination of aortic-septal displacement.[278] In this case, the aorta is displaced 1 mm anterior to the septum.

tricle. They measured the degree of posterior displacement of the septum from a line drawn along the plane of the interior surface of the anterior aortic wall at end-diastole, to a line drawn along the plane of the left ventricular side of the septum at end-diastole, determined at the level of the mitral valve (Fig. 48–5). They found that greater than 5 mm posterior displacement was a positive sign of true anatomic aortic or truncal overriding. Using this same method of measurement, Assad-Morell and colleagues[274] found that the range of aortic or truncal root overriding was 12 to 20 mm in 14 patients with tetralogy, 10 to 20 mm in 16 of 20 patients with truncus arteriosus, and 6 to 22 mm in 22 of 28 patients with pulmonary atresia with ventricular septal defect.

In addition to these technical problems of detecting an overriding aorta, there is a documented variability in the degree of aortic or truncal overriding that occurs in patients with tetralogy of Fallot and truncus arteriosus. Marked overriding is easily and reliably detected by echocardiography. However, in patients with less aortic or truncal overriding, echocardiographic, angiocardiographic, and even anatomic determination of overriding is more difficult to diagnose. A small number of these patients will show no overriding of the great vessel by echocardiography. Consequently, the failure to detect aortic or truncal overriding does not exclude the diagnosis of tetralogy of Fallot or truncus arteriosus.

Technical Hints. To avoid these multiple sources of error in the diagnosis of an overriding great vessel in tetralogy of Fallot and truncus arteriosus:
1. Diagnose an overriding aorta or truncus only if posterior septal displacement is abrupt, if it can be recorded from at least two intercostal spaces with careful, smooth M-mode scans, and if the aortic or truncal dimension is increased.
2. Record the anterior wall of the aorta or truncus and do not be misled by the diastolic closure line of the semilunar valve. Identify the full systolic opening of the semilunar cusps.

3. Measure the degree of overriding as stated above (Fig. 48–5). More than 5 mm of abrupt posterior displacement of the septum may be significant.

Because of the many factors that may produce the picture of "echo discontinuity" when no anatomic discontinuity is present and because anatomic discontinuity may exist without displacement, it has recently been proposed that the words "discontinuity" and "continuity" be abandoned as echo terms and reserved for anatomic descriptions.[279, 280] Instead of discontinuity and continuity, echocardiographers are asked to diagnose "displacement" and "lack of displacement," which is actually what they are observing. This displacement or lack of displacement may or may not be reflective of true anatomic discontinuity or continuity. Thus, aortic-septal discontinuity would become aortic-septal displacement and mitral-semilunar discontinuity would properly be read as mitral-semilunar displacement.

CASE 49

A 32-year-old engineer with the history of a cardiac murmur was catheterized in another state and told he had "a cardiomyopathy and WPW." He avoids participation in sports, but is asymptomatic. He is sent to the echo lab to characterize his heart disease.

MEASUREMENTS (Echo tracings *A* and *B* are continuous recordings)
Time lines = 200 msec

Make all pertinent measurements.

QUESTIONS

1. Which of the following abnormalities does this echo illustrate?

   (A) Decreased mitral E-F slope
   (B) Abnormal motion of the posterior mitral leaflet
   (C) Right ventricular dilatation
   (D) Mitral prolapse
   (E) Systolic anterior mitral motion
   (F) Large "a wave" of the pulmonic valve
   (G) Large tricuspid amplitude
   (H) Pericardial effusion
   (I) Paradoxic septal motion
   (J) Left ventricular dilatation

2. What is the most likely etiology of this patient's heart disease?

   (A) Mitral stenosis
   (B) Pulmonary hypertension
   (C) Hypertrophic subaortic stenosis
   (D) Atrial septal defect
   (E) Ebstein's anomaly
   (F) Pulmonic stenosis
   (G) Idiopathic cardiomyopathy
   (H) Marfan's syndrome

290

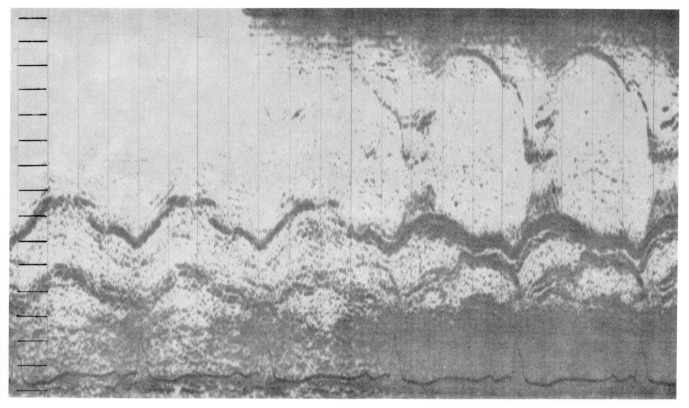

A

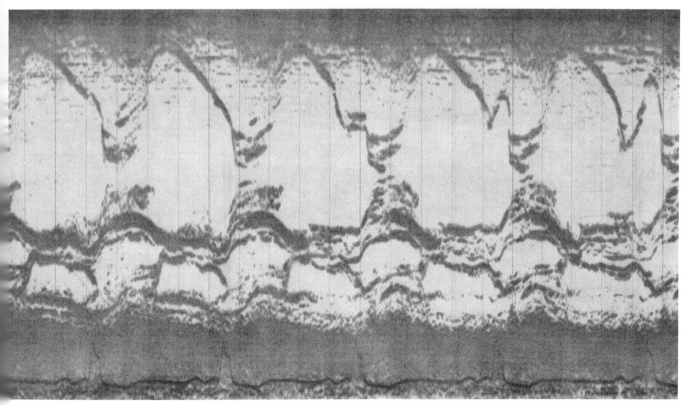

B

291

ANSWERS TO CASE 49
Ebstein's Anomaly

MEASUREMENTS

cf	= 1.50	"RV"	= 7.5
Ao	= 26 mm	EDD	= 2.0 cm
Mitral C-E amplitude	= 16 mm	IVS thickness	= 12 mm
Tricuspid C-E amplitude	= 44 mm		

ANSWERS

1. (A), (C), (G), and (I). 2. (E).

These tracings show the echo findings that may be recorded in Ebstein's anomaly of the tricuspid valve (Table 49–1).[258-265] Echo tracings A and B show an M-mode scan from the aortic root inferiorly to the mitral valve and left ventricle with a proper relationship demonstrated between the aorta, septum, and mitral valve. The mitral valve lies within a very small left ventricle and abuts against the septum during diastole, with a resultant low E-F slope. The lack of mitral thickening and the normal motion of the posterior leaflet exclude mitral stenosis. Anterior to the septum, a prominent tricuspid valve with markedly increased amplitude is recorded within a very dilated right ventricle. This tricuspid valve has a decreased E-F slope and remains abnormally anterior during diastole. The tricuspid and mitral valves are recorded simultaneously, and the tricuspid valve could easily be recorded with the transducer displaced very laterally on the chest wall. Also note the paradoxic, type A, abnormal septal motion. All these abnormalities have been described in Ebstein's anomaly. However, they are nonspecific signs, as they may also be recorded in some patients with marked right ventricular dilatation secondary to other causes.[3] We have observed all these findings, including the ability to record the tricuspid valve with marked inferolateral displacement of the transducer, in a patient who was found at surgery to have only a large atrial septal defect and no abnormality of his tricuspid valve. Furthermore, proved cases of Ebstein's anomaly have a great

TABLE 49–1. Echocardiographic Findings in Ebstein's Anomaly

Specific Finding:
1. Tricuspid closure follows mitral closure by at least 60 msec.

Nonspecific Findings:
1. Increased tricuspid amplitude.
2. Decreased tricuspid E-F slope.
3. Ability to record the tricuspid valve inferolaterally.
4. Ability to record tricuspid and mitral valves simultaneously.
5. Abnormal septal motion, Type A or B.

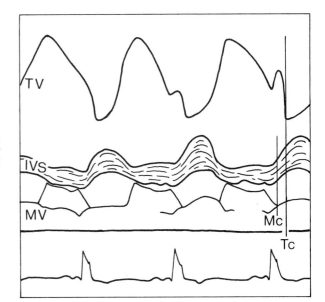

Figure 49–1 (Echo tracing *B*). Ebstein's anomaly, showing simultaneously recorded tricuspid and mitral valves. The delay of tricuspid closure (*Tc*) after mitral closure (*Mc*) is illustrated by the two vertical lines.

variability in the degree to which they show these nonspecific findings.[260, 263, 264] Some cases do not have a reduced tricuspid E-F slope. Others do not show grossly exaggerated tricuspid amplitude; some may even have reduced tricuspid excursion. Septal motion may also be normal in Ebstein's anomaly.

The only specific echo finding for Ebstein's anomaly is closure of the tricuspid valve at least 60 msec after mitral valve closure.[259, 260, 263, 264] On echo tracing *B*, if tricuspid closure is taken as the point where the tricuspid valve moves rapidly posterior at the beginning of systole, tricuspid closure occurs 60 to 70 msec after mitral closure in this case (Fig. 49–1).* Several workers have examined this delayed tricuspid closure in patients with Ebstein's anomaly. Lundstrom[259] reported that tricuspid closure exceeded mitral closure by greater than 60 msec in all 19 of the patients with Ebstein's anomaly in his series and that in all other cases of right bundle branch block, atrial septal defect, total anomalous pulmonary venous drainage, and pulmonary hypertension this value was less than 60 msec. Farooki and colleagues[263] found that in 14 of 16 patients with Ebstein's anomaly, tricuspid closure was later than mitral closure by at least 40 msec, whereas in all patients without Ebstein's anomaly tricuspid and mitral closure were closer. Milner and coworkers[264] reported delayed tricuspid closure for 65 msec after mitral closure in eight of 10 patients with Ebstein's anomaly and that all control groups with right bundle branch block, atrial septal defect, and pulmonary hypertension had less delay of tricuspid closure. From these last two studies, it is evident that a few patients with Ebstein's anomaly will even have the delay between tricuspid and mitral closure fall within the range that is seen in some other diseases. However, delay of tricuspid closure 60 msec or more after mitral closure is apparently specific for Ebstein's anomaly, as no other condition produces this much delay.

---

*In making this calculation, the variation in paper speed must be taken into account. On this echo tracing, 48 mm represents a time of 1000 msec. Thus, the 2.5 to 3 mm distance between mitral and tricuspid closure represents a time of 60 to 70 msec (41 mm/1000 msec = 2.5 to 3 mm/x; x = 60 to 70 msec). See page 11 of Echo Measurements and Calculations.

If tricuspid and mitral closure are not recorded simultaneously, the difference in timing between these two events can be calculated by reference to the electrocardiogram. The time from the Q wave of the electrocardiogram to tricuspid closure (Q-Tc) and mitral closure (Q-Mc) can be measured. The difference between these two values is the delay in tricuspid closure. For the most accurate measurements, recordings should be made at a paper speed of 75 or 100 mm/sec, rather than the usual 50 mm/sec.

Tricuspid closure, as represented by the C point of the tricuspid valve on echo, has been shown to correlate with the second component of the widely split first sound (T_1) that is the hallmark of the auscultatory findings in Ebstein's anomaly.[263]

Ebstein's anomaly of the tricuspid valve is characterized by an abundance of valvular tissue and by adherence of varying portions of the grossly abnormal septal and posterior leaflets to the right ventricular wall. This results in inferior displacement of the tricuspid valve and in formation of an "atrialized" portion of the right ventricle. One of the principal characteristics of Ebstein's anomaly is the wide spectrum of the degree of anatomic abnormality and resulting clinical expression of disease that occurs. This variability explains the wide spectrum and many differences in the echo findings recorded in Ebstein's anomaly. Some of the variation that may occur in the tricuspid E-F slope and amplitude and in the degree of prolonged anterior position of the tricuspid valve is to some extent a function of angulation of the transducer. This influence of the changing transducer angle is evident on the M-mode scan shown in this case. When the transducer is aimed more inferiorly, as on the right side of echo tracing B, the tricuspid E-F slope is not as reduced and the tricuspid valve does not remain so anteriorly during diastole compared with tracing A.

Late closure of the tricuspid valve in Ebstein's anomaly has been ascribed to mechanical obstruction created by the abnormal tricuspid valve.[260, 264] That delayed tricuspid closure is not due to right bundle branch block, as was previously assumed, has been shown by Tajik and colleagues.[261] They recorded a case of Ebstein's anomaly with delayed tricuspid closure who not only did not have right bundle branch block, but who even had pre-excitation of the right ventricle (WPW, type B). Although normal motion of the septum may rarely be recorded in Ebstein's anomaly, abnormal septal motion of either type A or B is the rule.[258-263] The cause of this abnormal septal motion is unclear, but it is probably secondary to either tricuspid regurgitation or an associated atrial septal defect.

The cardiac catheterization performed in this patient four years prior to this echocardiogram documented Ebstein's anomaly by simultaneous intracardiac pressure and electrocardiograms and by angiography. The patient has intermittent Wolff-Parkinson-White syndrome (type B).

CASE 50

This 18-year-old amateur boxer experiences a substernal, aching pain after his regular workouts, but denies any dizziness or syncope. He has known of a cardiac murmur "all his life," which at present is described as a grade 3/6 systolic ejection murmur at the base. The following echocardiogram is obtained.

MEASUREMENTS   (Echo tracings A-C)   **Time lines = 200 msec**

Make all appropriate measurements.

cf = 1.02 for echo tracings A and B.
cf = 2.10 for echo tracing C.

QUESTIONS

1. Which of the following observations are illustrated on this echocardiogram? More than one may apply.

   (A) Mitral–semilunar displacement
   (B) Asymmetric septal hypertrophy
   (C) Decreased opening of thickened aortic cusps
   (D) Partial early systolic closure of the aortic valve
   (E) Systolic anterior motion (SAM) of the mitral valve
   (F) Dilatation of the left ventricular cavity
   (G) Narrowing of the left ventricular outflow tract
   (H) Left ventricular hypertrophy
   (I) Pericardial effusion

2. What is the one best description of this echo?

   (A) Valvular aortic stenosis
   (B) Hypertrophic subaortic stenosis
   (C) Discrete subvalvular aortic stenosis
   (D) Left ventricular hypertrophy
   (E) Tetralogy of Fallot
   (F) Double outlet right ventricle

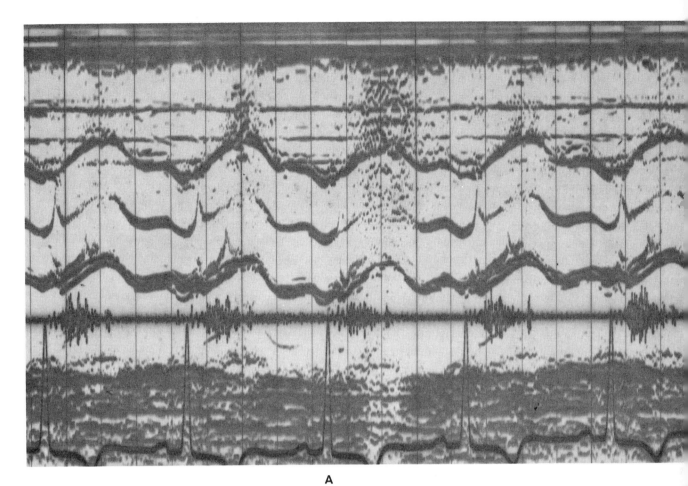

A

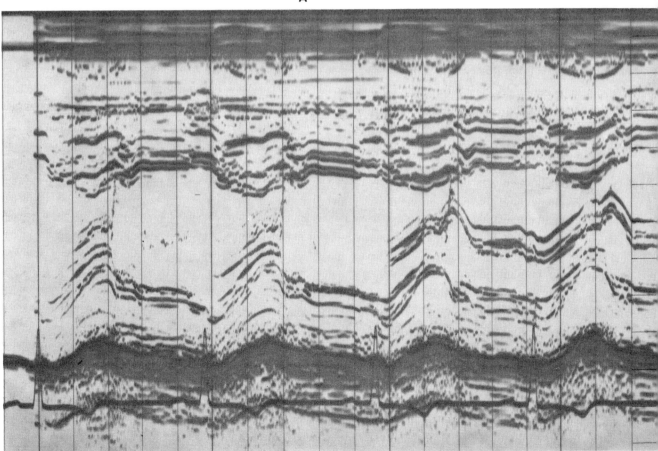

Illustration continued on page 299.

Figure 50C appears on the opposite page.

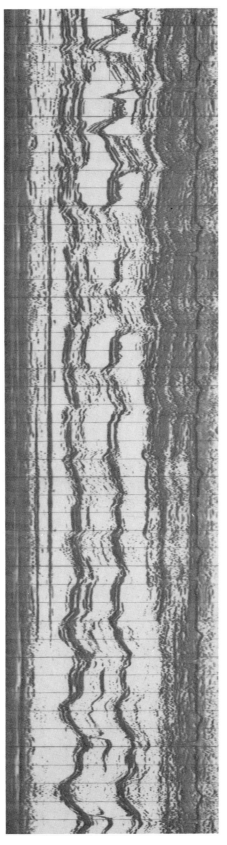

C

ANSWERS TO CASE 50
Discrete Subvalvular Aortic Stenosis

MEASUREMENTS

cf (For echoes A and B)	= 1.02	EDD	= 3.7 cm
cf (For echo C)	= 2.10	ESD	= 2.1 cm
Ao	= 33 mm	Ejection fraction	= 76%
Ao valve opening	= 1.7 cm	Percentage change	= 43%
LA	= 3.3 cm	IVS amplitude	= 6 mm
RV	= 1.5 cm	LVPW amplitude	= 14 mm
IVS thickness	= 13 mm		
LVPW thickness	= 14 mm		

ANSWERS

1. (D), (G), and (H). 2. (C).

This echocardiogram illustrates the two major findings reported in discrete sub-valvular aortic stenosis of the fibromuscular type.[281, 282, 284] On M-mode scan from the aorta to the tip of the anterior mitral leaflet on tracing C, narrowing of the left ventricular outflow tract just below the aortic valve is demonstrated. This area of narrowing, which measures 14 mm at end-diastole, is especially evident in comparison with the internal end-diastolic diameter of the aortic root (23 mm) measured at the level of the aortic cusps (Fig. 50–1). The range of the normal left ventricular outflow

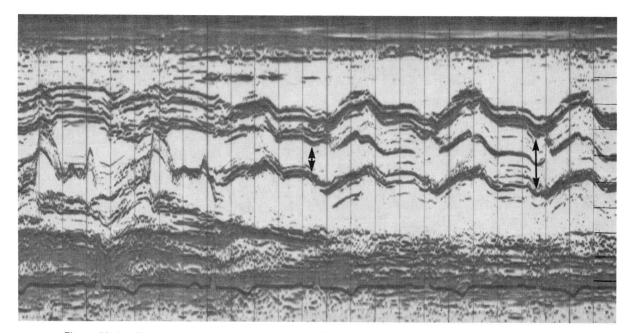

Figure 50–1. Discrete subvalvular aortic stenosis of a fibromuscular type with narrowing of the left ventricular outflow tract (LVOT). Measurement of the internal aortic diameter at the level of the aortic valve at end-diastole and of the left ventricular outflow tract (LVOT) below the level of the aortic cusps at end-diastole is illustrated.

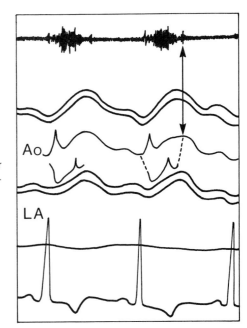

Figure 50–2 (Echo tracing *A*). Abnormal pattern of the anterior and posterior aortic cusps in discrete subvalvular aortic stenosis. See text for discussion.

tract is 20 to 35 mm.[251] This echo pattern was a consistent finding on multiple M-mode sweeps in this patient. Popp and colleagues[282] reported such a narrowed left ventricular outflow tract just below the aortic valve in three patients with discrete subvalvular aortic stenosis. Two of these patients had a fibromuscular type of subvalvular narrowing, and one patient had a predominantly membranous type.

Echo tracing *A* demonstrates the typical abnormality of the aortic cusps that Davis and coworkers[281] described in at least one of the aortic cusps of three patients with discrete subvalvular aortic stenosis. On this tracing, the anterior coronary cusp opens normally, but then, immediately in early systole, it abruptly moves to a partially closed position, where it remains for the rest of systole (Fig. 50–2). This premature closure is thought to be caused by obstruction to aortic flow produced by the bandlike fibrous subaortic tissue.

The echo of the aortic valve of the patient shown in this case is of particular interest in that it demonstrates a variation in the pattern of the aortic cusps that may occur in this disease. The posterior aortic cusp opens normally and remains in a normal position, even after the anterior cusp has moved to a partially closed position. However, in the last third of systole, this posterior cusp moves abruptly and rapidly toward a closed position for a brief period. It then rapidly reopens during the last one-third of systole prior to closing at the end of systole as defined by the second sound on a simultaneously recorded phonocardiogram. The systolic ejection murmur that is also recorded on the phonocardiogram diminishes as this posterior cusp reopens. This abnormality of the posterior aortic cusp undoubtedly is also caused by the subaortic tissue altering and distorting aortic flow. Thus, there may be a varying pattern of the aortic cusps seen in discrete subvalvular aortic stenosis. When premature systolic closure of an aortic cusp occurs in this entity, it may not occur in early systole, and the closure may not persist once it has closed, as has been previously reported.[281]

Although the echo pattern of aortic valve motion is helpful in suggesting the presence of discrete subaortic stenosis, it is a nonspecific finding and can be seen in other disorders such as hypertrophic subaortic stenosis, ventricular septal defect, and mitral insufficiency.[284] Narrowing of the left ventricular outflow tract on M-mode scan from the aorta to the mitral valve is the more specific finding in discrete subvalvular aortic stenosis. However, artifactual narrowing of this outflow tract can be produced on M-mode scan even when this entity is not present. This artifact can occur if the echo beam passes eccentrically through the outflow tract. To avoid this error, consistent significant narrowing of the left ventricular outflow tract should be demonstrated on multiple M-mode scans before the diagnosis of discrete subvalvular aortic stenosis is suggested. This source of error in the diagnosis of discrete subaortic stenosis is avoided with cross-sectional echocardiography.[284]

Because of many similarities, hypertrophic subaortic stenosis must be carefully excluded when considering the diagnosis of discrete subvalvular aortic stenosis. As Popp, et al.,[282] stressed, the narrowing of the left ventricular outflow tract in discrete subvalvular aortic stenosis is just below the aortic valve near the aortic annulus, whereas in hypertrophic subaortic stenosis the narrowing is most striking near the free edge of the mitral valve. In hypertrophic subaortic stenosis, the characteristic abnormality of the aortic valve is partial midsystolic closure with reopening prior to the end of systole. On the other hand, in discrete subvalvular aortic stenosis, the initial normal opening of the aortic valve usually is followed almost immediately by partial early systolic closure of at least one cusp, which usually remains in this closed position throughout systole. However, as discussed above, there are exceptions to this characteristic pattern. In addition, the interventricular septum in hypertrophic subaortic stenosis is disproportionately thickened in reference to the posterior left ventricular wall, whereas concentric left ventricular hypertrophy is present in discrete subvalvular aortic stenosis.

On the echograms performed postoperatively in patients with discrete subvalvular aortic stenosis, the aortic cusps appear to open more completely, although their pattern of motion usually remains abnormal.[282] The degree of narrowing of the left ventricular outflow tract may or may not be changed.[281, 284]

With cardiac catheterization and at the time of surgery, significant subvalvular aortic stenosis of a fibromuscular type was documented in this patient. At surgery, a fixed fibromuscular band was demonstrated 1 cm below the aortic valve with extension onto the anterior mitral leaflet and formation of a subvalvular aortic chamber. On a postoperative echocardiogram, there was no change in the degree of left ventricular outflow tract narrowing, although the anterior aortic cusp maintained a more open position during systole. This cusp showed only a slight degree of midsystolic closure, followed by reopening during the last third of systole. Abnormal closure of the posterior cusp in latter systole persisted.

In addition to discrete subvalvular aortic stenosis, the M-mode echocardiographic findings in supravalvular aortic stenosis with narrowing of the aorta above the valve have been described.[285-288] Echocardiography is, therefore, useful in evaluating left ventricular outflow obstruction of a valvular, supravalvular, hypertrophic, and discrete subvalvular nature.

CASE 51

A 47-year-old restaurateur is referred by his internist, who suspects that the patient has an atrial septal defect because of the widely split second heart sound, systolic murmurs at the base and apex, and a chest x-ray that demonstrates increased pulmonary vasculature. The patient is free of symptoms except for increasing fatigue noted at higher elevations.

MEASUREMENTS   (Echo tracings *A-E*)   **Time lines = 200 msec**

Make all appropriate measurements.

QUESTIONS

1. Which of the following echo abnormalities are present on these tracings?

   (A) Eccentric aortic valve closure
   (B) Abnormal pulmonic "a wave"
   (C) Right ventricular dilatation
   (D) Normal septal motion
   (E) Abnormal septal motion
   (F) Abnormal anterior motion of the tricuspid valve
   (G) Mitral prolapse
   (H) Abnormal mitral–septal approximation
   (I) Narrow left ventricular outflow tract

2. What diagnosis(es) is (are) best made from this echocardiogram?

   (A) Bicuspid aortic valve
   (B) Pulmonic stenosis
   (C) Secundum atrial septal defect
   (D) Primum atrial septal defect
   (E) Mitral valve prolapse
   (F) Cleft mitral valve
   (G) Ebstein's anomaly

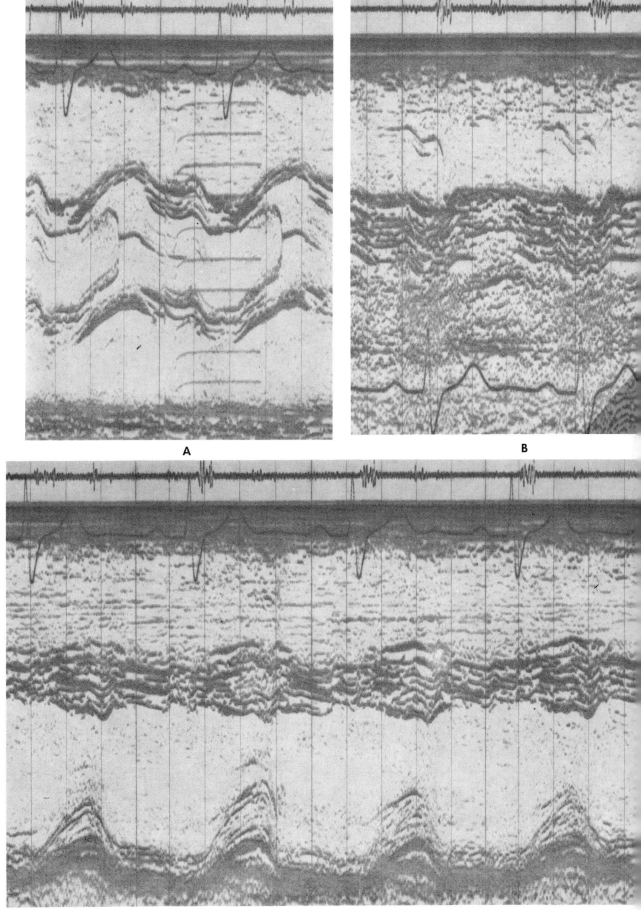

A

B

C

Illustration continued on the following page.

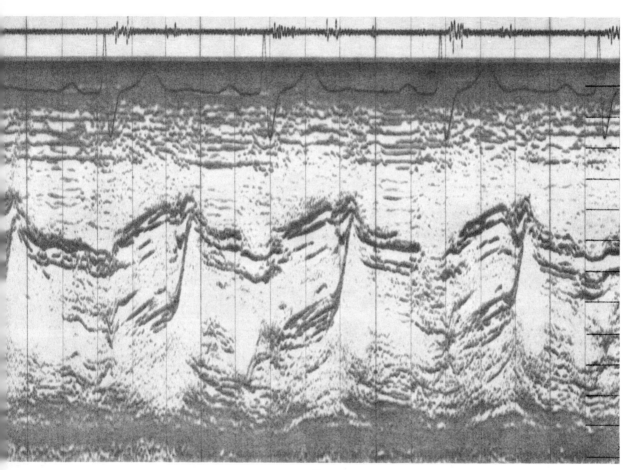

D

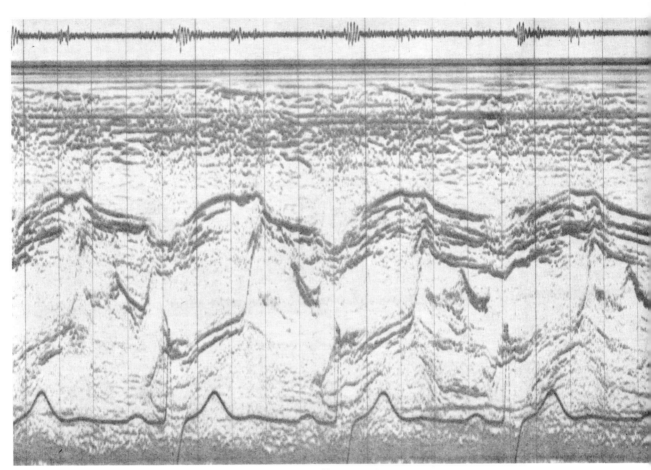

E

ANSWERS TO CASE 51
Endocardial Cushion Defect:
Ostium Primum Atrial Septal Defect
Cleft Mitral Valve with Mitral Regurgitation

MEASUREMENTS

cf	= 1.22	IVS thickness	= 12 mm
Ao	= 43 mm	IVS amplitude	= 5 mm
LA	= 3.7 cm	LVPW amplitude	= 18 mm
RV	= 3.7 cm	Pulmonic "a wave"	= 4 mm
EDD	= 4.9 cm	Minimal C point to	
		septal distance	= 13 mm
ESD	= 2.7 cm		

ANSWERS

1. (C), (E), (H), (I). 2. (D) and (F).

This echocardiogram shows the abnormality of the mitral valve seen in patients with ostium primum atrial septal defects, a form of endocardial cushion defect (Table 51–1).[251-257] The principal echo abnormality in this entity is abnormal approximation of the mitral valve to the septum during systole, resulting in narrowing of the left ventricular outflow tract. This narrowing is illustrated on echo tracings D and E and in Figures 51–2 and 51–3, where the C-D segment of the mitral valve is seen to be abnormally close to the septum. Gramiak and Nanda[251] found that the *minimal* C point to septal distance that could be recorded in ostium primum defects was always less than 20 mm. The normal range was 20 to 35 mm. Also in ostium primum defects, there is characteristically prolonged approximation of the anterior mitral leaflet and the septum during diastole. This results in the E-F portion of the mitral valve being recorded as overlapping the interventricular septum. Because it may be seen in other causes of marked right ventricular dilatation with compression of the left ventricle, this prolonged mitral-septal approximation in diastole is less specific for ostium primum defects than mitral–septal approximation in systole.[257] However, systolic narrowing of the left ventricular outflow tract can also be seen in mitral stenosis and hypertrophic subaortic stenosis.

Abnormal mitral motion in endocardial cushion defects results from abnormal attachment of the anterior mitral leaflet to the crest of the interventricular septum.[252, 253, 255] Because of this abnormal attachment, the anterior mitral leaflet is displaced anteriorly and inferiorly and its plane of motion in diastole is more perpendicular to the echo beam than parallel to it, as is normally the case. Consequently, the anterior mitral leaflet usually is best recorded close to the septum just below the aorta in the left ventricular outflow tract, rather than in its usual location. It tends to be seen best in systole and early diastole because it moves out of the echo beam for most of mid- and late diastole. Because of its abnormal attachment to the septum, the mitral valve narrows the left ventricular outflow tract, with the anterior mitral leaflet encroaching on the septum in diastole. This pattern is the echo equivalent of the "goose neck" deformity of the left ventricular outflow tract seen on angiography in patients with

TABLE 51–1. Echocardiographic Findings in Ostium
Primum Atrial Septal Defect

1. Mitral–septal approximation in systole with narrowing of left ventricular outflow tract (LVOT).
2. Prolonged mitral–septal approximation in diastole.
3. Right ventricular dilatation.
4. Abnormal septal motion (may be normalized by associated left ventricular volume overload—i.e., mitral regurgitation).

endocardial cushion defects. Multiple mitral echoes also are commonly seen in ostium primum defects, although this is a nonspecific finding.

Williams and Rudd[252] have stressed that mitral–septal approximation in endocardial cushion defects can best be demonstrated by a medially directed M-mode scan from the mitral valve to the left ventricular outflow tract (Fig. 51–1). The transducer beam is directed from the left ventricle in a superior and medial direction toward the outflow tract and superior part of the septum. Such a scan is directed more medially than the standard mitral valve-to-aortic scan. In endocardial cushion defects, the systolic portion of the mitral valve is thus recorded to be in a progressively more anterior position until it approximates the septum. Without abnormal attachment of the mitral valve to the septum, this pattern cannot be recorded. This type of medially directed scan is illustrated in the reverse direction in Figures 51–2 and 51–3 in two patients with endocardial cushion defects. Note that on the left of these tracings the systolic portion (C-D) of the mitral valve is abnormally close to the interventricular septum and that it narrows the left ventricular outflow tract. This abnormal mitral–septal approximation in systole is the most specific echo finding in endocardial cushion defect. However, in this entity, a standard M-mode scan from the mitral valve to the aorta usually will demonstrate a proper relationship of the anterior mitral leaflet and posterior aortic wall. Figure 51–2 shows both of these types of scan in a patient with an endocardial cushion defect.

This echocardiogram also shows right ventricular dilatation and an unusual, abnormal pattern of septal motion. The left side of the septum moves appropriately in a posterior direction during systole, but there is also abnormal, anterior systolic motion of the right side of the septum. Thus, this patient's septal motion falls in the spectrum between normal motion and abnormal type B motion.[240, 246] Usually in os-

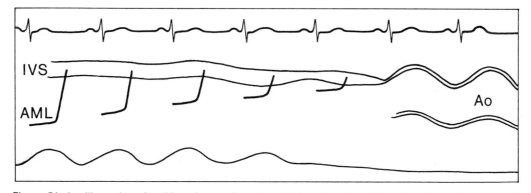

Figure 51–1. Illustration of an M-mode scan in endocardial cushion defect from the mitral valve superiorly and medially toward the left ventricular outflow tract and superior portion of the interventricular septum. Note that the systolic portion of the anterior mitral leaflet progressively approximates the interventricular septum just below the aorta.

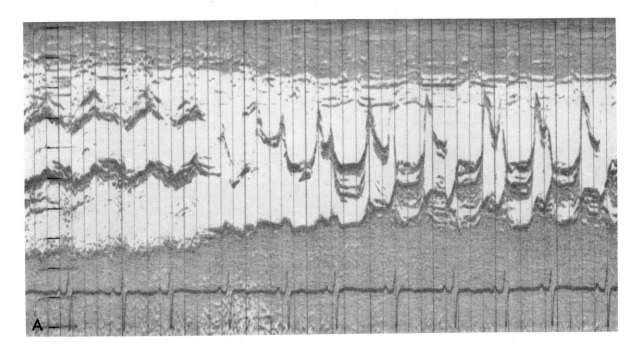

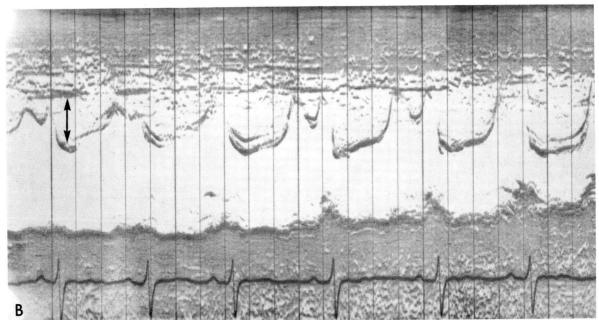

Figure 51–2. Echocardiograms of an 11-year-old patient with an endocardial cushion defect consisting of atrial and ventricular septal defects, and a typical "goose neck" deformity of the left ventricular outflow tract on angiography.

A, Standard M-mode scan from the aorta to the mitral valve. Note mitral-septal apposition in diastole with the E-F segment of the anterior mitral leaflet overlapping the septum. The posterior wall of the aorta and mitral valve have a proper relationship, although septal "drop-out" is evident in the superior part of the septum. (Paper speed is 25 mm/sec).

B, M-mode scan showing abnormal mitral-septal approximation during systole on the left, where the echo beam is directed medially into the left ventricular outflow tract. This abnormal approximation becomes less evident as the transducer is directed inferolaterally.

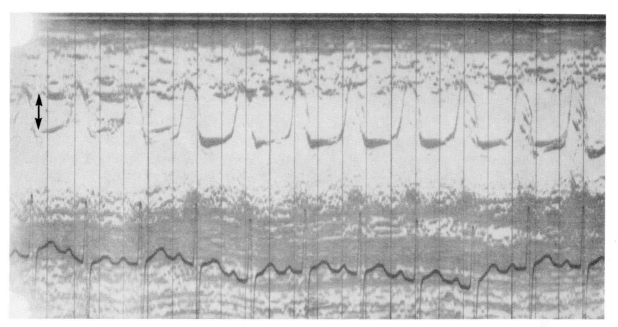

Figure 51–3. An M-mode scan from the left ventricular outflow tract inferolaterally to the mitral valve in an 11-month-old child with an endocardial cushion defect. Abnormal mitral-septal apposition in systole and in diastole is illustrated.

tium primum atrial septal defects, septal motion is abnormal, reflecting right ventricular volume overload.[251, 253-255] However, if significant mitral regurgitation secondary to a cleft mitral valve also is present, the resultant left ventricular volume overload may normalize septal motion. The mitral regurgitation present in the patient shown in this case apparently is having this effect on the septal motion. Significant left ventricular volume overload secondary to mitral regurgitation is a cause of normal septal motion in patients with atrial septal defects (Table 41–3).

Endocardial cushion defects are associated with a wide spectrum of anatomic abnormalities from an insignificant, partial cleft of the mitral valve to gross abnormality of the atrioventricular valves observed in complete atrioventricular canal. With minimal anatomic abnormality, the echocardiogram may be completely normal, or there may be nonspecific abnormalities of the anterior mitral leaflet if only a cleft mitral valve is present. In patients with complete atrioventricular canals, various other patterns of the mitral and tricuspid valves have been described.[252-257] The most specific finding in these complete forms is a common atrioventricular leaflet with wide excursion that crosses the interventricular septum from the left ventricle into the right ventricle during diastole.[252, 254] Abnormal mitral–septal approximation in systole and diastole, as described above in ostium primum defects, also may be seen in the more complete forms of endocardial cushion defect.

The patient in this case was found at cardiac catheterization to have an ostium primum atrial septal defect with a 3:1 pulmonic-to-systemic flow ratio. Angiography demonstrated moderate mitral regurgitation and a "goose neck" deformity of the left ventricular outflow tract, characteristic of endocardial cushion defects. At surgery, the patient had closure of his atrial septal defect and repair of the mitral cleft.

CASE 52

This 60-year-old motel manager with a long history of heart disease is admitted to the Coronary Care Unit following a prolonged episode of severe chest pain associated with the development of congestive heart failure. An arterial line and a flow-directed, pulmonary artery catheter are inserted. The central aortic pressure is 95/70 and the mean pulmonary artery wedge pressure is 26 mm Hg. With a grade 3/6 murmur of mitral regurgitation and prominent cardiomegaly noted on x-ray, an echocardiogram is ordered.

MEASUREMENTS   (Echo tracings *A* and *B*)   **Time lines = 200 msec**

cf	=	EDD	=
Ao	=	ESD	=
LA	=	Ejection fraction	=
E-F slope	=	Percentage change	=
C-E amplitude	=	PR-AC interval	=
D-E amplitude	=		
E-IVS distance	=		

QUESTIONS

1. What does the echo within the left atrium represent?

2. Which of the following diagnoses does this echo suggest?

   (A) Dissection of the aortic root
   (B) Aneurysm of sinus of Valsalva
   (C) Prolapsing aortic leaflet
   (D) Left atrial tumor
   (E) Right ventricular tumor
   (F) Ruptured chordae tendineae to the posterior mitral leaflet
   (G) Cardiomyopathy
   (H) Pericardial effusion

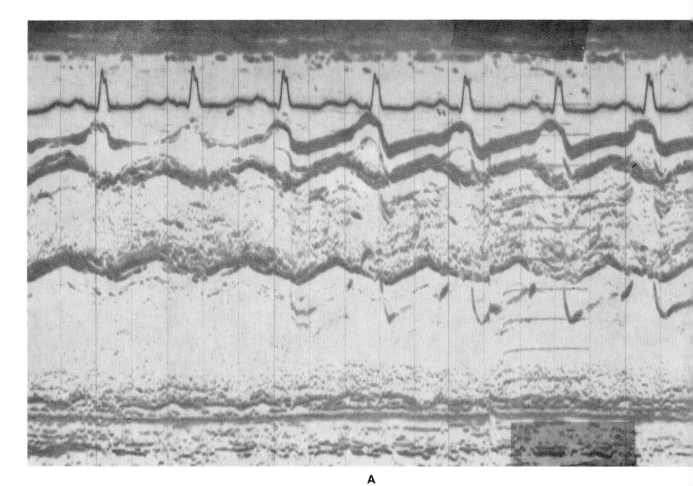

A

B

313

ANSWERS TO CASE 52
Reverberation from Pulmonary Artery Catheter
Cardiomyopathy

MEASUREMENTS

cf	= 1.23	EDD	= 7.4 cm
Ao	= 32 mm	ESD	= 5.9 cm
LA	= 4.6	Ejection fraction	= 40%
E-F slope	= 110 mm/sec	Percentage change	= 20%
C-E amplitude	= 23 mm	PR-AC interval	= 0.02–0.05 sec
D-E amplitude	= 20 mm		
E-IVS distance	= 26 mm		

ANSWERS

1. Within the left atrium on tracing *A*, a thin echo is recorded that appears to overlap the posterior aortic wall. This echo is a reverberation, or phantom echo, from the catheter that had been placed in the patient's pulmonary artery and that is recorded just anterior to the aorta on this tracing (Fig. 52–1). Immediately after removal of this catheter, the echo of the catheter and its reverberation within the left atrium disappeared.

The basis for this phenomenon of reverberation is illustrated in Figure 52–2. When echoes return to the transducer, the transducer surface itself may act as a reflecting surface. In such cases, part of the returning echoes may return to the original object and then again be reflected to the transducer. These re-reflected echoes (A′), which take twice as long to be sensed by the transducer, will be displayed on the oscilloscope and on the echo tracing as twice as far from the transducer as the

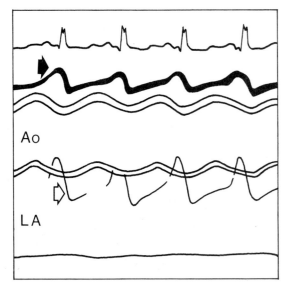

Figure 52–1 (Echo tracing *A*). Reverberation of echoes within the left atrium (*open arrow*) from a pulmonary artery catheter (*solid arrow*).

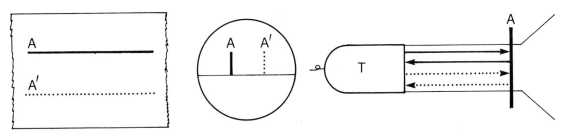

Figure 52–2. Illustration of reverberation of echoes from the surface of the transducer. Note that the re-reflected echoes (*A'*) travel twice as far as the original echoes (*A*) and are recorded as a weaker signal, twice as far from the transducer as the original echoes on the oscilloscope and on the echo tracing.

original echoes (A). Because their energy has been reduced, these reverberations are recorded as a weaker signal. In addition, if the object being recorded is moving, the distance moved by the reverberation will be twice as much as the original echo. For this reason, a reverberation will not have the exact pattern of motion as the original echo.

Reverberations are the source of the "heart behind a heart" and the "two mitral valves" that are occasionally recorded by echocardiography. If the depth of the echo tracing is too compressed, as may occur when an adult follows a child in the echo lab, such reverberations are more common. However, knowledge of reverberation and careful attention to the proper depth control for each patient should prevent this source of interpretative error and puzzling phenomena.

2. This patient has a markedly dilated left ventricle with decreased calculated ejection fraction and percentage change of the minor left ventricular diameter. The pattern of the mitral valve also suggests left ventricular dysfunction. It has a "double-diamond" configuration, an increaed E point-to-septal distance, a "B-bump," and an abnormal PR-AC interval (see Cases 32 and 33). Such echo abnormalities are most consistent with a cardiomyopathy, which by this patient's history and subsequent cardiac catheterization is secondary to coronary artery disease. There is no echo evidence of a pericardial effusion.

LIST OF CASES (AND ILLUSTRATIVE ECHOCARDIOGRAMS)

REFERENCES

Reference Books and Review Articles

1. Feigenbaum, H.: Echocardiography. Lea & Febiger, Philadelphia, 1972.
2. Gramiak, R., and Waag, R. C.: Cardiac Ultrasound. The C. V. Mosby Company, St. Louis, 1975.
3. Goldberg, S. J., Allen H. D., and Sahn, D. J.: Pediatric and Adolescent Echocardiography. Year Book Medical Publishers, Inc., Chicago, 1975.
4. Chang, S.: M-Mode Echocardiographic Techniques and Pattern Recognition. Lea & Febiger, Philadelphia, 1976.
5. Weissler, A. M.: Non-Invasive Cardiology. Grune & Stratton, New York, 1974, pp. 149–226.
6. Segal, B. L., et al.: Echocardiography: current concepts and clinical application. Am. J. Med. *57*:269, 1974.
7. Gramiak, R., and Shah, P. M.: Cardiac ultrasonography. A review of current applications. Radiol. Clin. North Am. *9*:469, 1971.
8. Joyner, C. R.: Echocardiography. Am. Heart J. *90*:413, 1975.
8a. Weyman, A. E., and Feigenbaum, H.: Echocardiography—where are we now and where are we going? Am. J. Med. *60*:315, 1976.
9. Feigenbaum, H.: Newer aspects of echocardiography. Circulation *47*:833, 1973.
10. Feigenbaum, H.: Clinical applications of echocardiography. Progr. Cardiovasc. Dis. *14*:531, 1972.
10a. Popp, R. L.: Echocardiographic assessment of cardiac disease. Circulation *54*:538, 1976.

Aortic Stenosis and Bicuspid Aortic Valve

11. Gramiak, R., and Shah, P.: Echocardiography of the normal and diseased aortic valve. Radiology *96*:1, 1970.
12. Yeh, H. C., Winsberg, F., and Mercer, E. M.: Echocardiographic aortic valve orifice dimension: its use in evaluating aortic stenosis and cardiac output. J. Clin. Ultrasound *1*:182, 1973.
13. Winsberg, F., and Mercer, E. N.: Echocardiography in combined valve disease. Radiology *105*:405, 1972.
14. Weyman, A. E., et al.: Cross-sectional echocardiography in assessing the severity of valvular aortic stenosis. Circulation *52*:828, 1975.
15. Nanda, N. C., et al.: Echocardiographic recognition of the congenital bicuspid aortic valve. Circulation *49*:870, 1974.
15a. Scovil, J. A., et al.: Echocardiographic studies of abnormalities associated with coarctation of the aorta. Circulation *53*:953, 1976.
16. Radford, D. J., et al.: Echocardiographic assessment of bicuspid aortic valves: angiographic and pathological correlates. Circulation *53*:80, 1976.
17. Edwards, J. E.: The congenital biscuspid aortic valve. Circulation *23*:485, 1961.
18. Johnson, M. L., et al.: Echocardiography of the aortic valve in non-rheumatic left ventricular outflow tract lesions. Radiology *112*:677, 1974.

Aortic Insufficiency

19. Mann, T., et al.: Assessing the hemodynamic severity of acute aortic regurgitation due to infective endocarditis. N. Engl. J. Med. *293*:108, 1975.
20. Hernberg, J., Weiss, B., and Keegan, A.: The ultrasonic recording of aortic valve motion. Radiology *94*:361, 1970.
21. Pridie, R. B., Benham, R., and Oakley, C. M.: Echocardiography of the mitral valve in aortic valve disease. Br. Heart J. *33*:296, 1971.
22. Botvinick, E. H., et al.: Echocardiographic demonstration of early mitral valve closure in severe aortic insufficiency, its clinical implications. Circulation *51*:836, 1975.
23. Winsberg, J., et al.: Fluttering of the mitral valve in aortic insufficiency. Circulation *41*:225, 1970.
24. Danford, H. G., et al.: Echocardiographic evaluation of the hemodynamic effects of chronic aortic insufficiency with observations on left ventricular performance. Circulation *48*:253, 1973.
25. Gray, K. E., and Barritt, D. W.: Echocardiographic assessment of severity of aortic regurgitation. Br. Heart J. *37*:691, 1975.

Vegetations

26. Dillon, J. C., et al.: Echocardiographic manifestations of valvular vegetations. Am. Heart J. *86*:698, 1973.

27. Martinez, E. C., Burch, G. E., and Giles, T. D.: Echocardiographic diagnosis of vegetative aortic bacterial endocarditis. Am. J. Cardiol. *34*:845, 1974.
28. Wray, T. M.: The variable echocardiographic features in aortic valve endocarditis. Circulation *52*:658, 1975.
29. Roy, P., et al.: Spectrum of echocardiographic findings in bacterial endocarditis. Circulation *53*:474, 1976.
30. DeMaria, A. N., et al.: Echography and phonography of acute aortic regurgitation in bacterial endocarditis. Ann. Intern. Med. *82*:329, 1975.
31. Hirschfeld, D. S., and Schiller, N.: Localization of aortic valve vegetations by echocardiography. Circulation *53*:280, 1976.
32. Wray, T. M.: Echocardiographic manifestations of flail aortic valve leaflets in bacterial endocarditis. Circulation *51*:832, 1975.
32a. Corrigall, D., Strunk, B. L., and Popp, R. L.: Phonocardiographic and echocardiographic features of ruptured aortic valvular cusp. Chest *69*:669, 1976.
33. Shahawy, M. E., et al.: Diagnosis of aortic valvular prolapse by echocardiography. Chest *69*:411, 1976.
34. Whipple, R. L., et al.: Echocardiographic manifestations of the flail aortic valve leaflet syndrome (Abstr.). Circulation *52*(Suppl. II):255, 1975.
35. Giuliani, E. R., et al.: Abnormal echo in the left ventricular outflow tract in bacterial endocarditis (Abstr.). Circulation *52*(Suppl. II):69, 1975.
35a. Yoshikawa, J., et al.: Cord-like aortic valve vegetation in bacterial endocarditis: demonstration by cardiac ultrasonography. Circulation *53*:911, 1976.
36. Gottlieb, S., et al.: Echocardiographic diagnosis of aortic valve vegetations in Candida endocarditis. Circulation *50*:826, 1974.

Aortic Root Dissection

37. Nanda, N. C., Gramiak, R., and Shah, P. M.: Diagnosis of aortic root dissection by echocardiography. Circulation *48*:506, 1973.
38. Krueger, S. K., et al.: Echocardiographic mimics of aortic root dissection. Chest *67*:441, 1975.
39. Brown, O. R., Popp, R. L., and Kloster, F. E.: Echocardiographic criteria for aortic root dissection. Am. J. Cardiol. *36*:17, 1975.
40. Kronzon, I., and Mehta, S. S.: Aortic root dissection. Chest *65*:88, 1974.
41. Millward, D. K., Robinson, N. J., and Craige, E.: Dissecting aortic aneurysm diagnosed by echocardiography in a patient with rupture of the aneurysm into the right atrium. Am. J. Cardiol. *30*:427, 1972.

Mitral Disease

Rheumatic Mitral Disease (Mitral Stenosis)

42. Edler, I.: Diagnostic use of ultrasound in heart disease. Acta Med. Scand. (Suppl.)*308*:32, 1955.
43. Edler, I.: Atrioventricular valve mobility in the living human heart recorded by ultrasound. Acta Med. Scand. (Suppl.)*370*:67, 83, 1961.
44. Joyner, C. R., Reid, J. M., and Bond, J. P.: Reflected ultrasound in the assessment of mitral valve disease. Circulation *27*:503, 1963.
45. Edler, I.: Ultrasoundcardiography in mitral valve stenosis. Am. J. Cardiol. *19*:18, 1967.
46. Zaky, A., Nasser, W. K., and Feigenbaum, H.: A study of mitral valve action recorded by reflected ultrasound and its application in the diagnosis of mitral stenosis. Circulation *37*:789, 1968.
47. Lundstrom, N. R.: Ultrasoundcardiographic studies of the mitral valve region in young infants with mitral atresia, mitral stenosis, hypoplasia of the left ventricle and cor triatriatum. Circulation *45*:324, 1972.
48. Laniado, S., et al.: A study of the dynamic relations between the mitral valve echogram and phasic mitral flow. Circulation *51*:104, 1975.
49. Segal, B. L., Likoff, W., and Kongsley, B.: Echocardiography—clinical application in mitral stenosis. J.A.M.A. *195*:99, 1966.
50. Gustafson, A.: Correlation between ultrasoundcardiography, hemodynamics and surgical findings in mitral stenosis. Am. J. Cardiol. *19*:32, 1967.
51. Effert, S.: Pre- and postoperative evaluation of mitral stenosis by ultrasound. Am. J. Cardiol. *19*:59, 1967.
52. Wharton, C. F. P., and Bescos, L. L.: Mitral valve movement: a study using an ultrasound technique. Br. Heart J. *32*:344, 1970.
53. Cope, G. D., et al.: A reassessment of the echocardiogram in mitral stenosis. Circulation *52*:664, 1975.
54. Henry, W. L., et al.: Measurement of mitral orifice area in patients with mitral stenosis by real time, two dimensional echocardiography. Circulation *51*:827, 1975.
55. Duchak, J. M., Chang, S., and Feigenbaum, H.: The posterior mitral valve echo and the echocardiographic diagnosis of mitral stenosis. Am. J. Cardiol. *29*:628, 1972.

56. Flaherty, J. T., Livengood, S., and Fortuin, N. J.: Atypical posterior leaflet motion in echocardiogram in mitral stenosis. Am. J. Cardiol. *35*:675, 1975.

57. Levisman, J. A., Abbasi, A. S., and Pearce, M. L.: Posterior mitral leaflet motion in mitral stenosis. Circulation *51*:511, 1975.

58. Ticzon, A. R., et al.: Echocardiographic manifestation of false mitral stenosis that was. Ann. Intern. Med. 83:503, 1975.

59. Quinones, M. A., et al.: Reduction in the rate of diastolic descent of the mitral valve. Echogram in patients with altered left ventricular diastolic pressure-volume relations. Circulation *49*:246, 1974.

60. McLaurin, L. P., et al.: An appraisal of mitral valve echocardiograms mimicking mitral stenosis in conditions with right ventricular overload. Circulation *48*:801, 1973.

61. Nanda, N. C., et al.: Mitral commissurotomy versus replacement, preoperative evaluation by echocardiography. Circulation *51*:263, 1975.

62. Lundstrom, N.: Echocardiography in the diagnosis of congenital mitral stenosis and in evaluation of the results of mitral valvotomy. Circulation *46*:44, 1972.

63. Nanda, N. C., et al.: Echocardiographic assessment of left ventricular outflow width in the selection of mitral valve prosthesis. Circulation *48*:1208, 1973.

64. Winters, W. L., Hafer, J., and Soloff, L. A.: Abnormal mitral valve motion as demonstrated by the ultrasound technique in apparent pure mitral insufficiency. Am. Heart J. 77:196, 1969.

65. Fischer, J. C., et al.: Echocardiographic determination of mitral valve flow. Am. J. Cardiol. *29*:262, 1972.

66. DeMaria, A. N., et al.: Mitral valve early diastolic closing velocity on echogram: relation to sequential diastolic flow and ventricular compliance (Abstr.). Circulation *50*(Suppl. III):144, 1974.

67. Shah, P. M., and Gramiak, R.: Echocardiographic recognition of mitral valve prolapse (Abstr.). Circulation *42*(Suppl. III):45, 1970.

Nonrheumatic Mitral Disease

68. Dillon, J. C., et al.: Use of echocardiography in patients with prolapsed mitral valve. Circulation *43*:503, 1971.

69. Kerber, R. E., Isaeff, D. M., and Hancock, E. W.: Echocardiographic patterns in patients with the syndrome of systolic click and late systolic murmur. N. Engl. J. Med. *284*:691, 1971.

70. Burgess, J., et al.: Echocardiographic findings in different types of mitral regurgitation. Circulation *48*:97, 1973.

71. Popp, R. L., et al.: Echocardiographic abnormalities in the mitral valve prolapse syndrome. Circulation *49*:428, 1974.

72. DeMaria, A. N., et al.: The variable spectrum of echocardiographic manifestations of mitral valve prolapse syndrome. Circulation *50*:33, 1974.

73. Greenwald, J. C., DeMaria, A. N., and Mason, D. T.: "Silent" mitral prolapse. Circulation *50*:1284, 1974.

74. Markiewicz, W., et al.: Mitral valve prolapse in one hundred presumably healthy females. Circulation *53*:464, 1976.

75. Sahn, D. J., et al.: Mitral valve prolapse in children, a problem defined by real-time cross-sectional echocardiography. Circulation *53*:651, 1976.

76. Roelandt, J., et al.: Resolution problems in echocardiography: a source of interpretation errors. Am. J. Cardiol. *37*:256, 1976.

77. Winkle, R. A., Goodman, D. J., and Popp, R. L.: Simultaneous echocardiographic-phonocardiographic recordings at rest and during amyl nitrite administration in patients with mitral valve prolapse. Circulation *51*:522, 1975.

78. Brown, O. R., and Kloster, F. E.: Echocardiographic criteria for mitral valve prolapse: effect of transducer position (Abstr.). Circulation *51*(Suppl. II):165, 1975.

79. Sweatman, T. W., Selzer, A., and Cohn, K.: Echocardiographic diagnosis of ruptured chordae tendineae. Am. J. Cardiol. *26*:661, 1970.

80. Weiss, A. N., et al.: Echocardiographic detection of mitral valve prolapse. Exclusion of false positive diagnosis and determination of inheritance. Circulation *52*:1091, 1975.

81. Brown, O. R., et al.: Aortic root dilatation and mitral valve prolapse in Marfan's syndrome. An echocardiographic study. Circulation *52*:651, 1975.

82. Spangler, R. P., et al.: Echocardiography in Marfan's syndrome. Chest *69*:72, 1976.

83. Duchak, J. M., Chang, S., and Feigenbaum, H.: Echocardiographic features of torn chordae tendineae. Am. J. Cardiol. *29*:260, 1972.

84. Gramiak, R.: American College of Cardiology Course, "Advanced Echocardiography," Indianapolis, Indiana, September 30–October 2, 1975.

85. Brown, O. R., Kloster, F. E., and DeMots, H.: Incidence of mitral valve prolapse in the asymptomatic normal (Abstr.). Circulation *52*(Suppl. II):77, 1975.

86. Procacci, P. M., et al.: Prevalence of clinical mitral-prolapse in 1169 young women. N. Engl. J. Med. *294*:1086, 1976.

86a. Malcolm, A. D., et al.: Clinical features and investigative findings in presence of mitral prolapse. Study of 85 consecutive patients. Br. Heart J. 38:244, 1976.

87. Hutter, A. M., et al.: Early systolic clicks due to mitral valve prolapse. Circulation *44*:516, 1971.

88. Mathey, D. G., et al.: The determinants of onset of mitral valve prolapse in the systolic click-late systolic murmur syndrome. Circulation *53*:872, 1976.

89. Hirschfeld, D. S., and Emilson, B. B.: Echocardiogram in calcified mitral annulus. Am. J. Cardiol. 36:354, 1975.

Tumors

90. Popp, R. L., and Harrison, D. C.: Ultrasound for the diagnosis of atrial tumors. Ann. Intern. Med. 71:1969.
91. Wolfe, S. B., Popp, R. L., and Feigenbaum, H.: Diagnosis of atrial tumors by ultrasound. Circulation 39:615, 1969.
92. Spencer, W. H., Peter, R. H., and Orgain, E. S.: Detection of a left atrial myxoma by echocardiography. Arch. Intern. Med. 128: 787, 1971.
93. Nasser, W. K., et al.: Atrial myxoma. II. Phonocardiographic, echocardiographic, hemodynamic and angiographic features in nine cases. Am. Heart J. 83:810, 1972.
94. Johnson, M. L., et al.: Echocardiographic diagnosis of a left atrial myxoma found attached to the free left atrial wall. J. Clin. Ultrasound 1:75, 1973.
95. Srivastove, T. N., and Fletcher, E.: The echocardiogram in left atrial myxoma. Am. J. Med. 54:136, 1973.
96. Martinez, E. C., Giles, T. D., and Burch, G. E.: Echocardiographic diagnosis of left atrial myxoma. Am. J. Cardiol. 33:281, 1974.
97. Sung, R. J., et al.: Hemodynamic features of prolapsing and nonprolapsing left atrial myxoma. Circulation 51:342, 1975.
98. Moscovitz, H. L., et al.: Simulated left atrial tumor. Am. J. Cardiol. 34:63, 1974.
99. Kerber, R. E., Kelly, D. H., and Gutenkauf, C. H.: Left atrial myxoma demonstration by stop action cardiac ultrasonography. Am. J. Cardiol. 34:838, 1974.
100. Potts, J. L., et al.: Varied manifestations of left atrial myxoma and the relationship of echocardiographic patterns to tumor size. Chest 68:781, 1975.
101. Pindyck, F., Peirce, E. C., and Baron, M. G.: Embolization of left atrial myxoma after transseptal cardiac catheterization. Am. J. Cardiol. 30:569, 1972.
102. Walton, J. A., Kahn, D. R., and Willis, P. W.: Recurrence of a left atrial myxoma. Am. J. Cardiol. 29:872, 1972.
103. Goldschlager, A., et al.: Right atrial myxoma with right to left shunt and polycythemia presenting as congenital heart disease. Am. J. Cardiol. 30:82, 1972.
104. Waxler, E. B., Kawai, N., and Kasparian, H.: Right atrial myxoma: echocardiographic, phonocardiographic and hemodynamic signs. Am. Heart J. 83:251, 1972.
105. Harbold, N. B., and Gau, G. T.: Echocardiographic diagnosis of right atrial myxoma. Mayo Clin. Proc. 48:284, 1973.
106. Farooki, Z. Q., Henry, J. G., and Green, E. W.: Echocardiographic diagnosis of right atrial extension of Wilms' tumor. Am. J. Cardiol. 36:363, 1975.
107. Farooki, Z. Q., et al.: Ultrasonic pattern of ventricular rhabdomyoma in two infants. Am. J. Cardiol. 34:842, 1974.
108. Allen, H. D., et al.: Echocardiographic demonstration of a right ventricular tumor in a neonate. J. Pediatr. 84:854, 1974.
109. DeMaria, A. N., et al.: Unusual echographic manifestations of right and left heart myxomas. Am. J. Med. 59:713, 1975.
110. Levisman, J. A., et al.: Echocardiographic diagnosis of a mobile pedunculated tumor in the left ventricular cavity. Am. J. Cardiol. 36:957, 1975.
111. Bass, N. M.: Left atrial myxoma diagnosed by echocardiography, with observations on tumor movement. Br. Heart J. 35:1332, 1973.
112. Child, J. S., Abbasi, A. S., and Pearce, M. L.: Echocardiographic differentiation of mediastinal tumors from primary cardiac disease. Chest 67:108, 1975.
112a. Tingelstad, J. B., McWilliams, N. B., and Thomas, C. E.: Confirmation of a retrosternal mass by echocardiogram. J. Clin. Ultrasound 4:129, 1976.
113. Felner, J. N., Fleming, W. H., and Franch R. H.: Echocardiographic identification of a pericardial cyst. Chest 68:386, 1975.

Hypertrophic Subaortic Stenosis

114. Henry, W. L., et al.: Echocardiographic measurement of the left ventricular outflow gradient in idiopathic hypertrophic subaortic stenosis. N. Engl. J. Med. 288:989, 1973.
115. Henry, W. L., Clark, C. E., and Epstein, S. E.: Asymmetric septal hypertrophy (ASH): the unifying link in the IHSS spectrum. Observations regarding its pathogenesis, pathophysiology and course. Circulation 47:827, 1973.
116. Abbasi, A. S., et al.: Echocardiographic diagnosis of idiopathic hypertrophic cardiomyopathy without outflow obstruction. Circulation 46:897, 1972.
117. Henry, W. L., et al.: Long-term effects of operation on obstruction and left ventricular hypertrophy in IHSS (Abstr.). Clin. Res. 21:425, 1973.
118. Henry, W. L., et al.: Differences in distribution of myocardial abnormalities in patients with obstructive and nonobstructive asymmetric septal hypertrophy (ASH): Echocardiographic and gross anatomic findings. Circulation 50:447, 1974.

119. Feizi, O., and Emanuel, R.: Echocardiographic spectrum of hypertrophic cardiomyopathy. Br. Heart J. 37:1286, 1975.

120. Henry, W. L.: American College of Cardiology Course, "Advanced Echocardiography," Indianapolis, Indiana, September 30–October 2, 1975.

121. Larter, W. E., et al.: The asymmetrically hypertrophied septum. Circulation 53:19, 1976.

122. Maron, B. J., et al.: Congenital heart malformations associated with disproportionate ventricular septal thickening. Circulation 52:926, 1975.

123. Henry, W. L., Clark, E. E., and Epstein, S. E.: Asymmetric septal hypertrophy, echocardiographic identification of the pathognomonic anatomic abnormality of IHSS. Circulation 47:225, 1973.

124. Rossen, R. M., et al.: Echocardiographic criteria in the diagnosis of idiopathic hypertrophic subaortic stenosis. Circulation 50:747, 1974.

125. Popp, R. L., and Harrison, D. C.: Ultrasound in the diagnosis and evaluation of therapy of idiopathic hypertrophic subaortic stenosis. Circulation 40:905, 1969.

126. Shah, P. M., Gramiak, R., and Kramer, D. H.: Ultrasound localization of left ventricular outflow obstruction in hypertrophic obstructive cardiomyopathy. Circulation 40:3, 1969.

127. Pridie, R. B., and Oakley, C. M.: Mechanism of mitral regurgitation in hypertrophic obstructive cardiomyopathy. Br. Heart J. 32:203, 1970.

128. Shah, P. M., et al.: Role of echocardiography in diagnostic and hemodynamic assessment of hypertrophic subaortic stenosis. Circulation 44:891, 1971.

129. Shah, P. M., et al.: Echocardiographic assessment of the effects of surgery and propranolol on the dynamics of outflow obstruction in hypertrophic subaortic stenosis. Circulation 45:516, 1972.

130. Henry, W. L., et al.: Mechanism of left ventricular outflow obstruction in patients with obstructive asymmetric septal hypertrophy (idiopathic hypertrophic subaortic stenosis). Am. J. Cardiol. 35:337, 1975.

131. King, J. F., et al.: Echocardiographic assessment of idiopathic hypertrophic subaortic stenosis. Chest 64:723, 1973.

132. Rossen, R. M., and Popp, R. L.: Mid-systolic AV closure in HSS. Circulation 51:1172, 1975.

133. Bolton, M. R., et al.: The effects of operation on the echocardiographic features of idiopathic hypertrophic subaortic stenosis. Circulation 50:897, 1974.

134. Morrow, A. G., et al.: Operative treatment in hypertrophic subaortic stenosis. Circulation 52:88, 1975.

135. King, J. F., et al.: Markedly abnormal mitral valve motion without simultaneous intraventricular gradient due to uneven mitral-septal contact in idiopathic hypertrophic subaortic stenosis. Am. J. Cardiol. 34:360, 1974.

136. Clark, C. E., Henry, W. L., and Epstein, S. E.: Familial prevalence and genetic transmission of idiopathic hypertrophic subaortic stenosis. N. Engl. J. Med. 289:709, 1973.

137. Rossen, R. M., et al.: Ventricular systolic thickening and excursion in idiopathic hypertrophic subaortic stenosis. N. Engl. J. Med. 291:1317, 1974.

138. Tajik, A. J., and Giuliani, E. R.: Echocardiographic observations in idiopathic hypertrophic subaortic stenosis. Mayo Clin. Proc. 49:89, 1974.

139. Johnson, A. D., Lanky, S. A., and Carleton, R. A.: Combined hypertrophic subaortic stenosis and calcific aortic valvular stenosis. Am. J. Cardiol. 35:706, 1975.

140. Cohen, M. V., Cooperman, L. B., and Rosenblum, R.: Regional myocardial function in idiopathic hypertrophic subaortic stenosis: an echocardiographic study. Circulation 52:842, 1975.

141. Shah, P. M.: American College of Cardiology Course, "Advanced Echocardiography," Indianapolis, Indiana, September 30–October 2, 1975.

142. Chung, K. J., Manning, J. A., and Gramiak, R.: Echocardiography in coexisting hypertrophic subaortic stenosis and fixed left ventricular outflow obstruction. Circulation 49:673, 1974.

143. Nanda, N. C., et al.: Echocardiography in the diagnosis of idiopathic hypertrophic subaortic stenosis coexisting with aortic valve disease. Circulation 50:752, 1974.

Left Ventricle

144. Hagan, A. D., et al.: Echocardiographic criteria for normal newborn infants. Circulation 48:1221, 1975.

145. Epstein, M. L., et al.: Great vessel, cardiac chamber and wall growth patterns in normal children. Circulation 5:1124, 1975.

146. Popp, R. L., et al.: Estimation of right and left ventricular size by ultrasound. Am. J. Cardiol. 24:523, 1969.

147. Popp, R. L., et al.: Effect of transducer placement on echocardiographic measurement of left ventricular dimensions. Am. J. Cardiol. 35:537, 1975.

148. Teichholtz, L. E., et al.: Problems in echocardiographic volume determinations: echocardiographic-angiographic correlations in the presence or absence of asynergy. Am. J. Cardiol. 37:7, 1976.

149. Pombo, J. F., Troy, B. L., and Russell, R. O.: Left ventricular volumes and ejection fraction by echocardiography. Circulation 43:480, 1971.

150. Fortuin, N. J., et al.: Determination of left ventricular volumes by ultrasound. Circulation 44:575, 1971.

151. Paraskos, J. A., et al.: A noninvasive technique for the determination of velocity of circumferential fiber shortening in man. Clin. Res. 29:610, 1971.

152. Fortuin, N. J., Hood, W. P., and Craige, E.: Evaluation of the left ventricular function by echocardiography. Circulation 46:26, 1972.
153. Cooper, R. H., et al.: Comparison of ultrasound and cineangiographic measurements of the mean rate of circumferential fiber shortening in man. Circulation 46:914, 1972.
154. Ludbrook, P., et al.: Comparison of ultrasound and cineangiographic measurements of left ventricular performance in patients with and without wall motion abnormalities. Br. Heart. J. 35: 1026, 1973.
155. Corya, B. C., et al.: Echocardiographic features of congestive cardiomyopathy compared with normal subjects and patients with coronary artery disease. Circulation 49:1153, 1974.
156. Quinones, M. A., Gaasch, W. H., and Alexander, J. K.: Echocardiographic assessment of left ventricular function with special reference to normalized velocities. Circulation 50:42, 1974.
157. Quinones, M. A., et al.: Echocardiographic determination of left ventricular stress-velocity relations in man. Circulation 51:689, 1975.
158. Rankin, L. S., Moos, S., and Grossman, W.: Alterations in preload and ejection phase indices of left ventricular performance. Circulation 51:910, 1975.
159. Karliner, J. S., and O'Rourke, R.: Usefulness and limitations of assessment of internal shortening velocity by ultrasound in man. Chest 68:361, 1975.
160. Hirshleifer, J., et al.: Influence of acute alterations in heart rate and systemic arterial pressure on echocardiographic measures of left ventricular performance in normal human subjects. Circulation 52:835, 1975.
161. Quinones, M. A., Gaasch, W. H., and Alexander, J. K.: Influence of acute changes in preload, afterload, contractile state and heart rate on ejection and isovolumic indices of myocardial contractility in man. Circulation 53:293, 1976.
162. Konecke, L. L., et al.: Abnormal mitral valve motion in patients with elevated left ventricular diastolic pressure. Circulation 47:989, 1973.
163. DeMaria, A. N., et al.: Mitral valve early diastolic closing velocity in the echocardiogram: relation to sequential diastolic flow and ventricular compliance. Am. J. Cardiol. 37:693, 1976.
164. Feigenbaum, H., et al.: Role of echocardiography in patients with coronary artery disease. Am. J. Cardiol. 37:774, 1976.
165. Betenkie, I., et al.: Assessment of left ventricular dimensions and function by echocardiography. Am. J. Cardiol. 31:755, 1973.
166. Feigenbaum, H.: American College of Cardiology Course, "Advanced Echocardiography," Indianapolis, Indiana, September 30–October 2, 1975.
167. Millward, D. K., McLaurin, L. P., and Craige, E.: Echocardiographic studies of the mitral valve in patients with congestive cardiomyopathy and mitral regurgitation. Am. Heart J. 85:413, 1973.
168. Linhart, J. W., et al.: Left ventricular volume measurements by echocardiography: fact or fiction? Am. J. Cardiol. 36:114, 1975.
169. Feigenbaum, H.: Echocardiographic examination of the left ventricle. Circulation 51:1, 1975.
169a. Rosenblatt, A., et al.: Echocardiographic assessment of the level of cardiac compensation in valvular heart disease. Circulation. 54:509, 1976.
169b. McDonald, I. G.: Echocardiographic assessment of left ventricular function in aortic valve disease. Circulation 53:860, 1976.
169c. McDonald, I. G.: Echocardiographic assessment of left ventricular function in mitral valve disease. Circulation 53:865, 1976.
169d. Clark, R., Rosenblatt, A., Kryda, W., Korcuska, K., and Cohn, K.: Serial echocardiographic evaluation of left ventricular function in aortic regurgitation (Abstract). Circulation 54 (Suppl. II):60, 1976.
170. Henning, H., et al.: Left ventricular performance assessed by radionuclide angiocardiography and echocardiography in patients with previous myocardial infarction. Circulation 52:1069, 1975.
171. Jacobs, J. J., et al.: Detection of left ventricular asynergy by echocardiography. Circulation 48:263, 1973.
171a. Joffe, C. D., et al.: Echocardiographic diagnosis of left anterior descending coronary artery disease. Am. J. Cardiol. 35:146, 1975.
172. Corya, B. C., et al.: Anterior left ventricular wall echoes in coronary artery disease—linear scanning with a single element transducer. Am. J. Cardiol. 34:652, 1974.
173. Chang, S., Feigenbaum, H., and Dillon, J.: Subxiphoid echocardiography. Chest 68:233, 1975.
174. Chang, S., Feigenbaum, H., and Dillon, J.: Condensed M-mode echocardiographic scan of the symmetrical left ventricle. Chest 68:93, 1975.
174a. Dillon, J. C., et al.: M-mode echocardiography in the evaluation of patients for aneurysmectomy. Circulation 53:657, 1976.
175. Stack, R. S., et al.: Left ventricular performance in coronary artery disease evaluated with systolic time intervals and echocardiography. Am. J. Cardiol. 37:331, 1976.
176. Ludbrook, P., et al.: Posterior wall velocity: an unreliable index of total left ventricular performance in patients with coronary artery disease. Am. J. Cardiol. 33:475, 1974.
177. Feigenbaum, H., et al.: Identification of ultrasound echoes from the left ventricle using intracardiac injections of indocyanine green. Circulation 41:615, 1970.
178. Abbasi, A. S., et al.: Left ventricular hypertrophy diagnosed by echocardiography. N. Engl. J. Med. 289:118, 1973.
178a. Abbasi, A. S.: Echocardiography in the differential diagnosis of the large heart. Am. J. Med. 60:677, 1976.
179. Feigenbaum, H., et al.: Ultrasound measurements of the left ventricle. A correlative study with angiocardiography. Arch. Intern. Med. 129:481, 1972.

180. Grossman, W., et al.: Wall thickness and diastolic properties of the left ventricle. Circulation *49*:129, 1974.
181. Troy, B. L., Pombo, J. F., and Rackley, C. E.: Measurement of left ventricular thickness and mass by echocardiography. Circulation *45*:602, 1972.
181a. Sjogren, A. L., Hytonen, I., and Frick, M. H.: Ultrasonic measurements of left ventricular wall thickness. Chest *57*:37, 1970.
182. Frishman, W., et al.: Non-invasive assessment of clinical response to oral propranolol therapy. Am. J. Cardiol. *35*:635, 1975.
182a. Winkle, R. A., Goodman, D. J., and Popp, R. L.: Echocardiographic evaluation of propranolol therapy for mitral valve prolapse. Br. Heart J. *38*:129, 1976.

Left Atrium

183. Hirata, T., et al.: Estimation of left atrial size using ultrasound. Am. Heart J. *78*:43, 1969.
184. Brown, O. R., Harrison, D. C., and Popp, R. L.: An improved method for echographic detection of left atrial enlargement. Circulation *50*:58, 1974.
184a. Yabek, S. M., et al.: Echocardiographic determination of left atrial volumes in children with congenital heart disease. Circulation *53*:268, 1976.

Pericardial Effusion

185. Feigenbaum, H., Waldhausen, J. A., and Hyde, L. P.: Ultrasound diagnosis of pericardial effusion. J.A.M.A. *191*:711, 1965.
186. Soulen, R. L., Lapayowker, M. S., and Gimenaz, J. L.: Echocardiography in diagnosis of pericardial effusion. Radiology *86*:1047, 1966.
187. Goldberg, B. B., Ostrun, B. J., and Isard, H. J.: Ultrasonic determination of pericardial effusion. J.A.M.A. *202*:927, 1967.
188. Pate, J. W., Gardner, H. C., and Normal, R. S.: Diagnosis of pericardial effusion by echocardiography. Ann. Surg. *165*:826, 1967.
189. Rothman, J., et al.: Ultrasonic diagnosis of pericardial effusion. Circulation *35*:358, 1967.
190. Feigenbaum, H., Zaky, A., and Waldhausen, J. A.: Use of reflected ultrasound in detecting pericardial effusion. Am. J. Cardiol. *19*:84, 1967.
191. Klein, J. J., and Segal, B. L.: Pericardial effusion diagnosed by reflected ultrasound. Am. J. Cardiol. *22*:57, 1968.
192. Feigenbaum, H.: Echocardiographic diagnosis of pericardial effusion. Am. J. Cardiol. *26*:475, 1970.
193. Kent, E., and King, D. L.: Pericarditis and pericardial effusion: radiologic and echocardiographic diagnosis. Radiol. Clin. North Am. *11*:393, 1973.
194. Horowitz, M. S., et al.: Sensitivity and specificity of echocardiographic diagnosis of pericardial effusion. Circulation *50*:239, 1974.
195. Feigenbaum, H., Zaky, A., and Grabhorn, L. L.: Cardiac motion in patients with pericardial effusion. A study using reflected ultrasound. Circulation *34*:611, 1966.
196. Ratshin, R. A., Smith, M., and Hood, W. P.: Possible false-positive diagnosis of pericardial effusion by echocardiography in the presence of a large left atrium. Chest *65*:112, 1974.
197. Casarella, W. J., and Schneider, B. O.: Pitfalls in the ultrasonic diagnosis of pericardial effusion. Am. J. Roentgenol. Radium Ther. Nucl. Med. *110*:760, 1970.
198. Abbasi, A. S., Ellis, N., and Flynn, J. J.: Echocardiographic M-scan technique in the diagnosis of pericardial effusion. J. Clin. Ultrasound *1*:300, 1973.
199. Schiller, N. B., and Botvinick, E. H.: Right ventricular compression: a reliable echographic sign of cardiac tamponade. Circulation *51*(Suppl. II):942, 1975.
200. D'Cruz, I. A., et al.: Diagnosis of cardiac tamponade by echocardiography. Circulation *52*:460, 1975.
200a. Morris, A. L.: Echo evaluation of tamponade. Circulation *53*:746, 1976.
201. Warren, B. H., Lynn, R. R., and Allen, F. H.: Echocardiographic observation of ventricular volume changes and swinging septal position in massive pericardial effusion. J. Clin. Ultrasound *3*:283, 1975.
202. Lemire, F., et al.: Further echocardiographic observations in pericardial effusion. Mayo Clin. Proc. *51*:13, 1976.
203. Kisslo, J.: American College of Cardiology Course, "Advanced Echocardiography," Indianapolis, Indiana, September 30–October 2, 1975.
204. Levisman, J. A., and Abbasi, A. S.: Abnormal motion of the mitral valve with pericardial effusion: pseudo-prolapse of the mitral valve. Am. Heart J. *91*:18, 1976.
205. Owens, J. S., et al.: Pseudoprolapse of the mitral valve in a patient with pericardial effusion. Chest *69*:214, 1976.
206. Vignola, P. A., et al.: Correlation of echocardiographic and clinical findings in patients with pericardial effusion. Am. J. Cardiol. *37*:701, 1976.
207. Gabor, G. E., Winsberg, F., and Bloom, H. S.: Electrical and mechanical alternation in pericardial effusion. Chest *59*:341, 1971.
208. Usher, B. W., and Popp, R. L.: Electrical alternans: mechanism in pericardial effusion. Am. Heart J. *83*:459, 1972.

Interventricular Septum

209. Hagen, A. O., et al.: Ultrasound evaluation of systolic anterior septal motion in patients with and without right ventricular volume overload. Circulation 50:248, 1974.
209a. Assad-Morell, J. L., Tajik, A. J., and Giuliani, E. R.: Echocardiographic analysis of the ventricular septum. Progr. Cardiovasc. Dis. 17:219, 1974.
210. Pool, P. E., et al.: Echocardiographic manifestations of constrictive pericarditis. Chest 68:684, 1975.
211. Payvandi, M. N., and Kerber, R. E.: Echocardiography in congenital and acquired absence of the pericardium. An echocardiographic mimic of right ventricular volume overload. Circulation 53:86, 1976.
212. Burggrof, G. W., and Craige, E.: Echocardiographic study of left ventricular wall motion and dimensions after valvular heart surgery. Am. J. Cardiol. 35:473, 1975.
213. Miller, H. C., Gibson, D. G., and Stephens, J. D.: Role of echocardiography and phonocardiography in diagnosis of mitral paraprosthetic regurgitation with Starr-Edwards prostheses. Br. Heart J. 35:1217, 1973.
214. Brodie, B. R., et al.: Diagnosis of prosthetic mitral valve malfunction with combined echo–phonocardiography. Circulation 53:93, 1976.
215. Sawaya, J., Longo, M. R., and Schlant, R. C.: Echocardiographic interventricular septal wall motion and thickness: a study in health and disease. Am. Heart J. 87:681, 1974.
216. Burch, G. E., Giles, T. D., and Martinez, E.: Echocardiographic detection of abnormal motion of the interventricular septum in ischemic cardiomyopathy. Am. J. Cardiol. 57:293, 1974.
217. Dillon, J. C., Chang, S., and Feigenbaum, H.: Echocardiographic manifestations of left bundle branch block. Circulation 49:876, 1974.
218. McDonald, I. G., and Melb, M. D.: Echocardiographic demonstration of abnormal motion of the interventricular septum in left bundle branch block. Circulation 48:272, 1973.
219. Abbasi, A. S., et al.: Paradoxical motion of interventricular septum in left bundle branch block. Circulation 49:423, 1974.
219a. Ticzon, A. R., et al.: Interventricular septal motion during pre-excitation and normal conduction in Wolff-Parkinson-White syndrome. Am. J. Cardiol. 37:840, 1976.
219b. Chandra, M. S., et al.: Echocardiography in Wolff-Parkinson-White syndrome. Circulation 53:943, 1976.

Pulmonary Hypertension and Valve

220. Goodman, D. J., Harrison, D. C., and Popp, R. L.: Echocardiographic features of primary pulmonary hypertension. Am. J. Cardiol. 33:438, 1974.
221. Weyman, A. E., et al.: Echocardiographic patterns of pulmonic valve motion with pulmonary hypertension. Circulation 50:905, 1974.
222. Nanda, N. C., et al.: Echocardiographic evaluation of pulmonary hypertension. Circulation 50:575, 1974.
223. McLaurin, L. P., et al.: An appraisal of mitral valve echocardiograms mimicking mitral stenosis in conditions with right ventricular pressure overload. Circulation 48:801, 1973.
224. Nanda, N. C., et al.: Evaluation of pulmonary hypertension by echocardiography. J. Clin. Ultrasound 1:255, 1973.
225. Weyman, A. E., et al.: Echocardiographic patterns of pulmonic valve in valvular pulmonic stenosis. Am. J. Cardiol. 34:644, 1974.
225a. Weyman, A. E.: American College of Cardiology Course, "Advanced Echocardiography," Indianapolis, Indiana, September 30–October 2, 1975.
226. Weyman, A. E., et al.: Pulmonary valve echo motion in pulmonary regurgitation. Br. Heart J. 37:1184, 1975.
227. Weyman, A. E., et al.: Echocardiographic differentiation of infundibular from valvular pulmonic stenosis. Am. J. Cardiol. 36:21, 1975.
228. Hirschfeld, S., et al.: The echocardiographic assessment of pulmonary artery pressure and pulmonary vascular resistance. Circulation 52:642, 1975.
229. Gramiak, R., Nanda, N. C., and Shah, P. M.: Echocardiographic detection of the pulmonary valve. Radiology 102:153, 1972.
230. Weyman, A. E., et al.: Premature pulmonic valve opening following sinus of Valsalva aneurysm rupture into the right atrium. Circulation 51:556, 1975.

Congenital Heart Disease

General Articles

231. Meyer, R. A., and Kaplan, S.: Noninvasive techniques in pediatric cardiovascular disease. Progr. Cardiovasc. Dis. 15:341, 1973.
232. Chesler, E., et al.: Echocardiography in the diagnosis of congenital heart disease. Pediatr. Clin. North Am. 18:1163, 1971.
233. Solinger, R., Elbl, F., and Minhas, K.: Echocardiography in congenital heart disease. Lancet 2:1093, 1971.
234. Lundstrom, N. R., and Edler, I.: Ultrasound cardiography in infants and children. Acta Paediatr. Scand. 60:117, 1971.

235. Solinger, R., Elbl, F., and Minhas, K.: Echocardiography in the normal neonate. Circulation 47:108, 1973.
236. Sahn, D. J., et al.: Multiple crystal cross-sectional echocardiography in the diagnosis of cyanotic congenital heart disease. Circulation 50:230, 1974.
237. Solinger, R., Elbl, F., and Minhas, K.: Deductive echocardiographic analysis in infants with congenital heart disease. Circulation 50:1072, 1974.
238. Murphy, K. F., et al.: Ultrasound in the diagnosis of congenital heart disease. Am. Heart J. 89:638, 1975.
239. Moss, A. F., Gussani, C. C., and Isabel-Jones, J.: Echocardiography in congenital heart disease. West. J. Med. 124:102, 1976.
239a. Hagler, D. J.: The utilization of echocardiography in the differential diagnosis of cyanosis in the neonate. Mayo Clin. Proc. 51:143, 1976.

Atrial Septal Defect

240. Diamond, N. A., et al.: Echocardiographic feature of atrial septal defect. Circulation 43:129, 1971.
241. Meyer, R. A., et al.: Ventricular septum in right ventricular volume overload. An echocardiographic study. Am. J. Cardiol. 30:349, 1972.
242. Tajik, A. J., et al.: Echocardiographic pattern of right ventricular diastolic volume overload in children. Circulation 46:36, 1972.
243. Tajik, A. J., Gau, G. T., and Schattenberg, T. T.: Echocardiography in atrial septal defect. Chest 62:213, 1972.
244. McCann, W. D., Harbold, N. B., and Giuliani, E. R.: The echocardiogram in right ventricular overload. J.A.M.A. 221:1243, 1972.
245. Kerber, R. E., Dippel, W. F., and Abboud, F. M.: Abnormal motion of the interventricular septum in right ventricular volume overload. Circulation 48:86, 1973.
246. Radtke, W. E., et al.: Atrial septal defect: echocardiographic observations. Ann. Intern. Med. 84:246, 1976.
247. Paquet, M., and Gutgesell, H.: Echocardiographic features of total anomalous pulmonary venous connection. Circulation 51:599, 1975.
248. Tajik, A. J., et al.: Normal ventricular septal motion in atrial septal defect. Mayo Clin. Proc. 47:635, 1972.
249. Tajik, A. J., Gau, G. T., and Schattenberg, T. T.: Echocardiogram in atrial septal defect with small left to right shunt. Chest 63:95, 1973.
250. Tajik, A. J., Gau, G. T., and Schattenberg, T. T.: Echocardiographic "pseudo HSS" pattern in atrial septal defect. Chest 62:324, 1972.
250a. Weyman, A. E., Wann, S., Feigenbaum, H., and Dillon, J. C.: Mechanism of abnormal septal motion in patients with right ventricular volume overload. Circulation 54:179, 1976.

Endocardial Cushion Defect

251. Gramiak, R., and Nanda, N. C.: Echocardiographic diagnosis of ostium primum septal defect (Abstr.) Circulation 46(Suppl. II): 37, 1972.
252. Williams, R. G., and Rudd, M.: Echocardiographic features of endocardial cushion defects. Circulation 49:418, 1974.
253. Sahn, D. J., et al.: Multiple crystal echocardiographic evaluation of endocardial cushion defect. Circulation 50:25, 1974.
254. Pieroni, D. R., Homey, E., and Freedom, R.: Echocardiography in atrioventricular canal defect. Am. J. Cardiol. 35:54, 1975.
255. Eshaghpour, E., et al.: Echocardiography in endocardial cushion defects: a preoperative and postoperative study. Chest 68:172, 1975.
256. Lopez, J. M., et al.: Echocardiographic and pathologic correlations in a patient with common atrioventricular canal. Chest 68:721, 1975.
257. Komatsu, Y., et al.: Echocardiographic analysis of intracardiac anatomy in endocardial cushion defect. Am. Heart J. 91:210, 1976.

Ebstein's Anomaly

258. Kotler, M. N., and Tabatznik, B.: Recognition of Ebstein's anomaly by ultrasound technique (Abstr.). Circulation 43 and 44 (Suppl. II):34, 1971.
259. Lundstrom, N. R.: Echocardiography in the diagnosis of Ebstein's anomaly of the tricuspid valve. Circulation 47:597, 1973.
260. Kotler, M. N., and Lundstrom, N. R.: Tricuspid valve in Ebstein's anomaly. Circulation 49:194, 1974.
261. Tajik, A. J., et al.: Echocardiogram in Ebstein's anomaly with Wolff-Parkinson-White pre-excitation syndrome type B. Circulation 47:813, 1973.
262. Yuste, P., et al.: Echocardiography in the diagnosis of Ebstein's anomaly. Chest 60:273, 1974.
263. Farooki, Z. Q., Henry, J. G., and Green, E. W.: Echocardiographic spectrum of Ebstein's anomaly of the tricuspid valve. Circulation 53:63, 1976.
264. Milner, S., et al.: Mitral and tricuspid valve closure in congenital heart disease. Circulation 53:513, 1976.
265. Matsumoto, M., et al.: Visualization of Ebstein's anomaly of the tricuspid valve by two dimensional and standard echocardiography. Circulation 53:69, 1976.

266. Crews, T. L., et al.: Auscultatory and phonocardiographic findings in Ebstein's anomaly; correlation of the first heart sound with ultrasonic records of tricuspid valve movement. Br. Heart J. *34*:681, 1972.

266a. French, J. W., Baum, D., and Popp, R. L.: Echocardiographic findings in Uhl's anomaly with demonstration of diastolic pulmonary valve opening. Am. J. Cardiol. *36*:349, 1975.

Ventricular Septal Defect

267. King, D. L., Steeg, C. N., and Ellis, K.: Visualization of ventricular septal defects by cardiac ultrasonography. Circulation *48*:1215, 1973.

268. Assad-Morell, J. L., Tajik, A. J., and Giuliani, E. R.: Aneurysm of membranous interventricular septum. Mayo Clin. Proc. *49*:164, 1974.

268a. Sahn, D. J., Kirkpatrick, S. E., and Friedman, W. F.: Echocardiographic recognition of ventricular septal aneurysm—a case report. J. Clin. Ultrasound *3*:297, 1975.

268b. Sapire, D. W., and Black, I. F. S.: Echocardiographic detection of aneurysms of the interventricular septum associated with ventricular septal defect. Am. J. Cardiol. *36*:797, 1975.

268c. Matsumoto, M., et al.: Echocardiographic diagnosis of ruptured aneurysm of sinus of Valsalva; report of two cases. Circulation *53*:382, 1976.

269. Carter, W. H., and Bowman, C. R.: Estimation of shunt flow in isolated ventricular septal defect by echocardiogram (Abstr.). Circulation 38(Suppl. IV):64, 1973.

269a. Lewis, A. B., and Takahashi, M.: Echocardiographic assessment of left to right shunt volume in children with ventricular septal defects. Circulation *54*:78, 1976.

Tetralogy of Fallot

270. Morris, D. C., et al.: Echocardiographic diagnosis of tetralogy of Fallot. Am. J. Cardiol. *36*:908, 1975.

271. Chung, K. J., et al.: Echocardiographic findings in tetralogy of Fallot (Abstr.). Am. J. Cardiol. *31*:126, 1973.

272. Tajik, A. J., et al.: Echocardiogram in tetralogy of Fallot. Chest *64*:107, 1973.

273. Henry, W. L., et al.: The differential diagnosis of anomalies of the great vessels by real-time, two dimensional echocardiography. Am. J. Cardiol. *33*:143, 1974.

274. Assad-Morell, J. L., et al.: Echo-phonocardiographic and contrast studies in conditions associated with systemic arterial trunk overriding the ventricular septum. Truncus arteriosus, tetralogy of Fallot and pulmonary atresia with ventricular septal defect. Circulation *53*:663, 1976.

275. Chung, K. J., et al.: Echocardiography in truncus arteriosus, the value of pulmonic valve detection. Circulation *48*:281, 1973.

276. Chesler, E., et al.: Echocardiographic recognition of mitral-semilunar valve discontinuity. An aid to the diagnosis of origin of both great vessels from the right ventricle. Circulation *43*:725, 1971.

277. Strunk, B. L., et al.: Echocardiographic recognition of the mitral valve–posterior aortic wall relationship. Circulation *51*:594, 1975.

278. French, J. W., and Popp, R.: Variability of echocardiographic discontinuity in double outlet right ventricle and truncus arteriosus. Circulation *51*:848, 1975.

279. Sahn, D. J., et al.: Echocardiographic vs. anatomical discontinuity. Circulation *53*:200, 1976.

280. Williams, R. G., et al.: Discontinuity continued. Circulation *53*:202, 1976.

Discrete Subaortic Stenosis

281. Davis, R. H., et al.: Echocardiographic manifestations of discrete sub-aortic stenosis. Am. J. Cardiol. *33*:277, 1974.

282. Popp, R. L., et al.: Echocardiographic findings in discrete subvalvular aortic stenosis. Circulation *49*:226, 1974.

282a. Cooperberg, P., Hazell, S., and Ashmore, P. G.: Parachute accessory anterior mitral valve leaflet causing left ventricular outflow tract obstruction. Report of a case with emphasis on the echocardiographic findings. Circulation *53*:908, 1976.

283. Caudill, C. C., et al.: Membranous subaortic stenosis complicated by aneurysm of the membranous septum and mitral valve prolapse. Circulation *53*:581, 1976.

284. Weyman, A. E., et al.: Cross-sectional echocardiography in evaluating patients with discrete subaortic stenosis. Am. J. Cardiol. *37*:358, 1976.

Supravalvular Aortic Stenosis

285. Usher, B. W., Goulden, D., and Murgo, J. P.: Echocardiographic detection of supravalvular aortic stenosis. Circulation *49*:1257, 1974.

286. Bolen, J. L., Popp, R. L., and French, J. W.: Echocardiographic features of supravalvular aortic stenosis. Circulation *52*:817, 1975.

287. Nasrallah, A. T., and Nihill, M.: Supravalvular aortic stenosis. Echocardiographic features. Br. Heart J. *37*:662, 1975.

288. Shaub, M., Wilson, R., and Young, G.: Echocardiographic diagnosis of supravalvular aortic stenosis. A case report. J. Clin. Ultrasound *3*:143, 1975.

Miscellaneous

289. Lundstrom, N.: Ultrasoundcardiographic studies of the mitral valve region in young infants with mitral atresia, mitral stenosis, hypoplasia of the left ventricle and cor triatriatum. Circulation 45:324, 1972.
290. Meyer, R. A., and Kaplan, S.: Echocardiography in the diagnosis of hypoplasia of the left or right ventricles in the neonate. Circulation 46:55, 1972.
291. Chesler, E., et al.: Ultrasound cardiography in single ventricle and the hypoplastic left and right heart syndrome. Circulation 42:123, 1970.
292. Silverman, N. H., et al.: Echocardiographic assessment of ductus arteriosus shunt in premature infants. Circulation 50:821, 1974.
293. Nimura, Y., et al.: Noninvasive pre-operative diagnosis of cor triatriatum with ultrasonocardiatomogram and conventional echocardiogram. Am. Heart J. 88:240, 1974.
294. Goldberg, B. B.: Suprasternal ultrasonography. J.A.M.A. 215:245, 1971.
295. Clark, R., Rosenblatt, A., Kryda, W., Korcuska, K., and Cohn, K.: Serial echocardiographic evaluation of left ventricular function in aortic regurgitation (Abst). Circulation 54 (Suppl. II):60, 1976.
296. Popp, R. L.: Echocardiographic assessment of cardiac disease. Circulation 54:538, 1976.

Index

Page numbers in *italics* refer to illustrations; (t) indicates tables.